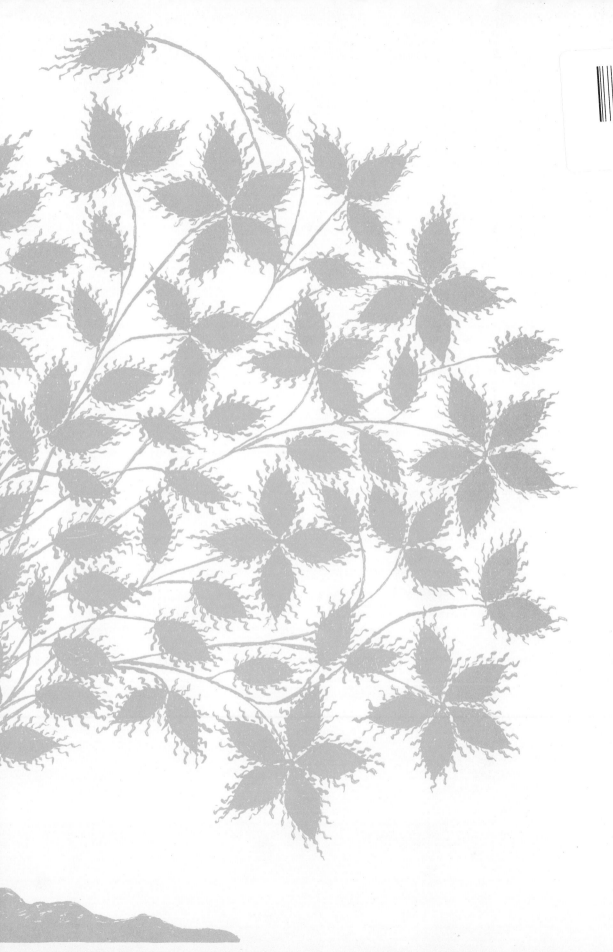

CW00547229

SHAKER
Medicinal
HERBS

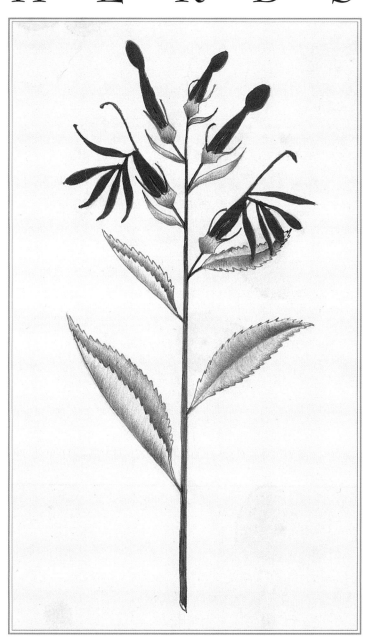

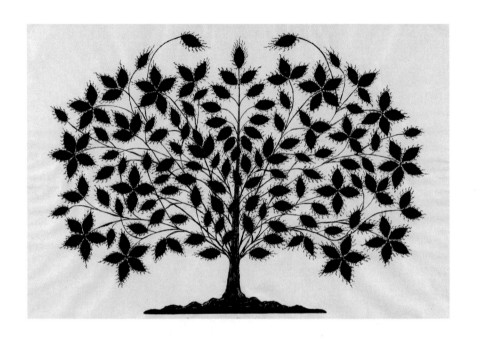

It is now the spring of the year, and you have all had the privilege of being taught the way of God; and now you may all go home and be faithful with your hands. Every faithful man will go forth and put up his fences in season, and put his crops into the ground in season, and such a man may with confidence look for a blessing.

— MOTHER ANN

SHAKER
Medicinal
HERBS

A COMPENDIUM *of* HISTORY, LORE, *and* USES

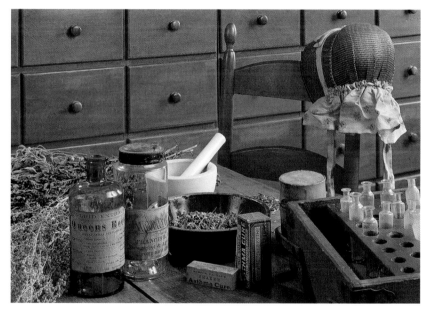

Amy Bess Miller

PUBLISHED IN ASSOCIATION WITH
HANCOCK SHAKER VILLAGE

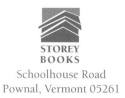

STOREY
BOOKS

Schoolhouse Road
Pownal, Vermont 05261

The mission of Storey Communications is to serve our customers
by publishing practical information that encourages personal independence
in harmony with the environment.

Edited by Deborah E. Burns
Section on the present-day Shaker herb industry at Sabbathday Lake, Maine,
    written by Stephen J. Paterwic
Cover design by Virginia Hand
Cover photographs taken at Hancock Shaker Village by Paul Rocheleau. Detail of
    "Tree of Light or Blazing Tree," collections of Hancock Shaker Village.
Art direction and text design by Cynthia McFarland
Production assistance by Susan Bernier, Eileen Clawson, and Ilona Sherratt
Editorial assistance by Dr. Magda Gabor-Hotchkiss, Stephen J. Paterwic,
    Aimee Poirier, and Marie Salter
Color botanical drawings by Sister Cora Helena Sarle © Canterbury Shaker Village,
    used by permission.
Black and white botanical illustrations by Beverly Duncan, Mallory Lake, Hyla Skudder,
    Charles Joslin, Pat Dailey, Louise Riotte, Alison Kolesar, Elayne Sears, Bobbi Angell,
    and Regina Hughes. For specific references, see page 215.
Photo credits may be found in the Notes section beginning on page 188.
Indexed by Randl W. Ockey, Writeline Literary Services

Copyright © 1998 by Amy Bess Miller

**The information in this book is intended to be read as a history of the Shaker medicinal herb industry.
Recipes and doctors' prescriptions are presented for their historical interest and are not intended to be
used by the reader for any other purpose such as treating illness or replacing the services of a physician.**

All rights reserved. No part of this book may be reproduced without written permission from the publisher, except
by a reviewer who may quote brief passages or reproduce illustrations in a review with appropriate credits; nor may any
part of this book be reproduced, stored in a retrieval system, or transmitted in any form or by any means — electronic,
mechanical, photocopying, recording, or other — without written permission from the publisher.

The information in this book is true and complete to the best of our knowledge. All recommendations are made
without guarantee on the part of the author or Storey Books. The author and publisher disclaim any liability in connection with the use of this information. For additional information please contact Storey Books., Schoolhouse Road,
Pownal, Vermont 05261.

Storey Books are available for special premium and promotional uses and for customized editions. For further information, please call the Custom Publishing Department at 800-793-9396.

Printed in Hong Kong by C & C Offset Printing Co., Ltd.
10 9 8 7 6 5 4 3 2 1

Library of Congress Cataloging-in-Publication Data

Miller, Amy Bess Williams.
        Shaker medicinal herbs : a compendium of history, lore, and uses / Amy Bess Miller.
            p.   cm.
        Includes bibliographical references and index.
        ISBN 1-58017-040-4 (alk. paper)
        1. Herbs—Therapeutic use. 2. Shakers. I. Title.
    RM666.H33M497   1998
    615'.321—dc21   97-50602
                                                                                                    CIP

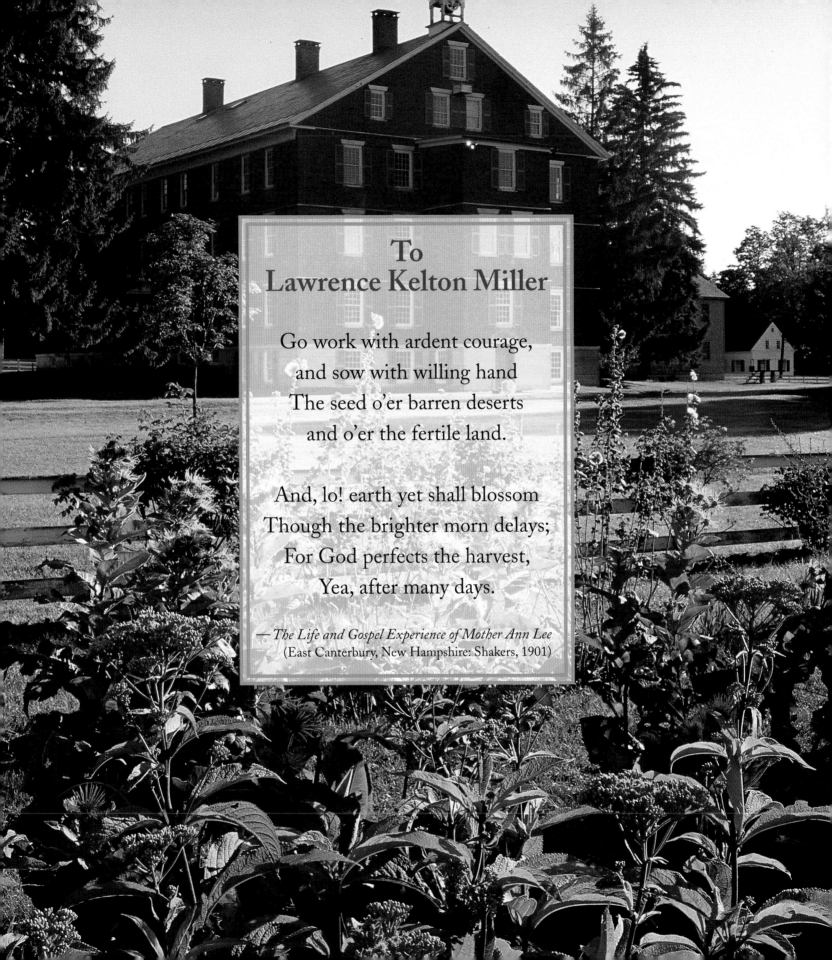

To
Lawrence Kelton Miller

Go work with ardent courage,
and sow with willing hand
The seed o'er barren deserts
and o'er the fertile land.

And, lo! earth yet shall blossom
Though the brighter morn delays;
For God perfects the harvest,
Yea, after many days.

— *The Life and Gospel Experience of Mother Ann Lee*
(East Canterbury, New Hampshire: Shakers, 1901)

SHAKER SOCIETIES

COMMUNITY	ESTABLISHED	DISSOLVED
Watervliet (Niskeyuna), New York	1787	1938
New Lebanon, New York*	1787	1947
Hancock, Massachusetts	1790	1960
Harvard, Massachusetts	1791	1918
Enfield, Connecticut	1792	1917
Canterbury, New Hampshire	1792	1992
Tyringham, Massachusetts	1792	1875
Alfred, Maine	1793	1931
Enfield, New Hampshire	1793	1923
Shirley, Massachusetts	1793	1909
Sabbathday Lake (New Gloucester), Maine	1794	Still active
Union Village, Ohio	1805	1910
Watervliet (Beulah), Dayton, Ohio	1806	1900
Pleasant Hill, Kentucky	1806	1910
South Union, Kentucky	1807	1922
West Union (Busro), Indiana	1807	1827
White Water, Ohio	1822	1916
North Union, Cleveland, Ohio	1822	1889
Groveland, New York	1836	1892

*The name was changed to Mount Lebanon after November 1861, when the first federal post office was installed. The Canaan Shakers were also part of this society.

TABLE OF CONTENTS

Shaker Societies vi

Acknowledgments viii

The History 1

    1 • Watervliet, New York 5

    2 • Home of the Central Ministry .19
       New Lebanon, New York (1787–1860)
       Mount Lebanon, New York (1861–1947)

    3 • Groveland, New York 53

    4 • The Hancock or Second Bishopric 55
       Hancock, Massachusetts 56
       Tyringham, Massachusetts 58
       Enfield, Connecticut 60

    5 • The Harvard or Eastern Bishopric 63
       Harvard, Massachusetts 64
       Shirley, Massachusetts 76

    6 • The New Hampshire Societies 79
       Canterbury, New Hampshire .80
       Enfield, New Hampshire 88

    7 • The Maine Societies 91
       Alfred, Maine 92
       Sabbathday Lake, Maine 93

    8 • The Western and Southern Societies 101
       Union Village, Ohio 102
       North Union, Ohio 113
       Pleasant Hill, Kentucky 114
       South Union, Kentucky 119

The Herbal Compendium 123

Notes 188

Glossary 197

Bibliography for the History 200

Bibliography for the Herbal Compendium .203

Index of Herbs 204

General Index 212

Photo credits may be found in the Notes section beginning on page 188.

Illustration credits may be found on page 215.

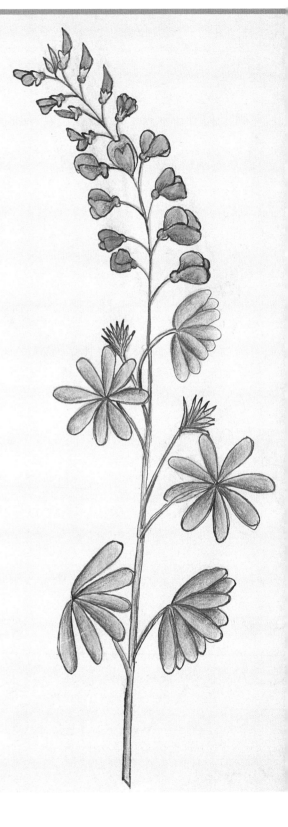

ACKNOWLEDGMENTS

I am deeply indebted to the members of the staffs of these institutions for their patience, helpful suggestions and encouragement:

The American Antiquarian Society, Worcester, Massachusetts; The Berkshire Athenaeum, Pittsfield, Massachusetts; Cleveland Public Library, Cleveland, Ohio; The Filson Club, Louisville, Kentucky; Fruitlands, Harvard, Massachusetts; Kentucky Library and Museum, Western Kentucky University, Bowling Green, Kentucky; The Emma B. King Library of the Shaker Museum, Old Chatham, New York; Library of Congress, Washington, D.C.; Library of the Francis H. du Pont Museum, Winterthur, Delaware; Library of Hancock Shaker Village, Inc., Hancock, Massachusetts; New York Botanical Garden, New York City; New York Public Library, New York City; Pleasant Hill, Shakertown, Kentucky; The United Society of Shakers, Sabbathday Lake, Maine; University of Kentucky, Lexington, Kentucky; Western Reserve Historical Society, Cleveland, Ohio; and Williams College Library, Williamstown, Massachusetts.

In addition, deepest thanks go to Eldress Gertrude M. Soule, Eldress Bertha Lindsay, and Sister Miriam Wall, then residing at Canterbury, New Hampshire, and to Charles E. Thompson for permission to use the beautiful colored drawings by Cora Helena Sarle in the first edition.

Thank you also to Mr. and Mrs. Donald E. Richmond, Julia Neal, and Elmer R. Pearson; Mr. and Mrs. William Henry Harrison at Fruitlands; and Robert F. W. Meader of the Shaker Museum.

In addition, I am grateful to Douglas Bogart, Persis Wellington Fuller, Veola Lederer, and John Ott, as well as Nancy Epley, Joelle Caulkins, Phyllis Rubenstein, and Philip L. Clark.

Note on the Revised Edition

The editor wishes to thank Dr. Magda Gabor-Hotchkiss, Coordinator of Library Collections at Hancock Shaker Village; Dr. M. Stephen Miller, eminent collector and author; and Stephen J. Paterwic, Shaker scholar and author, for extraordinary assistance in the revision of this book. In addition, many thanks to Mark Miller; Lawrence Yerdon, Director of Hancock Shaker Village; Sharon Koomler, Curator at Hancock Shaker Village; Rebecca Petrie, Museum Shop Manager at Hancock Shaker Village; Dr. Scott T. Swank, Director of Canterbury Shaker Village; Brother Arnold Hadd of the United Society of Shakers at Sabbathday Lake, Maine; Leonard Brooks and Gay Marks, Librarian and Archivist at the United Society of Shakers, Sabbathday Lake, Maine; and Wendy Liebenow, former herbalist at Hancock Shaker Village. For help finding photographs, thanks also to Galen Beale, Martha H. Boice, Mary Ryan M. Allen, and the staffs at the Shaker Museums at Pleasant Hill and South Union, Kentucky.

> **Please note** that one formatting change has been made to the longer diary excerpts that appear in this book. The diary entries are now gathered into paragraphs according to months, even though in their original form they appeared on separate lines or even on separate pages.

The History

On earth 'tis a heaven
By Providence given
And on its rich bounties
My soul doth regale.
ENFIELD, CONNECTICUT
HYMN, 1886

SINCE THE BEGINNING OF TIME humans have depended upon herbaceous plants to cure their ailments and diseases. Hippocrates, the Greek physician living in the fourth century B.C. (460–377), became an herbal practitioner in an attempt to dissociate medicine from the supernatural. In his writings he names about four hundred herbs for their medical value. This was a significant contribution, for up to his time the records of the great nations of antiquity showed that the Sumerians, Egyptians, Assyrians, Persians, Native Americans, and Chinese believed that it was the gods who first possessed the knowledge of plants and their healing properties.

The first-century herbal written by the Greek Dioscorides, said to have been Antony and Cleopatra's private physician, includes as many as six hundred medicinal plants and was accepted as an almost infallible authority throughout the Middle Ages. For more than sixteen centuries it was regarded as one of the authoritative works on medical botany and formed the main source of the herbals written after his time. Scores of Latin editions of Dioscorides' work were printed during the period of the Renaissance, and they were translated into many European languages. Yet, strangely enough, there was no modern edition in English until 1934.

From the time of the ancients onward, in each century and in every country, each generation has produced its herbalists and their herbals. Even in eighteenth-century England, that time of "enlightened" scientific rationalism, herbal remedies were much used by all classes. There was a remedy for gout, for example, that went by the name of the Duke of Portland's Powder. The duke had been cured by this mixture and had the formula printed and distributed for the benefit of other sufferers. It was composed of gentian root and the leaves of germander, birthwort, and centaury. All of these were herbs used by the Shakers in their remedies.

In England until the nineteenth century illnesses and wounds were treated at home, usually by the mother of the family or by some woman especially skilled in the making and application of plaster, ointments, and

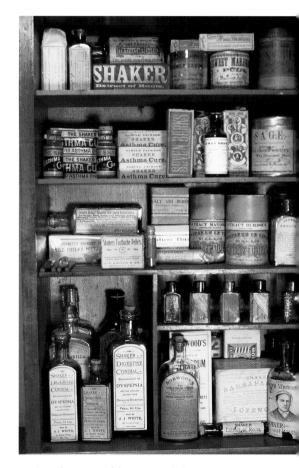

△ Apothecary cabinet containing herbal products from Shaker communities at New Lebanon, Canterbury, Sabbathday Lake, Harvard, Enfield (New Hampshire), and Watervliet (New York).

1

By 1800 eleven Shaker communities had been organized in the northeastern states, and thereafter they expanded to the west. By mid-century the Shakers attained their largest number of members — around four thousand.

Although Watervliet was the Shakers' first settled home, New Lebanon was the home of the Central Ministry. For decades the rules and regulations governing all aspects of Shaker life, spiritual and material, emanated from this source. Among the material aspects, the pharmaceutical industry began there and developed rapidly. Other Shaker communities at Watervliet, Harvard, and Canterbury soon took up this trade as well. Of the western societies the one to carry on the largest medicinal herb business was the Society of Believers at Union Village, near Lebanon, Ohio. At the height of its population this village numbered 600 members with some 4,500 acres of land.

medicines. In early America as well it was the housewife's business to prescribe for her household and to provide the necessary remedies, most of which were herbal. The stillroom was usually located as close to the kitchen as possible. Here the mistress distilled her medicines and fragrant cosmetics and concocted healing salves and syrups.

Putting Down Roots in a New Land

The Shakers originated in Manchester, England, in the late 1760s. Their little group practiced celibacy, their leader was a woman, and when they worshipped they danced, twirled, and trembled in wild ecstasy. They suffered much persecution for these unconventional views and practices. Ann Lees (the "s" was later dropped), their leader, had a vision that their faith would take root across the ocean in America.

In May 1774 Mother Ann sailed from Liverpool with eight followers aboard the ship *Mariah*, arriving in New York in early August. The men in the party traveled north up the Hudson to Niskeyuna, later named Watervliet, about seven miles northwest of Albany. This was to become the first home of the Shakers in America. The next spring Mother Ann and the women joined them, and that summer they worked hard clearing the land, cultivating the soil, and building houses, often working all night.

It was a time when the wilderness seemed inexhaustible and large sites for farming were easily available. The Shakers would not start a community unless water and sufficient timber were available. The virgin forest also produced vast amounts of botanical herbs. With these natural resources the Shakers built up profitable farms on rich and productive land.

Shaker Medicine

The Shakers were no different from their fellow countrymen and neighbors in their dependence upon herbal remedies. Like the earlier colonists they brought their herbal lore and craft with them. Encountering new and unfamiliar herbs in the fields and meadows around their communities, they drew upon the plant knowledge of Native Americans to become self-sufficient in maintaining good health by the use of herbs.

Medicines for large numbers of people required immense amounts of herbal material and its careful preparation. At first the Shakers gathered plants in the fields and woodlands; later they grew certain varieties in "physic gardens" to supply the family. If they harvested more than they needed themselves, they sold the herbs or preparations to buy other medicines that the family could not produce itself. In a very short time, outside demand for the herbs grew. From this modest beginning, born of necessity, the Shakers became the first people in the United States to produce herbs on a scale large enough to supply the pharmaceutical market.

Succeeding in an Age of Quackery

Healing in the eighteenth century was a ready field for the sharper, the quack, and the flamboyant purveyor of nostrums and cure-alls. But the Shakers, whom many regarded as "religious quacks," brought herbal medicine to a plane of probity and respectability and, of course, their business in pure herbs accordingly became the source of enormous profit to the order. Relying on the account books and journals kept in the medicine departments of the larger Shaker societies, we can make some calculation of the profitability of this business. During the seventy-five years when it was at its height, the business at just five Shaker communities (Watervliet and Mount Lebanon, New York; Harvard, Massachusetts; Canterbury, New Hampshire; and Union Village, Ohio) was averaging an aggregate gross of at least $150,000 annually.

The annual gross income under seedsman Jefferson White's direction at Enfield, Connecticut, was in excess of $30,000 before the Civil War, and a good part of this was from the sale of herbs and herb seeds. It seems conservative to estimate that the industry in the smaller societies was producing an annual gross of at least $50,000 for a total yield of over $200,000, a business that today would be reckoned at upward of $2 million.

Even after the height of the herb business had passed, the members at Enfield, New Hampshire, could send a note to *The Manifesto* dated December 1889 stating that:

> The Brethren have finished the drying of the Dock root and have shipped some forty-four thousand pounds to the firm of J. C. Ayer and Co., Lowell, Mass. Of this quantity the Second Family raised 27,856 lbs., the First Family 11,139 lbs. and the North Family 5,031 lbs.

Dock root was selling at around 50 cents per pound at this time.

Writing Their Own History

The Shakers are their own best historians. We know as much as we do about their life in the United States during the past two centuries because of what they have told us in their journals and letters, the printed testimonies of their disciples, their monthly publications, and their own literature. This is not by chance. Their Millennial Laws very clearly set forth orders concerning "Books, Pamphlets and Writings in General" and state that "two family journals should be kept by, or by the order of the Deacons and Deaconesses, in which all important occurrences, or business transactions should be registered." Therefore a vast amount of

△ Journal of the Harvard Shakers, July and August 1865.

manuscript material exists that covers every aspect of Shaker life dating from the earliest records in the late 1700s.

Without fail, the state of a community's health was given in some detail, as well as the weather and the success or failure of crops. These were obviously the important concerns of the community, and it was especially important to protect the health of every individual. There were few Shakers, and an epidemic disease could cause a disastrous setback. The Millennial Laws accordingly provided for the care of Believers by physicians and nurses: "As the natural body is prone to sickness and disease, it is proper that there should be suitable persons appointed to attend to necessary duties in administering medical aid to those in need." Those appointed were required to give the elders a full account of their proceedings regarding the administration of medicine. Well-appointed, efficiently managed infirmaries were organized in each community and, of course, extensive records were kept of medicines given, the course of treatment followed, and whether or not it was effective.

Charles Nordhoff was the first outsider to give a detailed account of the communitarian societies in the United States. He wrote at length about the Shakers in 1875 after a visit to the Mount Lebanon Society where he met Elder Frederick Evans.

> He gave me a file of the Shaker, a monthly paper, in which the deaths in all the societies are recorded; and I judge from its reports that the death rate is low, and the people mostly long-lived. In nine numbers of the Shaker, in 1873, twenty-seven deaths are recorded. Of these, Abigail Munson died at Mount Lebanon, aged 101 years, 11 months and 12 days. The ages of the remainder were 97, 93, 88, 86, 82, six above 75, four above 70, 69, 65, 64, 55, 54, 49, 37, 31, and two whose ages were not given.

> We look for a testimony against disease [Evans said] and even now I hold that no man who lives as we do has a right to be ill before he is sixty; if he suffer from disease before that, he is in fault. My life has been devoted to introducing among our people a knowledge of true physiological laws; and this knowledge is spreading among all our societies. We are not perfect yet in these respects; but we grow. Formerly fevers were prevalent in our houses, but now we scarcely ever have a case; and the cholera has never yet touched a Shaker village.

The concern for the good health and the well-being of their followers was passed on from Mother Ann to those who immediately succeeded her and thereafter from "lot to lot" of the ministry. She knew from bitter experience the utter misery of the sick and poor, and it was to create a new and better life that her heavenly visions had led her to a new country.

SHAKER FAMILIES

Each Shaker community was divided into individual "families," governed by elders. The Church, First, or Center Family was the founding unit, the geographic center, and the location of the meeting-house. The West, East, Second, and other families were added later and often formed in a rough cross around the center. Families sometimes took on different roles such as "gathering" newcomers or operating a specific industry, but this varied from community to community.

CHAPTER 1

Watervliet, New York

ELDER JOHN HOCKNELL, WHO CAME TO AMERICA with Mother Ann in 1774 at age fifty-two, told one of his contemporaries that he started out one day from Albany to purchase land for the Shakers to settle on and that during the course of his search his hand was forcibly stretched out in the direction of Watervliet. It remained in that position, resisting all efforts to draw it in, until he reached the spot the Shakers later called Wisdom's Valley. His hand fell to his side, and he knew it was the place appointed for the work. Elder John bought the land and settled the small Shaker colony in 1776.

Watervliet was the only community settled by the Shakers under Mother Ann's leadership, and it was her first home in America. Although it was the oldest of the communities, it was the second, after New Lebanon, to be formally organized (in 1787).

All of the early colonists to America brought with them a dependable knowledge of herbs from their homelands, but they were unfamiliar with many of the plants of the New World. This was true of the Shakers, too. They discovered and sampled the flora of their new habitats in their search for food. They learned also from the Native Americans, from neighbors, and from their own converts, who generally were residents of the area and knew what grew locally. Many plants were known or discovered to have medicinal properties, but there are also frightening accounts from those who experimented carelessly with poisonous plants. In fact, many plants later employed by the Shakers were deadly in all but small doses.

The first step to greatness is to be honest.

THE MANIFESTO, JANUARY 1887

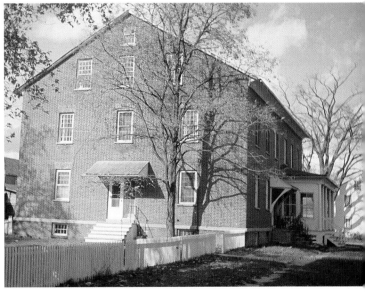

△ Brick shop, South Family, Watervliet.

To ensure top quality, exact rules, vigorously enforced, governed the gathering of herbs:

1. Only one variety was picked at a time. One herb in the morning, another in the afternoon, but not both at the same time.

2. Tow sheets fifteen feet square were used to collect the more fragile plants, and baskets were used for roots.

3. Material was collected "in season" when it was dry and ripe, before the sun had hit it but after the dew had evaporated. If flowers or seeds were to be gathered, "in season" meant in full flower with leaves fully developed.

4. Tree bark was collected during the spring, when the sap was rising and the bark peeled off easily. Bark was generally brought in as needed; orders were permitted to accumulate and then filled as soon as the material was processed.

5. Roots were dug up when the plants had matured and finished growing. They had to be clean, free of all extraneous matter, and then dried.

Although the Shakers of Watervliet did not offer their first printed catalog of medicinal plants and vegetable medicines until 1830, account books exist that record the sale of herbs and extracts to dealers, agents, pharmaceutical firms, and doctors as early as 1827. In this year Brother Harvey Copley listed 129 herbs and roots, and seven extracts: *Hyoscyamus niger* (black henbane), *Solanum nigrum* (garden nightshade), *Datura stramonium* (thorn apple or jimson weed, which was discovered at Jamestown in 1620), *Taraxacum officianale* (dandelion), *Atropa belladonna* (belladonna), *Conium maculatum* (cicuta, poison hemlock), and *Trifolium pratense* (red clover). Oil of pumpkin seed, oil of juniper, and bottles of sarsaparilla syrup were sold in addition to the extracts, as were moss by the box, metheglin by the gallon, and gallons of peach and rose water. Several journals from 1827 and 1830, in addition to Brother Harvey's, record the increasing diversity of the business in herbs, roots, barks, and seeds.

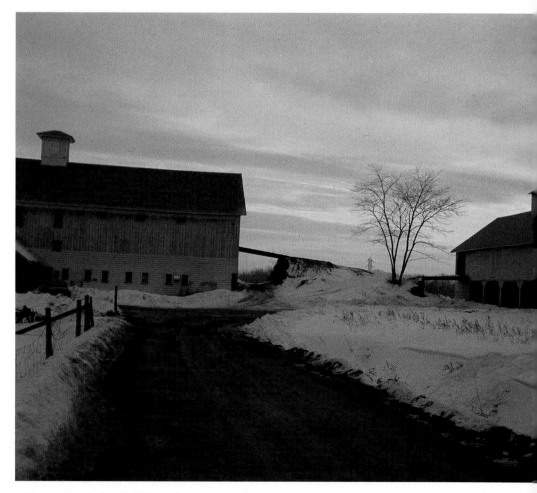

△ Barns, South Family, Watervliet, New York.

Catalogs

The Shakers published catalogs, advertisements, flyers, and broadsides of medicinal plants, vegetable medicines, and herb and garden seeds from 1830 to sometime after 1880. These publications, covering more than fifty years of the industry, give a complete picture of its growth and also of the medical needs of that time.

The first of these catalogs was printed in Albany by Packard and Van Benthuysen and dated 1830. On its cover it asked:

> *Why send to Europe's bloody shores*
> *For plants which grow by our own doors?*

It was eight pages in length and listed 120 varieties of wild herbs, which, with the roots, barks, berries, and seeds of many plants, brought the total items offered to 142. The common name, botanical name, and price per pound were given. A note said that the common names in the catalog "are such as are in general use in the cities of New York, Albany and Troy, etc. The Botanical names are from Eaton's *Manual of Botany*, last editions," and further informed that "orders for samples should be forwarded early in the season, as this will give an opportunity for their collection in their proper season. Orders for such indigenous plants or vegetable preparations as are not in the catalogue, will be attended to with care and fidelity."

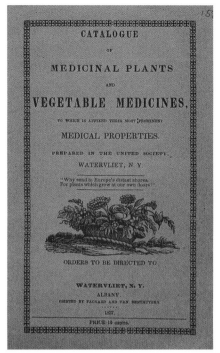

△ 1837 catalog of the Watervliet, New York, Shaker community.

A REMARKABLE DIVERSITY

A journal kept in 1848 listed orders for the following: motherwort, peppermint, spearmint, thoroughwort, catnip, pennyroyal, thyme, butternut, henbane, saffron, boneset, white root, dandelion, bloodroot, spikenard root, belladonna, elder flower, lobelia, wintergreen, Solomon's seal, skullcap, comfrey root, blackberry bark and root, sage, wormwood, southernwood, blue cardinal flower, bittersweet, marshmallow, tansy, thyme, hyssop, lemon balm, slippery elm, horehound, foxglove, summer savory, sweet bugle, sweet marjoram, lettuce, sweet fern, rue, ground ivy, chamomile flower, double tansy, dwarf elder root, liverwort, skunk cabbage root, angelica seed, burdock root, pleurisy root, mugwort, coltsfoot, male fern root, buckthorn berries, bayberry bark, smallage, cranesbill, stramonium, frostwort, sweet flagroot, Moldavian balm, goldthread, poppy flowers, poppy seed, poppy capsules, mullein, cleavers, cohosh root, yarrow, thorn apple, mayweed, coriander seed, elecampane, hemlock and oak barks, mandrake root, cranberry bark, caraway seed, indigo root, balm-of-Gilead buds, hickory ash bark, wild turnip, snakehead, golden seal root, bethroot, crawley root, cicuta, calamus root, sweet basil, rose willow bark, rose leaves, celandine, marigold flowers, garden and wild lettuce, datura, garget, lady's slipper, marsh rosemary root, princess pine, oak of Jerusalem, avens root, larkspur seed, vervain, yellow dock, life everlasting, white lily root, feverfew, queen of the meadow, horseradish, prickly ash, savin, *Lactuca virosa* (poison lettuce), scabbish, maidenhair fern, scurvy grass, bladderroot, St. John's-wort, and elderberry wine.

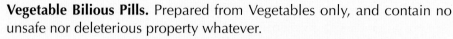

SHAKER MEDICINAL PREPARATIONS

In addition to listing herbs for sale in bulk, the Watervliet Shakers offered twelve medicinal preparations, giving the disorders they were supposed to cure and the price per box or by the dozen. These preparations were curatives for the basic ailments and were carried in nearly every edition of Watervliet catalogs, sometimes with additions and improvements. Seldom, however, were any of the twelve dropped.

Vegetable Bilious Pills. Prepared from Vegetables only, and contain no unsafe nor deleterious property whatever.

That medicine which goes slowly along the intestines, permitting the nutriment to be taken up by the absorbents, and gently stimulating the intestines, is the one to which we should have recourse in all bilious disorders. That this is the operation of the above Pills, has been abundantly proved by experience. They are a safe and valuable medicine in all bilious complaints, diseased liver, stomach and bowels, loss of appetite, foetid breath, piles and costiveness.

Their use as a cathartic, prevents or removes bilious fevers and inflammations in their forming stages. As an alternative, they can be taken without regard to diet or hindrance of business. Price 33 cents a box, or $3. a dozen.

Cephalic Pills. For periodical and nervous headache, chronic lameness and nervous debility.

These pills are prepared from vegetables only, and contain no mineral, nor narcotic substance whatever. They have been in use in our society for more than thirty years, and from a practical knowledge of their virtues, are confidentially recommended as a safe and efficacious remedy, in the above complaints. Price 50 cents a Box, or $4. a dozen.

Digestive Pills. For indigestion or dyspepsia, sourness of the stomach, loss of appetite and liver complaints.

These pills are made of the extracts of our indigenous plants, and have proved very useful in curing the above complaints, even after the failure of various approved remedies. Price 50 cents a Box, or $4. a dozen.

Vegetable Balsam. Prepared from pterospora and *Populus balsamifera*.

This medicine is found by experience to be a safe and excellent remedy for pain in the breast, coughs, and a faintness of the stomach, attended with debility and partial sweats.

Concentrated Syrup of Liverwort (*Hepatica triloba*)

A new safe, and valuable medicine for cough spitting of blood and consumption.

Compound Concentrated Syrup of Sarsaparilla (*Aralia nudicaulis*)

This medicine, taken in doses of an ounce, four or five times a day will fulfill every indication that the boasted panaceas and catholicons can perform; is free from the mercureal poisons such nostrums contain; and is much more safe and efficient as a medicine for cleansing and purifying the blood.

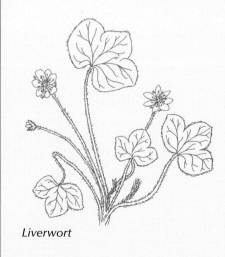

Liverwort

Compound Syrup of Black Cohosh *(Cimicifuga racemosa)*

The black cohosh is one of the most powerful deobstruents and alternatives in the vegetable kingdom; and as such has proved an effectual remedy in rheumatism, gout, chronic lameness; and in scrofulous, glandular and eruptive diseases.

N.B. The formulae and preparation of the above medicine is known and approved by the first physicians in our country.

Laurus Eye Water. A valuable remedy for chronic and acute inflammation of the eyes, weakness of sight, and morbid dryness of the eyes.

In inflammation of the eye, the motions of the eye are rendered painful, by an unnatural roughness of the parts; arising from an enlargement of the cutaneous vessels of the eye, or from small granulations on the inner surface of the eye-lids.

This eye-water contains a most delicate vegetable mucilage, which lubricates the eye and renders its motions easy and natural, while its tonic properties restore the vessels of the eye to healthy action. Price 25 cents a bottle, or $2. a dozen.

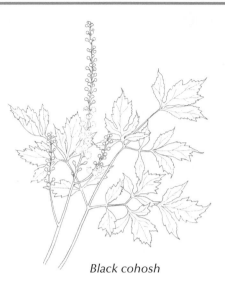

Black cohosh

Oil of Wormseed

The Oil of Wormseed is considered as the most innocent as well as the most powerful vermifuge yet known: If properly managed and genuine (as this is warranted to be) it scarcely ever fails.

N.B. The Oil of Wormseed is a powerful antispasmodic, and may be given with perfect safety and advantage, in most cases of fits and convulsions in children. In such cases, the doses should be one-third larger than the above.

Rose Water

Double distilled, very fragrant, equalling the English.

Superfine Flour of Slippery Elm *(Ulmus fulva)*

This flour is applicable to a variety of important uses. Experience, and the concurrent testimony of the most eminent physicians, prove it to be a valuable medicine, in all inflammations of the mucous membranes; such as colds, influenza, pleurisy, quinsy, dysentary, stranguary [slow and painful urination], and inflammation of the stomach or bowels. It is also a pleasant, salutary medicine and diet in consumption.

Powder of Whiteroot *(Asclepias tuberosa)*. Also called pleurisy root and cholic root, from its use in these disorders.

This root is highly recommended by the first physicians in our country, as a safe and valuable remedy in pleurisy, and diseased lungs attended with cough and a dryness of the mucous membranes. Also in fevers, where a sudorific is required; and in diseases of the digestive organs, flatulency, etc. See Barton, Bigelow, Thacher; Rafinesque's Medical Flora, and various Materia Medicas.

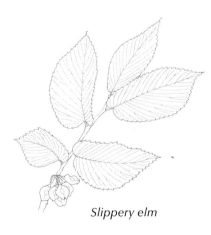

Slippery elm

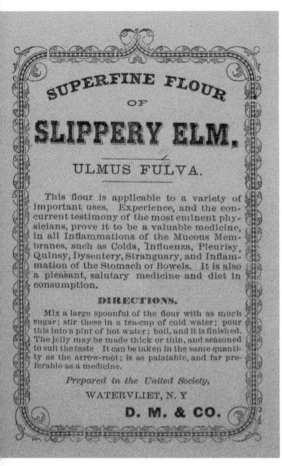

△ Wrapper for an herb cake, 1840–1860.

Peach Water and Cough Drops

Another eight-page catalog was issued in 1833 (printed date) carrying 137 herbs, most of the same pills and compounds, but adding PEACH WATER, "Very valuable as a perfume, and in eruptive diseases." A vegetable cough drop was also included and the manual proclaimed that it was "a safe and approved remedy for pulmonary complaints, asthma and for the prevention of consumption." Extracts of boneset, butternut, cicuta, cow parsnip, dandelion, henbane, hop, lettuce (both garden and wild), nightshade (both garden and deadly), and thorn apple appeared for the first time, as did four ointments: elder, marshmallow, savin, and thorn apple.

Filling the Orders

The more substantial orders were placed in the fall between October and December, and again in the spring from March to the end of May. Smaller orders came in and were filled monthly during the year. The two catalogs issued by 1835 generated as much business as the Shakers could handle. One hundred and thirty herbs and twenty-five other items were sold to twenty-two agents, ten doctors, and fourteen "individual purchasers." A Dr. Mary Entwistle was a regular customer, the only woman doctor listed. Orders came from Albany, Utica, Hudson, New York City, several hospitals in Philadelphia, and some from even farther afield. Two hundred pounds of material was shipped to San Francisco, California. The bill was $184.36 plus $6 for freight.

On November 4, 1857, one of the largest orders to be filled from Watervliet went to Butler and McCullock, Liverpool, England. It consisted of garden seeds and herbs, and the total cost including "freight, carriage and custom house charges" amounted to $175.46. The herbs sent were basil, sage, lavender, rue, mandrake, lobelia, mint, lemon and Moldavian balms, vervain, and poppy seed.

Another order went to Hopper and Company, Central Avenue, Covent Garden Market, London, England, on October 20, 1860, comprising "One hundred forty-one and a half pounds of sweet basil; $29.00 including box." The total amount of herbs processed, pressed, and delivered as recorded in this particular account book for 1859 and 1860 was 15,100 pounds. Several books for the previous year indicate a very good season, but only one gives a total. The trustee who kept the accounts wrote: "Several new plants this year, ozier, boxwood flowers, red cardinal, peony flower and blue violet. End of fiscal year 1859 for this one [meaning himself] 2,825 pounds, a tidy sum."

Cautions Included

Very often the order book also recorded observations about the plant being sent. When filling a large order in 1832 for "Hemlock plant" *(Conium maculatum),* the clerk noted: "Grows high, 6 feet." The brother keeping the book, William C. Brackett, also noted of *C. maculatum:* "Good to ease pain in open cancer which it does more powerfully than opium. Produces sweat and urine, but this plant is so very poisonous that it is imprudent to eat. It ought not to be administered by those unskilled in medicine." He also gives the "dose of the leaves in powder and extract" and concludes, "great care ought to be taken to distinguish this plant from water hemlock for the latter is a deadly poison."

The account books throughout show a constant concern for accuracy and a professional knowledge of the material being handled. On March 22, 1852, "lobelia sent to Geo. Belay, Crown Chambers Red Cross at Liverpool, England. $83.10, lobelia is too dangerous for internal use by unskilled. 408 pounds at $.20; $81.60 and boxes, $1.50."

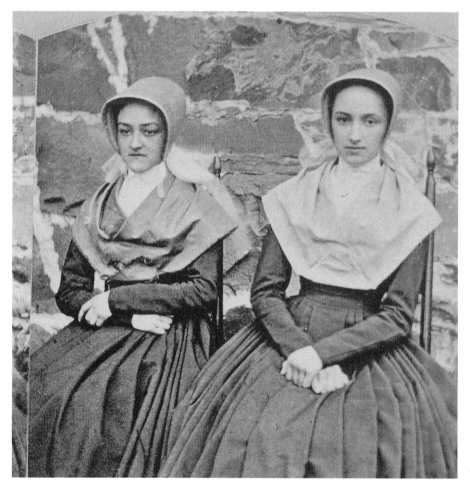

◁ Two Watervliet Shaker sisters.

DISCOUNTS . . . AND DISCONTENT

The Shakers offered the first discount, of 6 percent, in 1832 and thereafter offered discounts of from 25 to 50 percent to the larger and older accounts. At the same time, a charge for packing was instituted. By 1847 most bills were discounted, but still this was not allowed consistently, as an entry of November 1846 indicates: "To Hibbard: Vervain, sculcap, comfrey root, elderflowers, marshmallow root, foxglove, and rue, less 50%, hyssop and lobelia in bulk no %." As in all businesses, there were complaints; material was returned and much bookkeeping had to be adjusted. "November 26, 1846, Cutler returned herbs, roots and extracts: $152.58 with sharp letter."

Competitive Marketing

The market in which the Shakers competed to sell their herbs was flooded with exotic elixirs and extracts, "remedies for every malady," and there were few, if any, controls over them. The situation became so serious that the House of Representatives made a report to the Second Session of the 30th Congress in 1849 stating that "the increase of impiricism and of patent medicines within the 19th century is an evil over which the friends of science and humanity can never cease to mourne."

The Shakers built up confidence in their business in many ways. First of all they emphasized the purity of their herbs, which became well known, and their reliance on *Eaton's Manual of Botany* and *Rafinesque's Medical Flora* for identification of the wild herbs must have been most reassuring.

MARKETING TO PHYSICIANS

In these excerpts from their 1837 catalog the Shakers appealed for the first time directly to the medical profession.

Notice to Physicians — The foregoing compounds are recommended with confidence, as being selected from the best remedial agents that our knowledge of medical science can produce. The names of the active or leading articles of which they are composed accompany the medicines, and also plain directions for using, so that every person who understands the materia medica, can judge of their fitness for fulfilling the indications intended.

The attention of medical men is also particularly invited to the following samples:

Bugle [Bugleweed] *Lycopus virginicus*

In spitting of blood and similar diseases, it is, perhaps, the best remedy known. It is a sedative, and tonic, and appears to equalize the circulation of the blood. It is an active ingredient in the comp. syp. of Liverwort, and in cough and diseases of the lungs, should be taken along with that medicine, in cold infusion. The strength of an ounce of the bugle may be taken in one pint of infusion daily.

Button Snake-Root *Liatris spicata*

A powerful diuretic, well adapted to cases of stranguary, in cases of partial paralysis of the secreting vessels. Dose, 1 gill of the decoction made by boiling 1 oz. of the bruised root in 1 pint of water, 15 minutes. Saturated tincture, dose half an ounce.

Golden Seal *Hydrastis canadensis*

Tonic and gently laxative. Promotes the biliary secretions and removes jaundice. Dose of the powder, 10 to 20 grains three times a day. For dyspepsia combine ginger one quarter, and take as above.

Gravel Plant *Epigaea repens*

Diuretic. Infuse an ounce in 1 quart of boiling water. Drink freely. Has often cured where the catheter had to be habitually used.

Goldenseal

The catalogs became increasingly useful, for the Shakers included more material and information in each new edition. In the issue of 1837, on page one, twenty-five properties were listed and then ascribed to the 119 herbs within its eight pages. Terms were stated for the first time, although we have seen that they were noted in the account books: "A discount of twenty-five per cent from the catalog or retail prices, is made to those who purchase 25 dollars worth or more. Payments to be made once or twice a year, generally in the fall."

The 1837 catalog continued to offer the same extracts, but prince's pine, sarsaparilla, wormwood, and "inspissated juices generally double the price of Extracts" were added. The same four ointments (elder, mallow marsh, savin, and thorn apple) were listed, "and any other kinds made to order, and strictly according to the Pharmacopaeia." Taraxacum Blue Pills, having "nearly double the effect upon the liver and its secretions as the

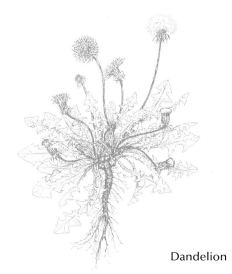

Dandelion

Indian Hemp *Apocynum* and *Rosaemifolium [Apocynum androsaemifolium]*

Diuretic, tonic and vermifuge. Is a powerful remedy in dropsy. Dose, 1 ounce of the infusion every four hours, or as often as the stomach will bear without nausea. A vinous tincture is also proper, where there is attendant debility. The extract is excellent in dyspepsia. Dose, 5 grains three times a day.

Pleurisy Root *Asclepias tuberosa*

In all inflammations of the chest this is an invaluable medicine. It is sudorific, anodyne and expectorant. Dose of the powder, 10 to 15 grains. Decoction, 1 oz. Combined with a tea of Skunk Cabbage, it is given in pleurisy with great relief.

Sweet Gale *Myrica gale*

Schirrous tumors have been removed by the use of this medicine. The strength of an ounce of it should be taken daily as a tea, and the patient rigidly confined to a diet of water biscuit or crackers. No other food or drink is allowed for 40 or 50 days. A compress of silk, or a mild discutient plaster is to be worn on the tumor. The Myrica seems to promote absorption and keep up the strength.

Thimble Weed *Rudbeckia laciniata*

In wasting diseases of the kidneys, this plant has proved an excellent medicine. It is diuretic and balsamic. Its properties were first learned by noticing its effect on a sheep that had lost the use of its hind legs. This animal daily dragged itself to this plant, and eat of it, when to the astonishment of all who noticed its situation, it recovered. By shepherds and herdsmen it has since been used in happy effects in stranguary and similar diseases. It is given in decoction, without much nicety as to dose.

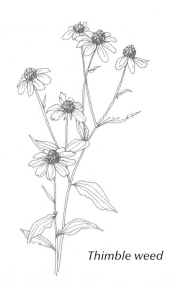

Thimble weed

BAYBERRY BARK,

Myrica Cerifera.

D. M. & Co.,

WATERVLIET, N. Y.

common blue pill," were added, and also Alterative Syrup for Purifying the Blood, and Tooth Wash and Cosmetic, "a superior article for cleansing and preserving the teeth and gums, and removing diseases of the skin." Cephalic Snuff, "a powerful remedy for pain and dizziness in the head, palsy, etc." was a new item, and five double-distilled and fragrant waters were added to the original rose and peach. They were cherry, sassafras, peppermint, spearmint, and elder flower.

6

VEGETABLE BILIOUS PILLS,

Prepared from vegetables only, and contain no unsafe nor deleterious property whatever.

They are a safe and valuable medicine in all bilious complaints, loss of appetite, foetid breath, piles, and costiveness.

Their use as a cathartic, prevents or removes bilious fevers and inflammations in their forming stages. As an alterative, they can be taken without regard to diet or hindrance of business.

Price 38 cents a box, or $3 a dozen.

CEPHALIC PILLS,

For periodical and nervous headach, chronic lameness and nervous debility.

These pills are prepared from vegetables only, and contain no mineral nor narcotic substance whatever. They have been in use in our society for more than thirty years, and are confidently recommended as a safe and efficacious remedy in the above complaints.

Price 50 cents a box, or $4 a dozen.

DIGESTIVE PILLS,

For indigestion or dyspepsia, sourness of the stomach, loss of appetite and liver complaints.

These pills are made of the extracts of our indigenous plants, and have proved very useful in curing the above complaints, even after the failure of various approved remedies.

N. B. A formulae for making the pills, with each box.

Price 50 cents a box, or $4 a dozen.

TARAXACUM BLUE PILLS,

Have nearly double the effect upon the liver and its secretions as the common blue pill.

Price 25 cents the oz.

COMPOUND VEGETABLE COUGH BALSAM,

Prepared from Lycopus Virginicus, Corallorhiza, Populus Balsomifera, &c.

This medicine is found by experience to be a safe and excellent remedy for pain in the breast, coughs, and faintness of the stomach, attended with debility and partial sweats.

Price 50 cents a bottle, or $4.50 a dozen.

CONCENTRATED SYRUP OF LIVERWORT,

Prepared from Sanguinaria, Lycopus, Pothos and Hepatica.

A new, safe and valuable medicine for cough, spitting of blood and consumption.

Price $1 a bottle, or $9 a dozen.

VEGETABLE COUGH DROPS,

A safe and approved remedy for pulmonary complaints, asthma, and for the prevention of *consumption.*

Price 75 cents a bottle, or $6 a dozen.

COMPOUND CONCENTRATED SYRUP OF SARSAPARILLA,

Of twice the medicinal strength of the common syrup of the shops.

Price $1 a bottle, or $9 a dozen.

7

COMPOUND SYRUP OF BLACK COHOSH.

(ACTEA RACEMOSA.)

The black cohosh is one of the most powerful deobstruents and alteratives in the vegetable kingdom; and as such has proved an effectual remedy in rheumatism, gout, chronic lameness; and in scrofulous, glandular and eruptive diseases.

Price $1 a bottle, or $9 a dozen.

ALTERATIVE SYRUP FOR PURIFYING THE BLOOD.

Prepared from the most efficient vegetable remedies of our country.

Price $1 a bottle, $9 the dozen.

TOOTH WASH AND COSMETIC,

A superior article for cleansing and preserving the teeth and gums, and removing diseases of the skin.

Price 50 cents a bottle, or $4 the dozen.

CEPHALIC SNUFF,

A powerful remedy for pain and dizziness in the head, palsy, &c.

Price 12¼ cents a phial, or $1 a doz.

DOUBLE DISTILLED AND FRAGRANT WATERS.

	Per gallon.
Rose,	$1 25
Peach,	0 75
Cherry,	0 75
Sassafras,	0 75
Peppermint,	0 50
Spearmint,	0 50
Elder flower,	0 50

And various other kinds.

LAURUS EYE WATER.

Price 25 cents a bottle, or $2 a dozen.

—

NOTICE TO PHYSICIANS.—The foregoing compounds are recommended with confidence, as being selected from the best remedial agents that our knowledge of medical science can produce. The names of the active or leading articles of which they are composed accompany the medicines, and also plain directions for using, so that every person who understands the materia medica, can judge of their fitness for fulfilling the indications intended.

The attention of medical men is also particularly invited to the following simples:

BUGLE.—*Lycopus Virginicus.*

In spitting of blood and similar diseases, it is, perhaps, the best remedy known. It is a sedative and tonic, and appears to equalize the circulation of the blood. It is an active ingredient in the comp. syp. of Liverwort, and in cough and diseases of the lungs, should be taken along with that medicine, in cold infusion. The strength of an ounce of the bugle may be taken in one pint of infusion daily.

△ 1837 catalog of the Watervliet Shaker Society.

New Herbs and New Products

The catalogs for 1843, 1845, and 1857 carried additional varieties of herbs and several new extracts and pills, but held to the same twenty-five properties and terms. In 1843, sage, summer savory, sweet marjoram, and thyme were offered for the first time, pulverized "for culinary and other use," and a journal entry for September 1846 recorded that the Hibbard Company printed 1,000 eight-page medicinal catalogs for the society for $30.

In 1845, in addition to 166 herbs, 73 garden seeds were included toward the end of the book. The Shakers included another notice to physicians:

The foregoing compounds are recommended with confidence, as being selected from the best remedial agents that our knowledge of medical science can produce. The names of the active or leading articles of which they are composed accompany the medicines, and also plain directions for using, so that every person who understands the materia medica can judge of their fitness for fulfilling the indications intended.

Again, the Shakers were well aware of the fiercely competitive patent medicine industry. They remained convinced of the purity of what they offered and did not hesitate to promote it.

The 1847 catalog offered the same items for sale as in preceding years, but there were advertisements for four different products sold by R. F. Hibbard and Company, 98 John Street, New York, on the last two pages. On the back cover the names of fifteen agents were listed; distributors in New York City, Albany, Utica, and Troy, and agents in the cities of Syracuse, Rochester, Buffalo, Watertown, Ogdensburg, and Rome were also included. This is an interesting publication, as it is a real selling piece of R. F. Hibbard Company, which nevertheless indicates that the herbal materials it uses in the four medicines offered are "Raised, Prepared and put up in the most careful manner by the United Society of Shakers, Watervliet." The medicines advertised under the Hibbard label were: Wild Cherry Bitters, Carminative Salve, Vegetable Family Pills, and Circassian Balm.

Catalogs Expand for a Growing Market

The 1850 catalog differed from earlier ones in that eighteen new herbs and their properties were listed, bringing the total to forty-three. Again the printer was Charles Van Benthuysen. One hundred and eighty-six herbs were listed, twenty-seven extracts, four ointments, five pulverized herbs for cooking, and composition powders. Also, the Shakers offered the same seventy-three garden seeds and one snuff.

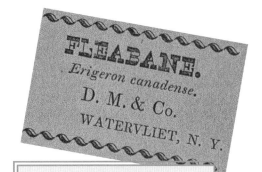

NATIVE REMEDIES

There are many other kinds worthy of trial of physicians, such as Bellwort, for curing the poison of rhus, and removing apthous sore throat; Cohosh, for rheumatism; Flea Bane, essential oil in haemorrhage; Ladies' Slipper and Skunk Cabbage, as antispasmodics; Snakehead, in jaundice, etc. etc. For a full description of the properties of these and many other active medicinal plants indigenous to our country, see Rafinesque's Medical Flora, Bigelow's and Barton's Medical Botanies, American Dispensatories, etc. etc. where it will be found that the use of many of our foreign drugs may be advantageously superseded by our own native remedies.

1837 CATALOG, WATERVLIET

The Shakers printed and distributed many flyers and broadsides during the years when the catalogs were published. These advertised medicines for the relief of nervous headaches, chronic lameness, piles, dimness of vision, inflammation of the eyes, and morbid weakness of sight, along with medicines for coughs and consumption. They also printed broadsides that showcased garden seeds, brooms, brushes, and other products.

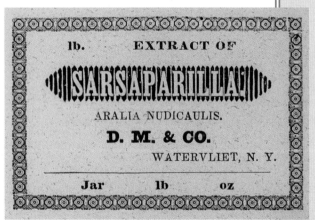

THE APPEAL OF SARSAPARILLA

Compound concentrated syrup of sarsaparilla was made and sold in the Watervliet society even before the Shakers listed it in the catalogs. The product was described in one or two sentences, and usually priced at $1 a bottle, $9 a dozen, until 1847, when the Shakers included a notice extolling its merits and successes. As a skillful example of selling appeal it is included here:

Compound Concentrated Syrup of Sarsaparilla

Price 75 cents a bottle. We are aware that the public are not only burdened, but in many instances have been imposed upon, with the almost endless variety of compound Medicines, whose virtues only exist in their boasted name.

But the Compound Syrup of Sarsaparilla having been used with peculiar success in our community for many years, as a restorative, laxative, tonic, diuretic, and alternative, we are able to present to the public a medicine possessing real merit, and one which has been used with universal success in cases of Chronic, Inflammation of the digestive organs, Saltrheum, Diarrhoea, Cutaneous Eruptions, Acute and Chronic Rheumatism, Dropsy, Dyspepsia, Scrofula, Erysipelas, Headaches of every kind, General Debility, Mercurial Diseases, and all diseases arising from an impur state of the Blood, and in the first stages of the consumption.

This medicine is also a Preventive against diseases, as it strengthens and cleanses the system, and has given general satisfaction to those who have used it in the cure of the above and many other complaints; and from the observation of competent medical judges, not of our community, it is found to be fully equal to any medical preparation offered to the public for the Syphillis.

It is not our aim to rate a thing above or below its merits, or to rival or monopolize in the presentment of this medicine. But as we desire the happiness of our fellow mortals, we solicit the afflicted to prove for themselves the trust of the above.

Brother Chauncey Miller, a Church Family trustee, issued the 1860 catalog, which is one of the most comprehensive and interesting in this category of Shaker literature. He greatly enlarged it, in comparison to earlier catalogs, in herbs listed and information; it was twenty-two pages in length. This was the first new catalog to be printed in ten years, and it would be the last of the complete formal catalogs issued by the Watervliet society.

Trustee Miller entitled the new catalog "Catalogue of MEDICINAL PLANTS, Barks, Roots, Seeds and Flowers, with their therapeutic qualities and botanical names, also, PURE VEGETABLE EXTRACTS, and Shaker Garden Seeds, Raised, prepared, and put up in the most careful manner, by the UNITED SOCIETY OF SHAKERS, Watervliet, (near Albany) N.Y." All orders were to be directed to Chauncey Miller, Shaker Village (Albany Post Office), New York. The catalog listed forty-four properties of the herbs offered for sale, one more than in previous years. The new property was "Antlithlic (A-lith) which was to be used to prevent the formation of calculus matter."

The 1860 catalog listed 292 herbs, 25 extracts, 73 garden seeds, and, for the first time, a list of 168 synonyms by which the herbs were commonly known. The extracts were boneset, burdock, butternut, cicuta, clover (red), dandelion, dock (yellow), fleabane, foxglove, gentian, henbane, horehound, hop, lettuce (garden), lobelia, mandrake, nightshade (deadly), poke, poppy, princess pine, sarsaparilla, savin, thorn apple, tomato, and wormwood. They were introduced by this statement signed by Chauncey Miller:

Pure Vegetable Extracts

It is a matter of eminent importance to the interested and benevolent physician, to be able to calculate with certainty, on the effect of any drug or medicine he may administer. This he cannot do, unless he be able to judge of its purity, condition, and carefulness of preparation. Perhaps no class of medicines present so many difficulties, and certainly none which have given such universal dissatisfaction on this point, as vegetable extracts and some of our best physicians have nearly abandoned their use on this account.

This is not surprising, when we consider the rude and imperfect means generally employed for evaporating, and the want of suitable knowledge and carefulness in the whole process of manufacture. Indeed, it requires much experience and consummate skill, in addition to the most perfect apparatus, to produce extracts that will be uniform and certain in their effects, — as much depends on the freshness of the vegetable operated upon, maturity, season of collection, and influence of climate.

To remedy the difficulties complained of, and furnish the profession with the article they so earnestly requested of us — pure and reliable extracts — we have directed our attention to this end, and spared no expense to procur the

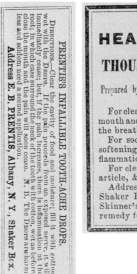

△ Front and side panels for a bottle label.

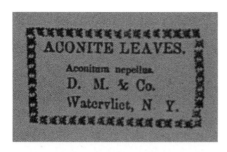

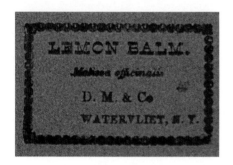

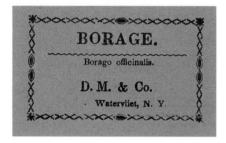

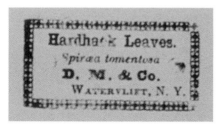

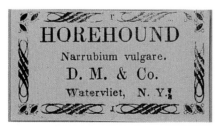

best information and conveniences for the purpose. Our former experience and observations, of thirty years, have been of value; and the possession of large botanic gardens gives us important advantages in the collection and freshness of the vegetables.

Having built a new laboratory, and furnished it with very complete fixtures for the various manipulations, among which is a vacuum pan for evaporation, embracing the late improvements of Benson and Day, and others peculiarly our own, built expressly for the purpose, we have succeeded in producing extracts which meet the approval of the faculty, from whom we are receiving very flattering encomiums of praise.

Thankful for past favors, and soliciting a continuance of the same, we subscribe in behalf of the Society,

Chauncey Miller.

The Herb Business Ends

Gradually the community at Watervliet declined, and its herb and medicine business gave way to other activities. In 1938 the three remaining sisters, all that was left of the oldest community of Shakers, moved to other societies.

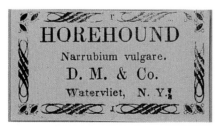

CHAPTER 2

Home of the Central Ministry

New Lebanon, New York (1787–1860)

Mount Lebanon, New York (1861–1947)

ON A LOVELY MOUNTAINSIDE IN NEW LEBANON, NEW YORK, the largest, most prosperous, and most influential of all the Shaker communities was settled and considered in complete "order" by 1792. The community began in the 1780s on a few small neighboring farms and grew to become a property of about 3,000 acres and 125 buildings in 1839. At its height in the 1870s its holdings increased to 6,000 acres, and the population reached 600 members.

The creation of the community had not been easy, however. In the backbreaking early days life was hard and the diet was scant as the first Shakers struggled to make a living from the new land. The community members often had only broth and bread to eat. For three years bread was rationed or "allowanced": A small piece was placed by each member's dish, with a piece of pie on special occasions. After a while potatoes and bean porridge became the staple, and a typical breakfast consisted of bread, sometimes a little butter, fried potatoes, fried gammon (a kind of bacon), and sage, celandine, or root tea. For coffee the root of water avens was used, or burnt rye or barley. In about 1800 pork, beef, mutton, eggs, turnips, and cabbage appeared.

No man who lives as we do has a right to be ill before he is sixty; if he suffer from disease before that, he is in fault.

ELDER FREDERICK EVANS,
NORTH FAMILY, MOUNT LEBANON

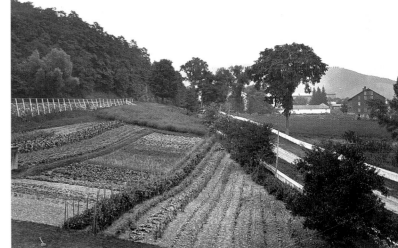

▷ Kitchen garden, North Family, Mount Lebanon, New York.

Travelers' Descriptions

In the next decades many travelers visited and wrote accounts of this dramatically placed village whose spiritual name, appropriately, was Holy Mount. In the autumn of 1819 Benjamin Silliman traveled from Hartford, Connecticut, to Quebec, Canada, and passed through New Lebanon. He recorded that:

We were indeed not clear of the mountain, before we found ourselves in the midst of their singular community. Their buildings are thickly planted, along a street of a mile in length. All of them are comfortable and a considerable proportion are large. They are, almost without an exception, painted of an ochre yellow, and, although plain, they make a handsome appearance.

The utmost neatness is conspicuous in their fields, gardens, court yards, out houses, and in the very road; not a weed, not a spot of filth, or any nuisance is suffered to exist. Their wood is cut and piled, in the most exact order; their fences are perfect; even their stone walls are constructed with great regularity, and of materials so massy [sic], and so well arranged, that unless overthrown by force, they may stand for centuries; instead of wooden posts for their gates, they have pillars of stone of one solid piece, and every thing bears the impress of labour, vigilance and skill, with such a share of taste, as is consistent with the austerities of their sect. Their orchards are beautiful, and probably no part of our country presents finer examples of agricultural excellence. They are said to possess nearly three thousand acres of land, in this vicinity. Such neatness and order I have not seen any where, on so large a scale, except in Holland, where the very necessities of existence impose order and neatness upon the whole population; but here it is voluntary.

ONE WRITER'S VIEW

Charles Dickens visited the village in 1842 and, although not attracted to the community, was evidently impressed by its reputation among farmers.

They are good farmers, and all their produce is eagerly purchased and highly esteemed. "Shaker seeds," "Shaker herbs," and "Shaker distilled waters" are commonly announced for sale in the shops of towns and cities. They are good breeders of cattle and are kind and merciful to the brute creation. Consequently Shaker beasts seldom fail to find a ready market.

NORWOOD'S

Tincture of

VERATRUM VIRIDE

Prepared Expressly for Physicians

—*by the*—

MEDICAL DEPARTMENT

—*of the*—

UNITED SOCIETY OF SHAKERS

Mount Lebanon, N. Y.

For Sale by
WHOLESALE DRUGGISTS

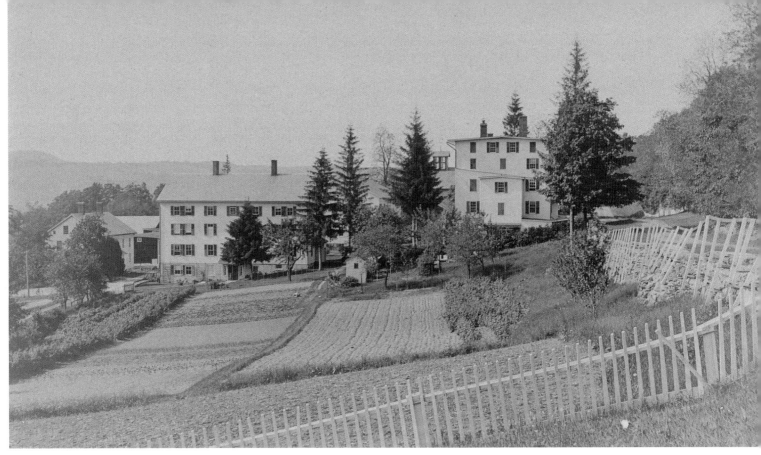

A Sister's Work

Journals, daybooks, diaries, and printed catalogs give a picture of the enormous botanical medicine business the New Lebanon Shakers developed. The sisters made numerous and continual excursions into the woods, swamps, and fields to gather thousands of pounds of wild herbs. The Shakers gathered only wild herbs until 1821, according to Sister Frances Carr of the Sabbathday Lake Shakers, but in January of that year they began selling herbs to the world. Later, "botanic gardens" were begun in which transplanted wild herbs and acres of herbs from seed were grown within the village for easier harvest.

Gathering Wild Botanicals

Because the Shakers and other early settlers gathered so many herbs and roots, it is easy to understand why so many wild botanicals have disappeared in certain areas and why so many are still on the protected lists of wildflower and Audubon societies today. The dandelion has never been in danger of extinction even though enormous quantities of its root were used in several Shaker remedies. (Its beneficial properties treated stomach and urinary disorders, and it was easy to gather and readily available.)

He who knows not what it is to labor knows not what it is to enjoy.

ELDRESS ANNA WHITE,
MOUNT LEBANON

The Shakers bought medicinal herbs from the outside whenever they could not gather material themselves. This is indicated by a letter to Edward Fowler from Horace Jennings, a peddler of Searsburg, Vermont, who wrote in August 1860:

I learnt by a man geathering Hearbs for you you Bought Balmony [snakehead] Sculcap wake Robin etc I am gethering Some of these kinds I have of Balmony 300 Pounds well Sorted & Dried in house on Racks what do you Pey for it Some was gethered in bud Some in blow I cannot make it look as well as Skulcap what is Evens Root worth . . . Dwarf Elder is plenty on my rout wild Latice [lettuce] Pipsiaway mountain Ash Sassafras etc. . . . My Balmony is Dry. . . .

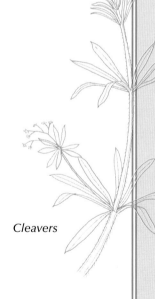

Cleavers

AN HERB-GATHERER'S GUIDE

As so much material was being processed, picked in the green state, and dried, a chart dated May 16, 1829, was hung up on the wall of the herb department office and also carried in one of the account books:

G. H. gathers 124 pound of green dandelions after dried 18½ lbs.

BUTTERNUT BARK when green weighs 35 lbs. And when dried 17 lbs.

CLEAVERS when green weigh 56 lbs. when dried 15 lbs.

ELDER FLOWERS when green weigh 289 lbs. when dried 56 lbs.

BURDOCK ROOTS when green weigh 50 lbs. when dried 6 lbs.

YARROW when green weighs 21 lbs. when dried 8 lbs.

HOARHOWN [horehound] when green weighs 45 lbs. when dried 16 lbs

BUGLE when green weighs 262 lbs. when dried 76 lbs.

STREMONIUM [Datura stramonium] when green weighs 15 lbs. when dried 2¾ lbs.

DEERWEED when green weighs 175 lbs. when dried 71¾ lbs.

SASAPRILLA when green weighs 27¾ lbs. when dried 15 lbs.

BITTERSWEET TOPS when green weighs 25 lbs. when dried 10 lbs.

SPIKNARD when green weighs 83¾ lbs. when dried 26½ lbs.

COMPHREY when green weighs 48 lbs. when dried 15½ lbs.

SOUTHERNWOOD when green weighs 32 lbs. when dried 13 lbs.

ELECOMPAIGN when green weighs 63 lbs. when dried 19¾ lbs.

Although not all those engaged in gathering material would pick the same amounts, it is interesting that "G. H." felt the above amounts were "common" enough to serve as a helpful guide.

The Shaker Digestive Cordial, however, required rarer varieties of plant material: blue flag, Culver's root *(Leptandra virginica),* stillingia, prince's pine and princess pine, and gentian. (These have all appeared on protected lists in the East.)

The New Lebanon sisters' journal, "A Journal of Domestic events and transactions; In a brief and conclusive form; Commenced January 1st, 1843; Kept by The Deaconesses, Church 2nd Order," was written for twenty-one years, until June 23, 1864. The deaconesses carefully recorded the activities of one family in supplying and preparing herbs:

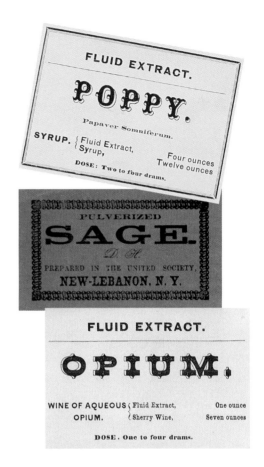

June 14th. George C. James L. Samuel W. go after meddow sweet, have good luck. June 27th. This morning a company of sisters start for Richmond swamp to gather tea. [Meadowsweet tea is steeplebush, Spiraea tomentosa, an astringent tonic for diarrhea.] George L. starts with the one horse waggon and James Gilbert takes the covered waggon. We start from home immediately after breakfast and arrived at 7 o'clock in the evening with a good load of meadow sweet tea. June 30th. Sisters go again after tea and have good luck. Get a meal of strawberrys for supper this is the first we have this year.

July 1st. This morning Abigail S. Lea, Phebe S. Elinor B. and James start on the mountain after Crosswort. [Crosswort is boneset, Eupatorium perfoliatum; this and meadowsweet were gathered in enormous quantities.] July 4th. Have pease for dinner, the first time. James L. prepares tea to the dry house. July 6th. Go after Elderflowers. Hannah A. and I go a strawburying, got a few, too. July 7. Their are 9 start to the sage place to cut sage, done about noon. . . . July 19th. Finishing preparing and pressing tea. July 20th. Go to empty the press and clean up. Have 307 lbs. of tea.

The Shakers strove to view the herbs they grew as strictly functional, not as sensual in any way. Children thus were taught not to cherish the vivid beauty of the blooms but to concentrate on the uses of the plant. One sister recalled her experiences with the Canaan Shakers at about the time of the Civil War:

Forty years ago it was contrary to the "orders" which governed our lives to cultivate useless flowers, but fortunately for those of us who loved them, there are many plants which are beautiful as well as useful. We always had extensive poppy beds and early in the morning before the sun had risen, the white-capped sister could be seen stooping among the scarlet blossoms to slit those pods from which the petals had just fallen. Again after sundown they came out with little knives to scrape off the dried juice. This crude opium was sold at a large price and its production was one of the most lucrative as well as the most picturesque of our industries.

The rose bushes were planted along the sides of the road which ran through our village and greatly admired by the passersby, but it was strongly impressed upon us that a rose was useful, not ornamental. It was not intended to please us by its color or its odor, its mission was to be made into rose water, and if we thought of it in any other way we were making an idol of it and thereby imperiling our souls. In order that we might not be tempted to fasten a rose upon our dress or to put it into water to keep the rule was that the flower should be plucked with no stem at all. We had only crimson roses [Rosa gallica] as they were supposed to make stronger rose water than the paler varieties. The rose water we sold, of course, and we used in the community to flavor apple pies. It was also kept in store at the infirmary, and although in those days no sick person was allowed to have a fresh flower to cheer him, he was welcome to a liberal supply of rose water with which to bathe his aching head.

Then there were the herbs of many kinds. Lobelia, Pennyroyal, Spearmint, Peppermint, Catnip, Wintergreen, Thoroughwort, Sarsaparilla and Dandelion grew wild in the surrounding fields. When it was time to gather them an elderly brother would take a great wagonload of children, armed with tow sheets, to the pastures. Here they would pick the appointed herb [each one had its own day, that there might be no danger of mixing] and, when their sheets were full, drive solemnly home again.

In addition to what grew wild we cultivated an immense amount of dandelion, dried the roots and sold it as "chicory." The witch hazel branches were too rough for women and children to handle, so the brethren cut them and brought them into the herb shop where the sister made them into hamamelis.

We had big beds of Sage, Thorn apple, Belladonna, Marigolds and Camomile, as well as of yellow Dock of which we raised great quantities to sell to the manufacturers of a well-known "sarsaparilla." We also made a sarsaparilla of our own and various ointments. In the herb shop the herbs were dried and then pressed into packages by machinery, labeled and sold outside. Lovage root we exported both plain and sugared and the wild flagroot we gathered and sugared, too. On the whole there was no pleasanter work than that in the "medical garden" and "herb shop."

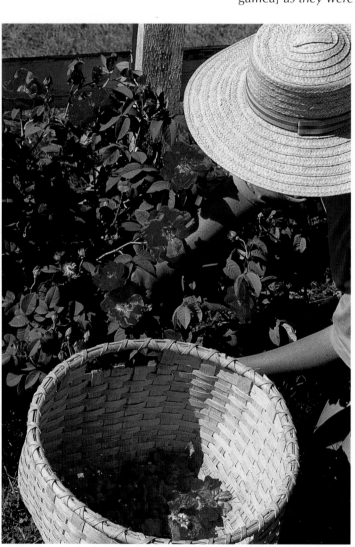

△ Roses were not supposed to be savored for their beauty but for their usefulness.

A Brother's Work

Philemon Stewart, an accurate and interesting journalist, introduces himself in this way in the first of his daybooks quoted here: "April 9, 1826, Philemon Stewart, a young man whose age will be 22 the 20th of the present month takes the business [peddling seeds and herbs] which the above mentioned Benj. Lyon a man of rather more than middle age has left. April 30, 1826 . . . Philemon Stewart relieved of peddling and is appointed to take care of the boys and as the garden is a suitable place for boys to work, he also takes [care of] the garden."

Accordingly, on March 29, 1831, he writes: "We set some glass in our sashes to cover our hot bed." There are many more entries regarding the hot bed which in the climate at New Lebanon was a great asset to the gardeners, and he feels certain that eventually he will also have "a glass house" near and between the "great garden."

April 11th. We are beginning to raise some strawberrys and gooseberrys. Graft peach trees. Gather raddish seed at herb house and finish sowing our raddish. We have two kinds here in the garden the scarlet turnip and the salmon. . . . April 20. Gardens too wet to work. . . . April 21. Peter and I sow some early peas. All forces is turned to setting out roots in the Great Garden. . . .

May 2, 1831. The boys go after cowslips this forenoon. . . . 5th. We gardners 4 in number go and help rake in the great garden. . . . May 6th. Sow carraway and parsley. . . . May 9th. It is very cold with repeated snow squalls through the day. We gardeners work here and there at this thing and that. . . . May 13th. Have made my alleys with poles for beans and brush for peas, the result pleases my eye. We pretty much finish planting our gardens. The weather is quite warm and pleasant. . . .

From many such records we know this was a large-scale operation, and it is not surprising that just over twenty years later (in 1852) an article appeared in the *American Journal of Pharmacy* describing a visit to the Shakers. The writer tells about his tour of the gardens, the "arrangements for drying and packing herbs and for making extract," and says that during the short visit a very hearty welcome was extended by "chief Trustee, Edward Fowler." Brother Edward gave an overview of the herb business, saying it had been operating for about fifty years and had increased rapidly, especially in the previous ten years.

There are now probably occupied as physic gardens in the different branches of our Society, nearly two hundred acres, of which about fifty are at our village. [The first number includes the settlements of Shakers in

"THE BEST OF ITS KIND"

They are honest, sober and industrious. There is a thoroughness of labor in many of their works which commands respect. Slovenly workmanship is a gross practical lie running through the world. The Shakers, limited in the extent of their manufactures, offer the best of the kind. The covers of their boxes fit, their brooms sweep, their packets of herbs are approved by the physicians, the products of their farms and dairies are sound and wholesome. This, with the fair and exact culture of their land, is a virtue before the world. Dealing simply with nature in their relations as agriculturists, in spite of constraint and their barren culture, beauty waits upon them. Their brimming water fountains by the roadside, for man and beast, the cleanliness and order of their farmyards and meadows, a certain grandeur (of a limited character) in their huge dwellings, the mountain simplicity of their retirement, are tributes to the spirit of Art.

EVERT A. DUYCKINCK, EDITOR
THE LITERARY WORLD

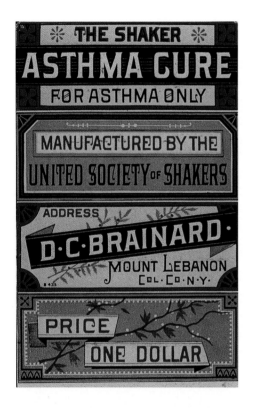

New England, Kentucky, Ohio, and New York.] *As we find a variety of soils are necessary to the perfect production of the different plants, we have taken advantage of our farms and distributed our gardens accordingly. Hyoscyamus, belladonna, tarazacum, aconite, poppies, lettuce, sage, summer savory, marjorum, dock, burdock, valerian, and horehound, occupy a large portion of the ground; and about fifty minor varieties are cultivated in addition, as rue, borage, carduus (Benedictus), hyssop, marsh-mallow, feverfew, pennyroyal, etc. Of indiginous plants we collect about two hundred varieties, and purchase from the South, and West, and from Europe, some thirty or forty others, many of which are not recognized in the Pharmacopoeia, or the dispensatories, but which are called for in domestic practice and abundantly used.*

The article described the herb house, storage rooms, and methods of drying various types of plant material before they were removed for pressing. The writer, obviously knowledgeable about these procedures, said: "Some plants which are very succulent or viscid, and which are difficult to properly cure, as conium, hyoscyamus, and garden celandine are desiccated in a drying room, constructed for the purpose where a temperature of about 115° Fahr. is maintained. Most of the roots are dried in this way, after being sliced." He approved of the double presses, each of which could press one hundred pounds daily and was in constant operation. Then he discussed the vacuum apparatus in the evaporating room and whether the Shakers or the Tilden Company of New Lebanon had it first.

The article went on to say:

WORLDLY COMPETITION

Because of their success, naturally the Shakers had competition. A circular was issued in 1849 by the Tilden Company, offering "Shaker Garden Seeds" on its front page, with its own list of roots, herbs, extracts, barks, ointments, and black and blue writing inks. Elam Tilden founded the company in 1824, and it was once hailed as the oldest pharmaceutical house in the nation. In a newspaper article written in 1969, six years after the company closed its doors, it was noted that "industrious, intelligent Elam Tilden discovered that the many beneficial poultices and brews made by the herb-growing Shakers on Mount Lebanon were truly beneficial to man, so he undertook their manufacture and sale."

Mr. Fowler informs us that the amount of extracts manufactured at their establishment annually was about six or eight thousand pounds, but since their improvements in apparatus and manipulations, this amount has been greatly increased, and the quality improved. Extract of taraxacum [dandelion] is in the greatest demand, their product in this article amounting the past year to 3700 pounds. Conium, hyoseyamus [henbane], and belladonna class next. They do not cultivate conium [poison hemlock], but collect that of spontaneous [wild] growth, believing it to be more active. Belladonna and hyseyamus, especially the latter, require a rich deep soil and abundance of strong animal manure.

They find henbane a very precarious crop, as when young it is almost impossible to keep it from being destroyed by insects, and some years they have entirely lost it, notwithstanding their best endeavors to protect it. The biennial variety of henbane is alone cultivated, and when not destroyed by insects, etc., has under the most favorable circumstances yielded at the rate of 1300 pounds of good extract from an acre of plants.

Catalogs and Cures

In 1815, some unknown Shaker wrote in a small leather-bound notebook seventy medical recipes and "cures" for the "Nurse Shop for the Church Family at New Lebanon: The Strengthening Sirrups and Cordials; the Elixirs; the Cleansing Bitters; concoctions for The Nerves' Consumption, for The Salt Rume, for The Rumatism, for The Gravel, For the Lungs, For Faintness, For the Use of the blue Violet Root; To Make Clove Water, To Make Liquid Landemon; A Beer to Cleanse the Blood." These brews, with directions for making the many kinds of wines that presumably rendered the dose more palatable, were the forerunner of the dozens of preparations put out commercially by the medical department. This notebook for the infirmary was followed by printed catalogs, some of which carried recipes for medicines.

In 1836 the society issued its first dated catalog, offering medicinal plants and vegetable medicines. One hundred sixty-four herbs were listed as well as twelve extracts, four ointments, seven double-distilled and fragrant waters, four pills, a cough drop, two cough syrups, the compound concentrated syrup of sarsaparilla (offered by all the Shaker medical departments), a syrup of black cohosh for rheumatism and gout, a blood purifier, a "tooth wash and cosmetic," and "Laurus Eye Water."

The 1837 catalog was similar in many ways to that distributed in the previous year and identical to the one the Watervliet Shakers had issued the same year. The following year the Shakers of New Lebanon added a few more herbs, bringing the list to 170. One hundred seventy-two herbs, "and various other kinds indigenous to our country," were offered by the New Lebanon Shakers in 1841, with price per pound and the botanical name listed as well. Four pulverized culinary herbs, twenty-one extracts, four ointments — the same ones as in previous years — and the same listed pills, syrups, other medicines, and fragrant waters were included.

The catalogs of 1848 and 1850 were essentially the same as the earlier ones, but the content of the next four catalogs to be issued under the New Lebanon imprint was greatly increased (and the catalogs became increasingly useful as botanical manuals as well). There were many changes in the issue of 1851. The cover gave much more information as to the content of the book: "A Catalogue of Medicinal Plants, Barks, Roots, Seeds, Flowers and Select Powders with their Therapeutic Qualities and Botanical names; also Pure Vegetable Extracts, prepared in vacuo; Ointments, Inspissated Juices, Essential Oils, Double Distilled and Fragrant Waters, etc. etc., Raised, prepared, and put up in the most careful manner by the United Society of Shakers at New Lebanon, N.Y." Orders, it said, should be addressed to Edward Fowler.

The Shakers now described forty-four properties for 356 herbs, which was 184 more than ever offered before. The same pulverized culinary

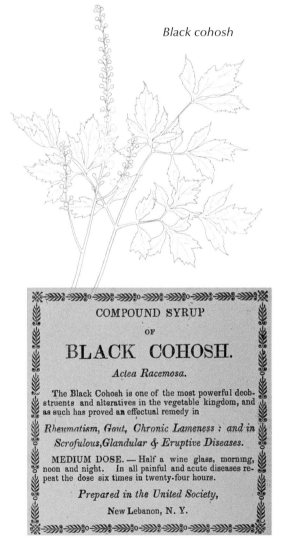

Black cohosh

COMPOUND SYRUP

OF

BLACK COHOSH.

Actea Racemosa.

The Black Cohosh is one of the most powerful deobstruents and alteratives in the vegetable kingdom, and as such has proved an effectual remedy in

Rheumatism, Gout, Chronic Lameness ; and in Scrofulous, Glandular & Eruptive Diseases.

MEDIUM DOSE. — Half a wine glass, morning, noon and night. In all painful and acute diseases repeat the dose six times in twenty-four hours.

Prepared in the United Society,

New Lebanon, N. Y.

herbs were listed, as well as 181 fluid extracts. Another list gave "pure inspissated alcoholic and hydro-alcoholic solid extracts, sixty-one in number as well as forty-eight ordinary extracts," twenty-two alkaloids and resins, ten ointments, and seven double-distilled and fragrant waters. "Also waters distilled *in vacuo*, from the expressed juice of Cicuta, Belladonna, Henbane, Sarsaparilla, Dandelion, Thorn Apple; and various others can be had by giving NOTICE in time of preparation, and are recommended to Physicians for trial, especially Cicuta, Dandelion, and Sarsaparilla for the cleansing of foul ulcers, etc." Nine essential oils and eighty-four powdered articles completed the list.

"Cheap, Fresh and Genuine"

This catalog also for the first time carried the following endorsement of Professor C. S. Rafinesque:

The best medical gardens in the United States are those established by the communities of the Shakers, or modern Essenians, who cultivate and collect a great variety of medical plants. They sell them cheap, fresh and genuine.

This was indeed high praise from a botanist of acknowledged national repute. There were also complimentary statements from H. H. Childs and Willard Clough, neighboring physicians in Pittsfield, Massachusetts.

Herbal Extracts, Ointments, and Syrups

The catalogs of 1860 and 1866 were identical to the 1851 issue and contained no new or additional material. But in 1867 a three-page list of fluid extracts manufactured by the Lebanon Shakers was issued announcing 182 fluid and 60 solid extracts of herbs, barks, and roots, among other things, with the common names followed by botanical names. Prices were stated for one-pound and five-pound bottles. The Shakers issued a second little booklet in the 1870s, listing 132 fluid extracts, along with pearls of

---

ALTERNATIVE COMMON NAMES

The society completed the 1851 book with, for the first time, a list of 264 synonyms or alternative common names. It was noted that "Difficulties have sometimes arisen from the use of the common name being applied to different plants in different localities, and also from the fact that druggists are frequently called upon for some article which they have, by a name distinct from that by which it is sold under, which they are not aware of, we have appended a list of synonyms, which the seller will please refer to before turning a customer away." The usual pills, snuff, and syrups — and, for the first time, seventy-four garden seeds — were listed.

A blade of grass — a simple flower,

Cull'd from the dewy lea;

These, these shall speak with touching power,

Of change and health to thee.

FROM THE NEW LEBANON SHAKERS' 1851 CATALOG

ether, pearls of chloroform, and pearls of turpentine, with a liberal discount to the trade; in 1872 they issued a wholesale price list of medicinal herbs and roots, giving the common names and prices of 358 herbs.

In 1874 a *Price List of Medicinal Preparations* was issued, listing 405 herbs, roots, seeds, and barks with botanical names and the prices for preparations in pulverized, fluid, or solid form. Six ointments, four pulverized culinary herbs, and three syrups were included. The syrups remained the best-sellers: bitter bugle, "a new and valuable medicine for coughs, spitting of blood and consumption"; sarsaparilla compound; and genuine syrup of buckthorn, used in rheumatism, gout, and dropsy. This number of herbs, exceeding 400, was the most ever offered for sale by this society or any of the others. It was extraordinary in view of the fact that in 1874 there were many commercial houses "in the world" giving the Shakers considerable competition.

The 1873 *Druggist's Handbook* was the last of the large catalogs, but the Shakers continued to publish price lists, broadsides, and testimonials advertising specific medicines, some several pages in length, for many years and even into the twentieth century. These will be examined in connection with the remedies they promoted, and the individuals who conceived them.

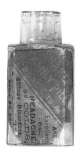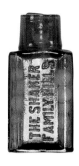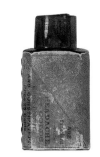

△ These bottles, 2⅛ inches high, contain white BB-sized pellets, called Shaker Family Pills.

Discount on Fluid and Solid Extracts.—On $10, 25 per cent.;—$20, 30;—$40, 35;—$50, 40;—$75, 45;—$100, 50.

April 1st, 1874.

SHAKERS' PRICE LIST
OF
MEDICINAL PREPARATIONS,

Mount Lebanon, Columbia Co., N. Y.

HERBS, ROOTS, BARKS AND POWDERS, NET PRICES.

FLUID AND SOLID EXTRACTS, DISCOUNT ACCORDING TO THE AMOUNT PURCHASED.

COMMON NAMES.	BOTANICAL NAMES.	Herb Price	Pulverized Price	Fluid Price	Solid Price	COMMON NAMES.	Botanical Names.	Herb Price	Pulverized Price	Fluid Price	Solid Price
ABSCESS ROOT	*Polemonium Reptans*	25				Buchu leaves	*Diosma Crenata*	60		2 50	
Aconite Leaves	*Aconitum Napellus*	25		1 90		Do. Comp				2 50	
Do. Root	" " *Radix*	22	30	2 00	4 50	Buck Bean	*Menyanthes Trifoliata*	36			
Agrimony	*Agrimonia Eupatoria*	20		1 75		Buckhorn Brake	*Osmunda Spectabilis*	36			
Alder Bark black	*Prinos Verticillatus*	20		1 50		Buckthorn berries	*Rhamnus Catharticus*	45		1 50	
Do. Berries, black	" " *Bacca*	30				Bugle	*Lycopus Virginicus*	18		1 25	
Do. red or tag		10		1 25		Burdock leaves	*Lappa Major, Folium*	13			
Aloes				2 75		Do. Root	" " *Radix*	17	22	1 50	3 00
Angustura				4 00		Do. Seed	" " *Semen*	18	24		
Aromatic Comp.	*Alnus Rubra*			2 25		Butternut Bark	*Juglans Cineria*	13		1 25	3 00
Alum Root	*Heuchera Pubescens*	22				CANADA Thistle Root	*Cirsium Arvense*				
Angelica Leaves	*Archangelica Atropurpurea*	15				Cancer Root Plant	*Epiphegus Virginiana*	22			
Do. Root		25		1 25		Canker Weed	*Nabalus Albus*	25			

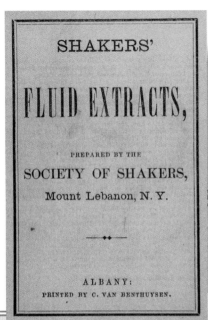

SHAKERS'

FLUID EXTRACTS,

PREPARED BY THE

SOCIETY OF SHAKERS,

Mount Lebanon, N. Y.

ALBANY:
PRINTED BY C. VAN BENTHUYSEN.

In presenting you a New Edition of our Catalogue, we would call especial notice to our Inspissated Juices and Superior Fluid Extracts, prepared in Vacuo.

Our particular attention has been directed to this branch of business for some years past, and we have procured very Perfect and Expensive Apparatus, and the Instructions and assistance of some of the Best Chemists and Pharmaceutists. We have been able to produce Extracts which we confidently believe are not inferior to any, and for which we have received high encomiums from many of the Medical Faculty and some of our Principal Colleges.

We wish to call the particular attention of the Medical Faculty to our SUPERIOR FLUID EXTRACTS, which we Manufacture from the Best Material according to the Established Principles of Pharmaceutical Science —PERFECTLY PURE—possessing all the Medicinal Properties of the Plant, from which they are manufactured, without the addition of Sugar, or any Saccharine whatever, as is the case with most Fluid Extracts now offered in market.

Our Society having been actively engaged in the business of Manufacturing Extracts over forty years, we claim the advantage of EXPERIENCE, and the rapidly increasing demands for SHAKER HERBS AND EXTRACTS, with their various Botanic Preparations, is satisfactory evidence of public approval and esteem.

We pledge ourselves to furnish articles of superior excellence, and are determined not to be surpassed in the Quality or Neatness of our Preparations.

New Lebanon, Shaker Village, N. Y.

FLUID EXTRACTS.

COMMON NAME.	OFFICIAL NAME.	DOSE.
Aconite	Aconitum napellus	4 to 8 drops
Angelica root	Archangelica utrop.	1 to 2 drams
Arnica	Arnica montana	10 to 40 drops
Balmony	Chelone glabra	1 to 2 drams
Bayberry	Myrica cerifera	1 to 2 drams
Barberry bark	Berberis	1 to 2 drams
Belladonna	Atropa belladonna	6 to 10 drops
Beth root	Trillium purpureum	1 to 2 drams
Bitter root	Apocynum audros.	10 to 20 drops
do	do tonic	2 to 5 drops
Bittersweet	Solanum dulcamara	20 to 30 drops
Black alder	Prinos verticilatus	1 to 2 drams
Blackberry	Rubus villosus	4 to 1 dram
Black cohosh	Macrotys rac.	7 to 12 drops
Black hellebore	Helleborus niger	8 to 20 drops
Blazing star	Aletris farinosa	5 to 15 drops
Bloodroot	Sanguinaria	8 to 10 drops
Blue cohosh	Caulophyllum thalic.	12 to 20 drops
Blue flag	Iris versicolor	10 to 40 drops
Boneset	Eupatorium perfoliatum	1 to 2 teaspfl.
Boxwood	Cornus florida	1 to 2 teaspfl.
Buchu	Barosma crenata	1 to 1¼ teaspfl.
do compound	do	¼ to 1 dram
Buckthorn	Rhamnus catharticus	¼ to 1 dram
Bugleweed	Lycopus virginicus	1 to 2 drams
Burdock	Lappa major	2 to 3 teaspfl.
Butternut	Juglans cinera	1 to 2 teaspfl.
Cayenne Pepper	Capsicum	6 to 18 drops
Chamomile	Anthemis nobilis	¼ to 1 dram

A BOOK OF EXTRACTS

As one of his many activities, Philemon Stewart worked with Elder Calvin Green and Brother Seth Wells to compile a book of extracts. This book listed 133 herbs with common and official names in extract form and with prices for one- and five-pound bottles. Doses were given for twenty-nine extracts, and three new preparations were advertised: pearls of ether, pearls of chloroform, and pearls of turpentine. Previous to the year 1841 the "Extracts both Inspissated and Boiled" were made by the sisters, but the business became more than they could handle and "the Brethren took sole burden of the work." The little booklet, eventually published in 1871, stated:

In presenting you a New Edition of our Catalogue, we would call especial notice to our Inspissated Juices and Superior Fluid Extracts, prepared in Vacuo.

Our particular attention has been directed to this branch of business for some years past, and we have Procured very Perfect and Expensive Apparatus and the Instructions and assistance of some of the Best Chemists and Pharmaceutists. We have been able to produce Extracts which we confidently believe are nor inferior to any, and for which we have received high encomiums from many of the Medical Faculty and some of our Principal Colleges.

We wish to call the particular attention of the Medical Faculty to our Superior Fluid Extracts, which we Manufacture from the Best Material according to the Established Principles of Pharmaceutical Science. Perfectly Pure — possessing all the Medicinal Properties of the Plant, from which they are manufactured, without the addition of Sugar, or any Saccharine whatever, as in the case with most Fluid Extracts now offered in market.

Our Society having been actively engaged in the business of Manufacturing Extracts over forty years, we claim the advantage of Experience, and the rapidly increasing demands for SHAKER HERBS AND EXTRACTS, with their various Botanic Preparations, is a satisfactory evidence of public approval and esteem.

We pledge ourselves to furnish articles of superior excellence and are determined not to be surpassed in the Quality or Neatness of our Preparations.

New Lebanon Shaker Village.

Medical Care among the Shakers

The Shaker families maintained large, efficient "nurse houses" — or infirmaries — as well as the botanic gardens and vegetable medicines necessary for the care of the ill and aged. According to a New Lebanon journal for 1789, the entry for May 23 establishes an apothecary in residence: "To dressing a hat for the apothecary 2 shillings, 3 pence." An early physician was "Dr." Eliab Harlow, who, with Brother Garrett Keatin Lawrence, was credited with establishing the scientific standards for the medical gardens that gave them such a good reputation.

Benjamin Gates kept a diary starting October 1, 1827, when he was working in the "new taylers shop," in which he describes how varied the chores were in the community and in Brother Garrett's medical department. On the 8th, he goes

a chestnutting with Joseph Fearey and finish Amos Jewetts drawers. On the 15-16-17th, pick apples, work with Issac Youngs on the Meeting house.
May 1828 the 13th through the 21st, I work in the medical garden with Garrett Lawrence. 22nd, work in seed garden. 23rd, work Issac Young's drawers.
June 7th help cut slippery elm bark. 9th medical garden with G. K. L. 11th, 12th. work in seed garden. 23rd. to strawberrying.
July 1 and 2 work in physic garden with Gideon.
October 10th helped about culling tobacco. Broken time [different kinds of chores all mixed up] from now on.

In 1829 he starts his diary on April 8 digging horse "raddish." He then records miscellaneous chores until midsummer.

July 14, 15th working in physic garden, here a little, and there a little, but don't fail.
August — gathering herbs here and there — go on west hills after lobelia. 26 and 27th work in medical garden. 30 and 31st gathering bugle here and there.
Sept. 1830 spend this month gathering herbs and roots here and there, up hill and down. 2nd 23, 24th. down to Sheffield after blue cohosh. 28th on the mountain after maidenhair.

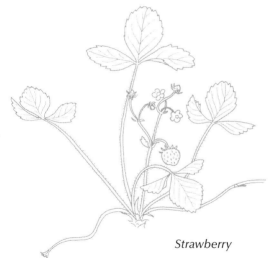

Compound Concentrated Syrup
OF
SARSAPARILLA,
Aralia Nudicaulis.

THIS medicine, taken in doses of an ounce, four or five times a day, will fulfil every indication that the boasted Panaceas and Catholicons can perform ; is free from the mercurial poisons such nostrums contain; and is much more safe and efficient as a medicine, for cleansing and purifying the blood.

PRICE ONE DOLLAR.
Prepared by   **J. ADAMS,**
United Society, New-Lebanon, N. Y.

Where are also prepared, Syrup of Cohosh for Rheumatism ; Compound Vegetable Cough Balsam for Pain in the Breast, Coughs, and Faintness of the Stomach ; Bilious and Cephalic Pills ; and various other vegetable medicines ; the formulæ of which are known and approved by the medical faculty of our country.

Strawberry

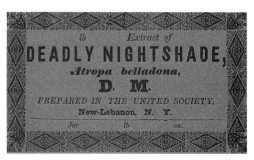

lb   *Extract of*
DEADLY NIGHTSHADE,
Atropa belladona,
D. M.
PREPARED IN THE UNITED SOCIETY,
New-Lebanon, N. Y.
Jar   lb   oz.

Blue cohosh

DIARY OF AN INVALID

Another diary was kept by Milton Homer Robinson of the South Union, Kentucky, society. He "went South to New Orleans" for his health. Eventually, after the long journey down the Mississippi River and by slow boat up the coast to Philadelphia, he took passage on a steamboat to New York with some New Lebanon Shakers he met in the City of Brotherly Love. His trip took him up the Hudson to Albany, where a wagon was hired for New Lebanon, and there he was put in the care of Brother Garrett Lawrence. The following excerpts from his diary demonstrate the Shakers' concern for health.

May 22, 1831. Pleasant weather. Brother Garrett Lawrence brought me a bottle of syrup to take for my cough. I took a glass and retired to my bed. May 23. Bro. Garrett Lawrence visited me and made some inquiries into the state of my health, how long I had been affected with the cough and Elder Brother John visited me again and desired that I would amuse myself by walking in Garrett's garden or to the House. Not to confine myself to close to the rooms. After breakfast Brother Daniel showed me the different gardens. May 26. 10 a.m. Brother Garrett K. Lawrence took me through a good bathing operation. Met John Wright brother of Lucy Wright our last Mother. Isaac also gave me council. Plans to return to New Orleans and then South Union cancelled, will stay now at 2nd Family and see how health improves. Some fears are apprehended that I would not be able to stand the journey home. Visited Garrett's gardens again and went through a sweating operation. May 31, 1831. 90°. I attended to Garrett's bees to watch and give notice when they would swarm. Issac N. Youngs measured me for a new pair of trousers.

June 1. Have done a considerable hoeing in Garrett's gardens today. I assisted Eliab Harlow about raising Elmbark. . . . Thurs. June 9th. Moderately warm. Gideon Kibby, Issac Knight and myself hived a swarm of bees this afternoon. Also Charlie Crosman and myself started at ½ after 3 o'clock p.m. with the 2 horse waggon to the mountain directly west of Bro. James Farnums family for a load of dogwood poles for the purpose of getting the bark as a medicine. . . . Received from the sisters a neat and pleasant summer hat and also a genteel and handsome frock for to wear to meetings at home and Sabbath evenings. June 11th. Went a strawberrying west of the medical garden. June 15th Garrett went with the 2 horse waggon for a load of Elm bark. June 17, 1831. A group of brothers and sisters took a ride for recreation and health to Lebanon P.O. [post office] thence to town of Hancock a distance of 6 miles where we put up at Tussells Tavern and eat supper about 3 o'clock. We return to New Lebanon by way of Hancock [Shaker Village] we did not stop there. We arrived at home about 6 o'clock p.m. and I can say that there are few days of my life that I took so much real comfort and satisfaction as I have taken today. The day was uncommon pleasant, the roads good and the company agreeable and interesting.

June 27th. I attend to keeping the fire rekindled under Garrett's kittles [kettles] of liverwort syrup for the purpose of inhaling the steam arising there from for the benefit of my lungs. . . . This morning Elder Bro. Sam Johnson and myself went on a visit to Hancock [the Shaker Village, not the town of

Hancock]. Sometime after we arrived there we obtained leave to visit their new brick building accompanied by El. Br. William Deming. From there we went to where Comstalk Betts was engaged making the doors for the above mentioned building. While here Elder Nathaniel came to the door and beaconed to S. Johnson to accompany him to the Ministry shop. Comstalk then accompanied me to a shop where Deacon Daniel Goodrich was employed in pasting paper bags to hold garden seed. I took great comfort with Daniel, he was familiar and pleasant and manifested a great desire for my future happenings and safe return to South Union.

For a while it seemed as if Milton's health was really improving. At least his diary was not so much concerned with it, and for over a month the entries had to do with the herb industry:

July 12. *Clear and moderate. G. K. Lawrence went to Washington for a load of timber and also for the purpose of engaging the digging of 30 or 40 pounds of spikenard roots and to get some other herbs. July 14. This afternoon Issac Knight and myself went up on the mountain and gathered a Dearborn load of yarrow. Something diverting. July 15. Garrett and company have been cutting and hauling catmint all day. The sisters with my assistance have picked it all over ready for cutting fine. July 18. Bro. Garrett went to Hancock on his professional business [doctoring]. July 19. Clear and warm. This morning Garrett K., Lucy C. Sarah K. and Hannah Ann went in two horse waggon to Whitings pond for the purpose of gathering medical herbs in the lots about home such as yarrow and catmint. Have been engaged this p.m. picking over wormwood. This weather is a great hindrance to the brothers in getting in the hay.*

Day after day two-horse wagons brought in loads of whortleberries, of wormwood, of catnip, of lobelia, of senna, and of Indian tobacco. The herbs were picked over and dried. Great loads of elm bark were cut up at the machine shop and then he reports: "I am some unwell and take a sweat in the p.m. Aug. 6th. Went to the ministry shop with a letter I have prepared to send to Elder Benjamin [of South Union]. Brother Rufus spared no pains to comfort me and make my way as easy as possible."

The handwriting now is very weak, the letters small and pale. He is obviously very sick. He writes "THE END" in larger-than-usual letters. There are two pages accounting for letters written by him and those received by him from South Union. It is a record of his correspondence and the end of the book also. Brother Milton Robinson died at age twenty-five on October 19, 1832.

There were many conferences regarding Milton's health and whether or not he should return to South Union. Brother Garrett attended him with great concern, and Milton records the comings and goings of this greatly admired doctor with fidelity and in detail. He had a tedious day coughing but was able to go to the Second Family to "see them casting stove-plate." Saturday, June 27, he attended a meeting where "they spoke the Gospel in unknown tongues," he reported.

"Oh that I could give the reader some idea," he continued, "of the beauty and simplicity, the life and the zeal manifested in this meeting. Suffice me to say it was everything that is pretty and good."

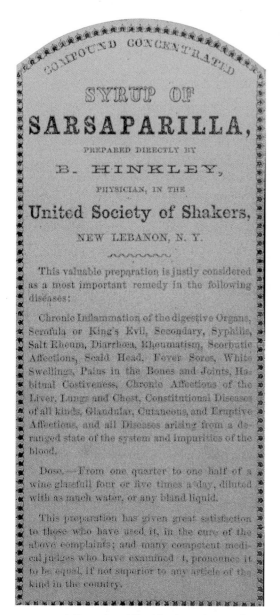

△ Barnabas Hinckley's testimonial can be seen on this label.

Notes of a Shaker Physician

These excellent journals are only the forerunners of one that is much fuller and gives more information about Brother Garrett. This is Barnabas Hinckley's account, written in 1836. He was the physician at the Church Family and conducted the herb industry after the deaths of Garrett Lawrence (1837) and Eliab Harlow (1840).

This record is important for many reasons. It gives a touching account of the love and affection felt for Brother Garrett as well as a real feeling of the activity of the medical herb department that was his business. It describes the business dealings in herbs that were carried on between societies, the visiting back and forth, and some of the medical practices.

May 16th. I commence working in the medical garden — sow to sage. . . .
17th. Scrape up and fix a bed and sow it to whiteroot and summer savory and set out some Butter Snakeroot. Continue plowing East. 19th. Rake and sow a bed — some sweet basil and Foxglove and Moldaven Balm. In the p.m. set out some rose bushes. May 20th. Garrett has a bad turn and I tend upon him beside ploughing the ground for peppermint and for I[Issachar]. Bates' willow slips. I. Bates and Eliab Harlow set out the slips. 21st. We set out the Hyssop bed in the alley and finish fixing the alley. Garrett gets some better so as to ride out with Levi Chauncey. 23rd. We commence setting out catnep. I. B. and E. H. and myself. 24th. We finish setting out catnep and I plough up the tanzy bed and set out some red rose bushes. 25th. We transplant some lemon balm and rake and fix a bed and set out some Lobelia Selfelettica [L. siphilitica]. 26th. Set out the peppermint and tanzy. 27th. Nothing down in the garden today, I put up some extract. 28th. We set out some chamomile and a row of lovage and marshmallow and sow three rows of poppy in the p.m. 31st. Help hoe out horehound.

June 1836. 1st. Sisters clean up the drying house. 3rd I assist Garret about this altorative [alterative] syrup and make some preparations for making a closet in the drying house. 13th. Transplant some horehound. 14th. I hold the plough to brake up east of the herb garden. 18th. We transplant the belladonna and Hysoscyamus and finish setting out horehound. 22nd. Garret and John Dean start out for Hoosic. Cut sage.

July 1st. Powder cicuta. 11th. Weed Foxglove south of the alley. 12th. Weed out the Time [thyme]. 14th. Transplant Foxglove. July 16th. Continue pounding Cicuta. G. L. goes after catnep. 28th. It rains today so I set out some sage.

August 23rd. I go with Charles Crossman to Albany. Aug. 24th. I got home about 4 o'clock with 500 and 45 lbs. of horehound from Sodus. 25th. Help Gideon cultivate his sage. 29th. Cut the belladonna and horehound.

Sept. 12th. G. K. Lawrence and John Dean start for New York. I pick over herbs. Elder Brother complains of being sick so I give him an emetic. 13th. Help cut sage. Eliab Harlow goes with N. Bennet out to Kinderhook after fleabane. 14th. Today I take a walk on the mountain with Elder Sister Ruth and Elder Sister Hannah Ann Treadway and I. Bates. We return home in good season and I steam Elder Brother and Gideon Turner who is some sick. 16th. Tend the sick. Help cut Summer Savory. 19th. Go on the mountain after Bugle and sculcap and other herbs. 21st. Do some chores and help the sisters gather Coltsfoot.

Between September 28 and October 4 Brother Barnabas describes a visit to Watervliet. Upon his return he resumes his record of daily activities.

Oct. 5. Back home. I grind some Hellebore and lady-slipper. Oct. 6th. Help pack herbs. Snowy today. 11th. Gather garden lettuce stalks for Extract. 24th. I cut some fox-glove and tend upon Jonathan Wood who is quite sick at the office.

[Nov.] 14th. Measles at the Second House. I get measles and feel sick. 16th. I feel better. My measles have turned and Garret H. Lawrence steam me and I begin to think about getting better. Nov. 21st. G. H. L. bottle up some sarsa-parilla syrup. 25th. Garret and I go over to Hancock to see George Wilerson who is sick with dropsey of the heart case. 28th. Garret and I pack some herbs for New York. 29th Garret goes to the Second House and commence a course of medicine to get prepared for tapping. Takes a dose of senna Jalap and cream a tartar and prepare some pills for Dr. Jonathan's doses.

Dec. 19th. Garret H. Lawrence moved into the south west room in the great house. Gideon and I tend upon him til the end.

Jan. 1. 1837. I commence again taking care of G. H. L. and continue thru his sickness with help of Dan Wood., after the 9th. 24th. Unwelcome event. Our beloved and useful brother GARRET H. LAWRENCE this morning departed this life at 10 mins. past 5 o'clock having passed thru a serious and lengthy sickness and hard sufferings. He has scarcely enjoyed any health since June 1833 at which time he has a severe attack of acute rheumatism.

[Feb.] 5. We tend the funeral at 2 o'clock p.m. 12 of the world, 6 males and 6 females attend.

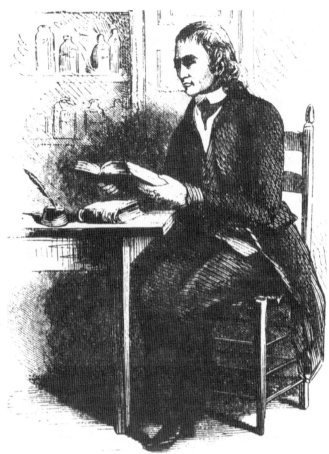

△ The physician at his desk was Barnabas Hinckley (1808–1861), a well-trained and careful doctor. He came to the Shakers in 1821 as a child and became their doctor in 1837, before he was even thirty years old. Later, after studying at the Berkshire Medical College in Pittsfield, Massachusetts, he received his degree in 1858, only three years before he died at fifty-three — young for a Shaker. He left a good medical library to the society.

THE CANAAN SOCIETY

The Shakers at Canaan, New York, three miles from Mount Lebanon, were fully organized in 1823 as the Upper and Lower Families. The Shakers considered the Canaan families to be two branches of the New Lebanon North Family.

Levi Shaw, a member of the Upper Canaan Family, wrote in his journal that he was born November 5, 1818, and came to the Shakers with his father after his mother died when he was six years old. "For the first six years after I came among Believers my occupation was chiefly in the Garden and Garden House, putting up Herbs in the summer season and at school in the winter season. In the fall of 1836 I was apprenticed to take charge of the fruit trees and fruit. In December 1836 I was apprenticed to take charge of the Boys there was then 5 of them in the order."

Diaries, journals, daybooks, and account books indicate that the Canaan Families assisted to a considerable extent in the herb department of the larger New Lebanon community. The Deaconesses' journal kept from 1843 to 1864 has numerous entries about gathering herbs at Canaan assisted by that family, and having them help out at Mount Lebanon.

May 1846. The 4th. Fruit trees in full bloom. Cherry, peach, Plum. 5th. Our dinner table today was graced with a noble plate of Pot Herbs, for the first time this season [cowslip greens]. 6th. The sisters not other ways engaged commenced cleaning elecompane roots. 13th. The sisters engaged in cleaning roots such as blue flag, angelica. 27th. Rhoda and Fanny go out with Canaan herbing after Squaw Weed.

June 3rd. Three sisters go with Joseph to Canaan after herbs. 10th. We go on the Mountain fishing. 11th. Joseph takes sisters to Canaan after herb and Shoemak [sumac] leaves.

July 1846. 3rd. Go after Johnswort to Canaan. 6th. To Canaan after Johnswort.

August 1st. 5 sisters spend chief of the day cutting Mayweed. 6th. We have a meeting commemorating our blessed Mother's landing in America. 11th. Go after Shoemake. 13th. Go after raspberry leaves. 19th. Sisters all engaged in cleaning roots. Canaan here helping. 20th. Go after laurel leaves. 24th. Clean roots. Canaan helps. 28th. After dinner 15 sisters are called to cutting sage, balm, etc. 29th. 5 sisters work in the garden picking leaves. 31st. Sisters pick leaves. Canaan here to help.

The South Union Ministry traveling in the spring and summer of 1869 recorded their visit to Canaan on August 4, 1869. The diarist commented on the fine sweet corn, pumpkins, and ice cream, and then remarked: "They have nearly abandoned the seed and herb business."

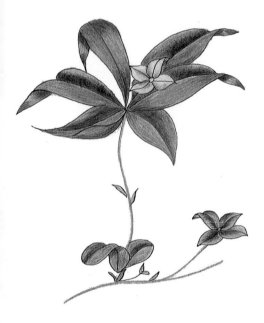

△ *Cornus canadensis,* drawn by Canterbury sister Cora Helena Sarle .

Visitors' Views

The travel journal of Eldress Betsy Smith gives us a concise picture of New Lebanon. The company from South Union, Kentucky, and Union Village, Ohio, arrived at Holy Mount on August 19, 1854, and stayed ten days:

Aug. 21. . . . Spent the forenoon in company with brothers Jonathan Wood [an herbalist] and Allen Reed, John Dean. . . . Came by the farm they recently purchased. Halted and went thro the Herb Garden. The lot & farms lying in the township of Lebanon. . . . The Believers carry on the herb and botanical business quite extensively. Raise a portion of the herbs themselves and buy a great many from the worlds people.

The sales in that business amounts to about $30,000 annually. Garden seed business carried on extensively and perhaps more Lucrative than the Botanic. In the afternoon we visited the second order, had an agreeable time of it with the good souls in that family, and returned to the office about dark, while there we went thro their herb and botanic establishment.

We were taken to bro Barnabas Hinckley medicine shop, saw many nice things & he made us a present of some nice candies of different kinds and gave each one of us a cologne bottle filled with cologne of their own manufacture. He covered some on the subject of medicine. Said he considers water is good in some case, but dont consider it a specific for all diseases. Uses medicine in some cases, and think's to advantage, and says he would make use in certain cases, any human remedy to mitigate pain. But at the same time he would be cautious about using strong medicines of all kinds, and not use them where one more simple would answer.

AIMING FOR SIMPLICITY

Had a visit with bro Henry DeWitt he prints all the herb laybills & seed bags saw him operate on the printing press. He thinks believers ought to avoid unnecessary embellishment in the printing, and instead of gaudy borders, use plain black lines.

FROM THE TRAVEL JOURNAL OF ELDRESS BETSY SMITH, AUGUST 1854

The Heart of the Shaker Herb Industry

Benson J. Lossing visited New Lebanon in 1857 and later that year, in *Harper's New Monthly Magazine,* published one of the best-detailed and best illustrated accounts of the Shaker herb industry. After meeting Elder Bushnell and Frederick Evans, he wrote, he had "an excellent supper" and returned to the family at the store, where he passed the night. The next day his investigation continued.

The chief business trustee of the Lebanon community, and whose name is best known abroad is Edward Fowler, a middle-sized man, about sixty years of age. With him I visited the various industrial establishments. These are situated in convenient places in various parts of the village. All of them are supplied with the best implements, and are conducted in the most perfect manner.

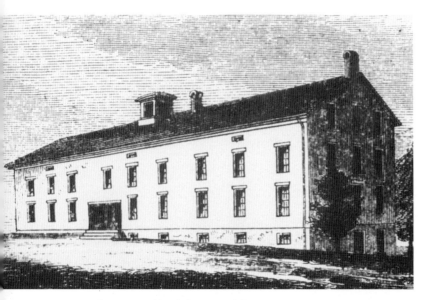

△ The original herb house of the Church Family was destroyed by fire in 1875. It contained all processes necessary to prepare, pack, and ship herbs. In 1870, the Second Order sisters cut more than a million labels in this building.

The Herb House

The Herb House, where the various botanical preparations are put up for market, is a frame building in the centre of the village, one hundred and twenty feet in length, and forty feet in width, and two stories and an attic in height. There are some spacious out-houses connected with it. The lower part is used for the business office, store-rooms, and for pressing and packing of herbs and roots. The second story and attic are the drying rooms, where the green herbs are laid upon sheets of canvas, about fourteen inches apart, supported by cords.

The basement is devoted to heavy storage and the horse-power by which the press in the second story is worked. That press, seen in the engraving, is one of the most perfect of the kind. It has a power of three hundred tons, and turns out each day about two hundred and fifty pounds of herbs, or six hundred pounds of roots, pressed for use. This performance will be doubled when steam shall be applied to the press. The herbs and roots come out in solid cakes, an inch thick, and seven and a quarter inches square, weighing a pound each. These are then taken into another room, where they are kept in small presses, arranged in a row, so as to preserve their form until placed in papers and labeled.

During the year 1855 about seventy-five tons of roots and herbs were pressed in that establishment. About ten persons are continually employed in his business, and occasionally twice that number are there, engaged in picking over the green herbs and cleansing the roots brought from the medicinal fields and gardens. The extra laborers are generally females. These fields and gardens cover about seventy-five acres, a portion of which is devoted to the cultivation of various herbs and vegetables for their seeds.

The Extract House and Laboratory

The Extract House, in which is the laboratory for the preparation of juices for medical purposes, is a large frame building, thirty-six by one hundred feet. It was erected in 1850. It is supplied with the most perfect apparatus, and managed by James Long, a skillful chemist, and a member of the Society. In the principal room of the laboratory the chief operations of cracking, steaming,

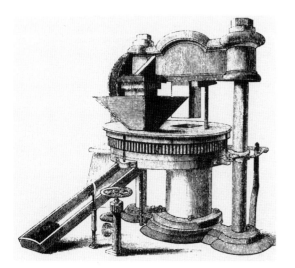

◁ The powerful hydraulic press, housed in the second story of the herb house, daily turned out 250 pounds of herbs and 600 pounds of roots pressed into solid pound cakes wrapped in dark blue paper.

and pressing the roots and herbs are carried on, together with the boiling of the juices thus extracted.

In one corner is a large boiler, into which the herbs or roots are placed and steam introduced. From this boiler, the steamed herbs are conveyed to grated cylinders, and subjected to immense pressure. The juices thus expressed are then put in copper pans, inclosed in iron jackets and the pans, and the liquid boiled down to the proper consistency for use. Some juices, in order to avoid the destruction or modification of their medical properties, are conveyed to an upper room and there boiled in a huge copper vacuum pan, from which, as its name implies, the air has been exhausted. This allows the liquid to boil at a much lower temperature than it would in the open air.

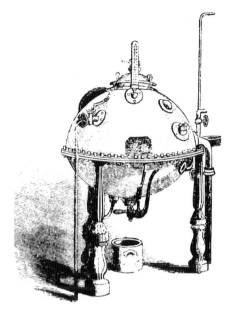

△ This vacuum pan gave added impetus to the herb industry in 1850. It was airtight, and herbal liquids were boiled in it at a low temperature. This piece of equipment attracted Gail Borden, and he perfected it in developing his evaporated milk. In 1931, it was purchased for $50 from Sister Emma J. Neale of the Church Family at Mount Lebanon by Borden's Milk Products Company, Inc. It is now in the collection of the Smithsonian Institution, Washington, D.C.

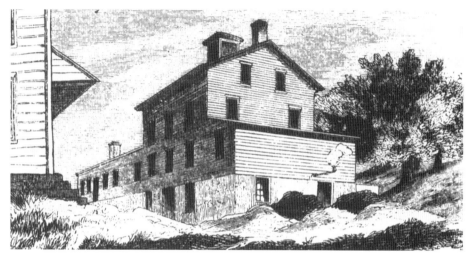

△ The extract house, erected in 1850, contained the laboratory for the preparation of juices for medicinal purposes. By 1855, various extracts were put up by the sisters, who prepared more than 75,000 pounds for market during one fifteen-year period.

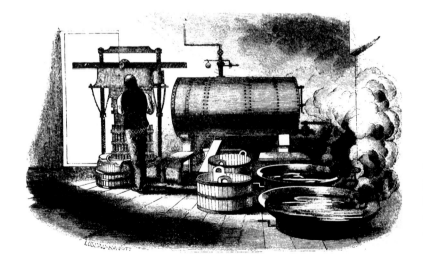

◁ Roots and herbs were cracked, steamed, and pressed in the laboratory of the extract house. The processes were carefully directed by skilled Shaker chemists. In 1861 and 1862, more than 100 different varieties, both solid and fluid, were manufactured.

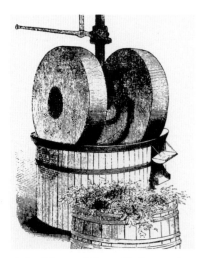

△ In this crushing mill, the roots and herbs, which were sold in powdered form, were first dried and then cracked and crushed.

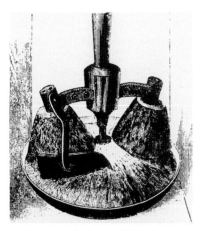

△ The powdering mill further reduced the crushed roots and herbs to the finest powder.

▷ The sisters worked in the finishing room wrapping and packing herbs. They attached beautiful labels printed on light blue, mint green, salmon, pale pink, nut brown, orange, and yellow paper, made by Crane and Company of Dalton, Massachusetts.

Extracting and Grinding

In a room adjoining the vacuum pan are mills for reducing dried roots to impalpable powder. These roots are first cracked to the size of "samp" [coarse hominy] in the room below, by being crushed under two huge discs of Esopus granite, each four feet in diameter, a foot in thickness and a ton in weight. These are made to revolve in a large vessel by steam power. The roots are then carried to the mills above. These are made of two upper and a nether stone of Esopus granite. The upper stones are in the form of truncated cones, and rest upon the nether stone, which is beveled. A shaft in the centre, to which they are attached by arms, makes them revolve, and at the same time they turn upon their own axes. The roots ground under them by this double motion are made into powder almost impalpable [so fine that it cannot be felt].

The Finishing Room

In a building near the Extract House is the Finishing Room, where the preparations, already placed in phials, bottles, and jars, are labeled and packed for market. This service is performed by two women; and from this room those materials, now so extensively used in the materia medica, are sent forth. These extracts are of the purest kind. The water used for the purpose is conveyed through earthen pipes from a pure mountain spring, an eighth of a mile distant, which is singularly free from all earthy matter. This is of infinite importance in the preparation of these medicinal juices. They are, consequently, very popular, and the business is annually increasing. During the year 1855 they prepared at that laboratory and sold about fourteen thousand pounds. The chief products are the extracts of dandelion and butternut. Of the former, during that year, they put up two thousand five hundred pounds; of the latter, three thousand pounds.

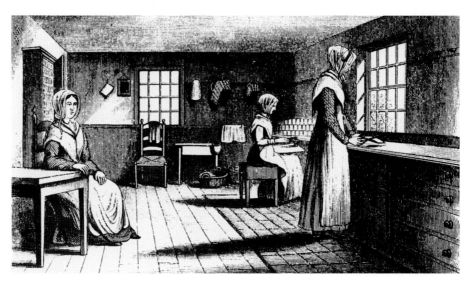

An Orderly System

Lossing was much impressed with the perfect order and neatness that prevailed. "System is every where observed," he wrote, "and all operations are carried on with exact economy. Every man, woman and child is kept busy. The ministry labor with their hands, like the laity, when not engaged in spiritual and official duties; and no idle hands are seen. Having property in common, the people have no private ambitions nor personal cares; and being governed by the pure principles of their great leading doctrines, they seem perfectly contented and happy. All labor for the general good, and all enjoy the material comforts of life in great abundance."

Lossing also mentioned an outstanding Shaker doctor.

The Medical Department, under the charge of Dr. Hinckley, appears to be perfect in its supplies of surgical instruments, and other necessaries. A large portion of the medicines are prepared by themselves; and Dr. Hinckley applies them with a skillful hand, under the direction of a sound judgment. He has a library of well-selected medical works; and the system which he most approves and practices is known as the Eclectic [a method of selecting what seemed best from various sources and systems].

Productivity and Prosperity

"They prospered in sales" was frequently said about the Shakers, and indeed, their meticulous accounts proved it. One daybook kept by the Church Family from 1860 to 1862 records that a prodigious amount of material was processed.

This diary gives an account of the production of extracts from May through December 1860. The output for May, June, and July totaled over 2,500 fluid pounds, from these herbs:

Quassia, bayberry, lady slipper, common dandelion, stillingia, sarsaparilla, yellow dock, rhubarb, senna, columbo, English valerian, henbane, jalap, belladonna, mandrake, butternut, goldenseal, stramonium, cicuta. Received 9 loads and obtained 8 barrels of juice.

In August the record continues.

1st. James makes 150 lbs. Stramonium ointment. 6th. Spread nine barrels of Golden Seal in kiln. Benj. Gates and Br. Daniel start West. 7th. Press out lobelia tintc. 130 lbs. from 45 lbs of herbs. Press out lady slipper, tintc. 140 lbs. from one bushel of roots. Press out Rhatany tinct., 271 lbs. from 10 lbs. of roots. 10th. Finished Scullcap. Put about 50 lbs. more or less Golden Seal to macerate. James making preparations to go to salt water [on vacation].

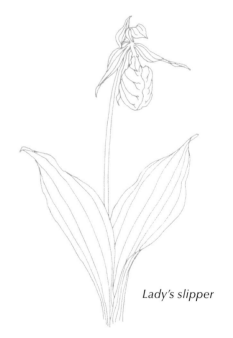

Lady's slipper

11th. Take up 194 lbs. pulverized Scullcap in 4 days. 24th. Work at the herb shop for Gabriel who goes after Feverbush and Black alder. 28th. Put in a chest full of sarsaparilla. 364 lbs. whole chopped, 92 lbs. chaff leavings off the ground, total 456 lbs. fill chest with water to top of the glass. Put 4 barrels of ground Scullcap in the kiln to pulverize. Receive also 5 bushels of Bayberry for a like purpose and 1 barrel about 98 lbs. yellow dock for fluid extract, 114 gross. 29th. Fire up and cook Sarsaparilla. 30th. Drain off liquor and press the Sarsaparilla. Put into chest 385 lbs. more Sarsaparilla. That being all they have. 31st. Finish evaporating Sarsaparilla, 140 lbs. and cook. SUMMARY 556 lbs. fluid extracts; 140 lbs. solid extracts; 150 lbs. Stramonium ointment; 194 pulverized scullcap.

At this time the Shakers were selling their fluid extracts for $1.25 a pound, but they charged more for pulverized material and ointments. The total output according to this book represents a sales value of at least $4,500 for the four months.

The same daybook continuing for September states on September 8, "Press Unicorn [star root, *Aletris farinosa* of the lily family, widely used for colic]. 11th. James stills cherries and gets between 2 and 3 gallons brandy. Alonzo and Henry C. [Clough] get 2 bushels of black cherries for S. A. Co."

For some reason October was skipped or perhaps recorded elsewhere. "November 20th. . . . Pulverize with West pair and try the new outlet which works like a charm." And then to start the year's last month:

Dec. 3, 1860. Benjamin [Gates] arrives about noon in company with the State Chemist, Prof. Charles H. Porter, James having reported that he had mislabelled the extracts. Dr. Porter takes a view of matters and gives his advice which amounts to rejecting a few bottles of medicine not adequately designated by their labels, 2 or 3 bottles being distributed. The fact is none of us believe the report to be anything but report, but are confident after a close scrutiny that all is right so far it concerns articles actually labelled. Dr. Porter leaves soon after dinner taking with him a bottle of Veratrum for examination, also some Aconite crystals and poppy deposites. Three days this week spent putting up extracts, one day spent in unpacking, cleaning and putting away up stairs 200 lbs. white jars. [These beautiful ceramic jars with a fine glaze had snug-fitting lids and held one pound of ointment.]

Dec. 8th. Press Bloodroot. Dec. 10th. Nearly one foot of snow on the ground. Try an experiment making Bloodroot tincture and conclude to resaturate the foot. 12th. Receive a keg of lard containing 90 lbs. hard fat for stramonium ointment. 13th. Alonzo goes to Albany with Benjamin to see the chemist. Find him absent. Take out some of the Quassia above mentioned to have it tested by Dr. Porter's assistant who was unable to detect any copper and gave his opinion that there was not copper enough in it to injure it. Dec. 31st. Pick over Bayberry.

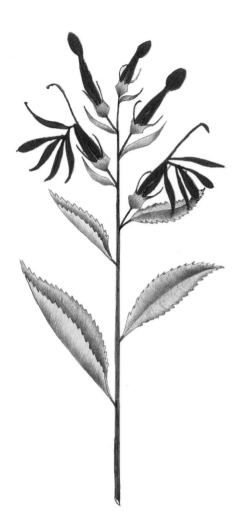

△ *Lobelia cardinalis,* drawn by Canterbury sister Cora Helena Sarle.

Shaker Medicines

The Shakers processed and sold a variety of products developed by outside physicians. Shaker gardeners could ensure quality: They usually propagated plants themselves from the best stock, they carefully tended their gardens, and they were able to harvest and process large quantities of herbs at the optimal moment.

Norwood's Veratrum

An example was tincture of hellebore, which sold under the name of "Norwood's Veratrum" because of the wide distribution and persistent advertising by Dr. W. C. Norwood, who maintained, "It is nervine, not narcotic." The manufacturers claimed that it was efficacious in treating "puerperal eclampsia, pneumonia, typhoid fever, hypertrophy of heart, dysmenorrhea, acute rheumatism, aneurism, scarlet fever, measles, etc., yellow fever, and other diseased conditions."

Dr. Norwood had originally produced this medicine, but, as the demand constantly increased, he employed the Shaker society at Lebanon for a number of years to make it under his direction. Before he died he turned the business entirely over to the Shakers. It was a powerful drug not to be administered heedlessly or by amateurs. The product carried the guarantee of the Food and Drug Act of June 30, 1906, Serial No. 3026.

Sister Marcia Bullard recalled that the sisters made thousands of paper boxes for use in sending out medicines. They also cut paper wrappers, which they made on a form just large enough to slip around a four-ounce bottle of Norwood's tincture.

The Shakers of New Lebanon published a booklet in eleven editions from the early 1850s to 1904 that extolled the powerful, but controllable, effects of tincture of *Veratrum viride* (white hellebore). Most of the booklet was devoted to specific cases submitted by doctors, the procedure followed in administering hellebore, and the results. Then several pages outlined specific diseases that could be treated effectively by using the medicine, and five pages contained testimonials from doctors.

ADVERTISEMENT

Having frequently visited the Laboratory and Botanic Gardens of the Shakers, at New Lebanon, Columbia County, New York, I can unhesitatingly recommend their Preparations, as the most pure and reliable Medicines manufactured in the country, as they spare no pains in doing their work on the most scientific and Pharmaceutical principles. Just such articles as the Practitioner wants to ensure him success in his Professional treatment; and as such I recommend them to the Medical Faculty.

DR. NORWOOD

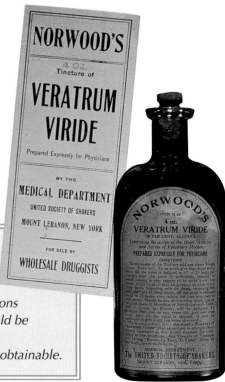

NORWOOD'S VERATRUM

In March 1934 the Shakers printed the formula for the tincture:

Take 200 lbs. of White Hellebore Roots put in container & cover with 52 gallons of 85% Alcohol, let stand 16 days in mash, then drain, press & strain. It should be 75% when ready to bottle.

This medicine prepared by the Shakers, is made from the purest materials obtainable.

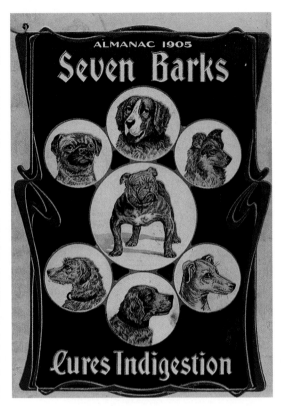

ALMANAC 1905

Seven Barks

Cures Indigestion

△ This is the last publication in a series of almanacs, published annually by Lyman Brown beginning in 1883.

The last three pages in the book listed seventy botanicals used in "Pure Vegetable Extracts, solid and fluid, Manufactured by the Shakers." This was preceded by a statement concerning the Shaker botanic gardens, the laboratory, and its very complete and expensive fixtures. It concluded with a point that had created some debate during the period:

It has been a matter of controversy among Apothecaries and Pharmaceutists, whether it was wise in the Inspissated juices, to retain the Chlorophylle and Albumen, so as to preserve the green color, as an index of its careful preparation; but the well conducted experiments of Mr. Solon have proved them to be nearly inert. Hence their presence only tends to enfeeble the proper extract; and by the recommendation of Professor Proctor of Philadelphia, and others, we shall in most cases reject them, unless otherwise desired by parties so ordering in time for preparing.

A Variety of Botanical Products

About this same time another preparation became popular and sold on a par with Brother Barnabas Hinckley's Syrup of Sarsaparilla. It was "The Genius of Beauty! Toilet Prize and Sufferer's Panacea or Imperial Rose Balm." It was claimed to be unequaled for cleaning the teeth, healing sore or spongy gums, and soothing the sore mouths of children. It was supposed to cure foul ulcers and pimples, ringworm, salt rheum, and chapped hands and face; it also could soothe burns, scalds, bruised skin, sunburns, and freckles. It was a beautiful and useful toilet soap for ladies and an excellent fluid for gentlemen to rub on their faces immediately after shaving.

Another Shaker medicine produced at Mount Lebanon in the 1880s was Seven Barks, manufactured exclusively for Dr. Lyman Brown. It contained blue flag, butternut, goldenseal, sassafras, lady's slipper, bloodroot, black cohosh, and mandrake. A second preparation called Pain King is mentioned in an undated letter by Benjamin Gates concerning these preparations: "Lyman Brown goes to Mexico. He has a good supply . . . at present [of Pain King and Seven Barks] so do not distress our good Sisters. Only think they put up in 3 days NINETEEN THOUSAND, TWO HUNDRED BOTTLES." Seven Barks was modified early in 1905 and eventually contained only one of the original barks — powdered sassafras.

The Shaker Asthma Cure, made at Lebanon, sold very well. The Shakers stated in its promotion that "No disease is harder to cure." And, "We offer the reasonable hope that the preparation will effect a cure, and a still greater possibility exists that it will procure at least so much relief that you can breathe air of heaven without distress and be able to lie down and find rest in sleep."

Shaker Hair Restorer also met with approval from a public who was informed that

The well-known Society of Shakers . . . has, for a century past been engaged in the cultivation of medicinal herbs and in this preparation of various essences, extracts and compounds, that are largely used in medical practice and by the public at large. The Society takes great pleasure in informing the public that they have added a HAIR RESTORA-TIVE to their already lengthy list of preparations. GRAY HAIR MAY BE HON-ORABLE, BUT THE NATURAL COLOR IS PREFERABLE.

Besides their efficacious qualities there was a charm and beauty to the herbal preparations of the Shakers. The labels for Extract of Dandelion, English Valerian, Syrup of Arnikate of Tannin, Shaker Family Cough Syrup, Vegetable Pills, Decoction of Rumex, Vegetable Cough Drops, Taraxacum Blue Pills (for the liver), Concentrated Syrup of Bitter Bugle (for consumption), and Vegetable Aromatic Cephalic Snuff (a powerful remedy for pain and dizziness in the head) were colorful and the products immaculately packaged. Labels for pressed herbs were printed on light blue, mint green, salmon, nut brown, orange, and yellow papers. Medicine labels were plainly printed with informative directions, given in simple English, and were easy to follow.

As the business grew it was necessary for the Shakers to have help in distribution. In the 1870s A. J. White of 319 Pearl Street, New York City, served them well — and himself, too, no doubt, as it was to be a most lucrative account. Mr. White solicited others to take on the selling and issued a pamphlet outlining the benefits the salesmen would enjoy. The Shakers also made "White's Curative Syrup" for this agent. He advertised that the Shakers had a worldwide reputation for gathering and curing roots, barks, and herbs and had been engaged in the business for "upwards of fifty years." He said that whatever the Shakers manufactured was anxiously sought by the public.

They are now engaged in making a medical preparation which has been placed in my hands for sale. For the purpose of enlisting your services in selling this Medicine, I send you this Circular, thinking perhaps that you may find it to your interest to take the Agency. The business is respectable, for all goods made by the Shakers are known to possess real merit. It can not be classed with the ordinary patent Medicines of the day, as there is no secret about its composition, the formula from which it is prepared being printed on each bottle.

PAIN KING

Brother Benjamin wrote out the original formula for Pain King:

20 gal. water. 10 lbs. Witch Hazel bark, stir well every-day for one week. 20 gall. strong alcohol — oils Spruce, Sassafras, Peppermint, Camphor gum, dissolve in separate portions of alcohol and mix all together — Opium, reduce to a miscible condition with warm water and Masher till all parts are accessible to alcohol and water, after the former mixture has been put together and well stirred. Or find out by Dispensatory, by The Pharmaceutical Journal, what is the proper strength of Alcohol to extract the active principle of Opium, and preceed accordingly. Then mix with the rest.

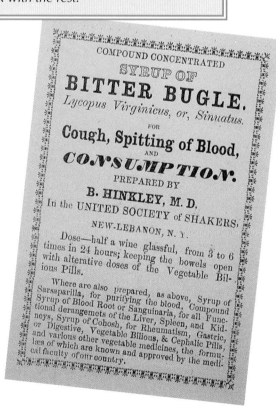

Some firms, however, found cause to complain that Shaker material was inferior — as in the following letter, dated 1877 — but this was not the general rule:

Edward Fowler
Friend

The Parsley Rt. and Sage leaves came to hand yesterday and on examination prove very unsatisfactory.
The root seems to be roasted inside and for our use worthless. The sage is all shrivelled up and discolored. We send in this mail samples of each.
We write to have you be more careful of the next lot you put on the kiln.
Send some of each prime quality immediately for we cannot use these. Also chicory and comfrey. The Parsley Leaves are prime.

Respectfully yours,
Peck and Velsor

The inferior quality was the result of improper drying in the kiln and not due to the choice of material gathered.

A TRUSTEE'S ERRAND

In August 1884, Benjamin Gates wrote to Henry Clough from the Windsor Hotel in Montreal, where he was on a mission of considerable importance to the society. The company making Smith Brothers Cough Drops had, it appeared, been using "Shaker" as a trademark in selling its product. Brother Benjamin and Agent White were trying to settle the problem:

Montreal. August 20th. 1884

Dear Bro. H. Clough. It looks a little like my having to go to Ottawa.
We find Smith Bros. have registered in Ottawa the name Shaker as their trademark. This we must have taken off from the Government records or it will stand for ages. Smith Bro. are poor and want us to purchase their Trademark "Shakers". How funny this looks. How Contemptable. Meaness boiled down!! A. J. White is disgusted and feels determined to uproot this business. I am quite willing to give him a lift in the good work.
Arn't that real Cheeky to ask us to purchase this Trade Mark. A name our Society has used for over one Hundred Years. What will come next?
I need not repeat how much I love thee. Only remember it and think of it often and all is right.

Your Bro. Benjamin G.

The matter was resolved in favor of the Shaker society according to subsequent references, but we do not know whether Brother Benjamin had to go to Ottawa.

The Mount Lebanon medicine department made a sarsaparilla under its own name as well as preparing quantities of the extract *in vacuo,* which was sold to other manufacturers. It was a medicine made by hundreds of companies and was quite naturally produced by the Lebanon Shakers, but never on as large a scale as that of the Canterbury or Union Village societies.

Other "best sellers" included Mother Seigel's Syrup (Extract of Roots), also sold by White but distributed by other companies as well.

Witch Hazel and Mother Seigel

There is considerable light-hearted correspondence from Benjamin Gates to Henry Clough during the 1880s. Generally the substance of the letters concerned sales, what firms had placed orders, and whether to ship the material by "Express" or "other means." Gates wrote on September 23, 1882: "Now for Witch Hazel. Br. Alonzo [Hollister] said to me there was a good supply on hand. Is he right? Rubber Gloves shall have full attention. The large Corks for Sister Cornelia were shipped long ago. So says our friend Lyman [Brown]. No matter how things go I love THEE still. Your best friend, Benjamin."

On a selling trip in New York City, Benjamin Gates wrote on October 31, 1885: "Dear Henry, The Prophet, The Wheelman, The Dude. I have secured orders as follows: 4800 Doz. Mother Seigel done in Spanish Labels. 4800 Doz. in English for London. Now is the time to make Hay while the Sun Shines. Don't let them Slumber. Your Br. B. G."

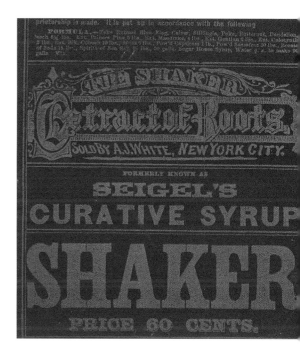

Native American Plant Knowledge

As has been shown, the sisters and brothers did most of the picking of the herbs and roots, but on occasion they were helped by others. A letter dated 1807 from "David at New Lebanon, to the world," says: "The Indians are here helping, mostly bringing botanics from the fields and woods."

An 1842 journal kept at New Lebanon records Native Americans attending meetings and concludes:

Nov. 30th. All now sat down in a ring and the Indians felt they had a great
    privilege. Gave baskets of all sizes and showed Elder Sister how to make
    them. Also blankets, leather pieces and hides and fur skins of animals.
    Nice large amounts of berries, dried very well and wild roots especially
    prized at this time by our Physicians it being now the beginning of the
    cold season. We have made an understanding that the wild produce will
    be coming to us in regular amounts as their picking is clean and material
    is not cut into or marred. L. G. [Lawrence Garrett] is pleased to have this
    extra source and will guide them as to the general variety of roots and
    herbs he needs from their woods which are rich in resources.

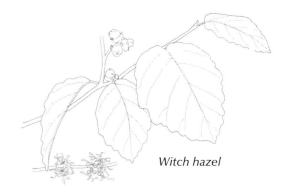

Witch hazel

Another entry describes Native Americans who brought cornmeal they had ground:

But being of a clean and nice consistency we enjoyed it and gave some fruits[,] in exchange[,] for their children. There were 5 large baskets of roots for the herb house and in a sack many barks all kept apart and easy for us to determine and use. The brothers are very pleased now to have Indians understand and separate properly.

A Prodigious Output

James Vail kept a record of his business in the herb shop at New Lebanon covering the years from 1841 to 1857, and the book was continued by Alonzo Hollister through 1902. According to these records, Vail began pressing herbs in the winter of 1841, and each year he felt constrained to press a greater amount until his activity built up to a production in 1853 of 400 days (he worked some nights all through and included the time as "days"). He gathered and cleaned roots and herbs, made extracts and ointments, and cut labels for the packages — a total of 98,179 pounds for the market, or just over 245 pounds a day.

Continuing his summary Vail says: "1854 covering same material less in pounds and only 160 days worth, but next year 405 days work and about the same pounds as 1853 and in 1857 these new items added: Blue flag, Comfrey, Polewort, Pole Cat Weed, Skunk Cabbage, Hyssop, Nettle blows, Buskbean, Canada Snakeroot, yarrow, Lovage, Strawberry Leaves, total for 1858, 18552 pounds. Total for the past 7 years $57,290."

He also wrote that on "January 17, 1851, herbalists borrowed the printing press from Watervliet from which was dirived the plans and execution of the press upon which the printing is now done for the Herb Extract and Seed business."

Blazes . . . and Recovery

On February 6, 1875, eight buildings were burned in New Lebanon. In November 1890, the Church Family lost its drying kiln by fire, worth about $4,000. On September 18, 1894, a midnight blaze destroyed a number of buildings belonging to the same family. One contained a year's store of roots, alone valued at $1,500. These buildings were at the East Farm. Like the previous fires at Mount Lebanon, it was the work of an incendiary.

Despite these catastrophic events, the medicine department made a strong comeback every time, for the orders continued to pour in and were promptly filled. A typical small order from "Friend W. H. Barnes" dated May 9, the year after the fire of 1875, was filled by Edward Fowler and

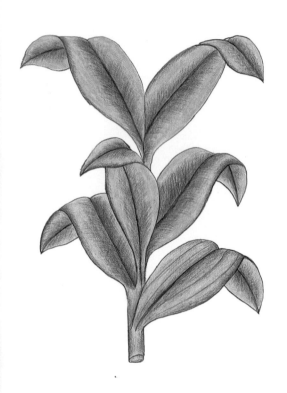

△ False hellebore *(Veratrum viride)*, drawn by Canterbury sister Cora Helena Sarle.

amounted to $75 before discount. It included the following fluid extracts: bugle weed, cherry bark, cleavers, cotton root, hydrangea, motherwort, pleurisy root, Virginia snakeroot, stone root, wahoo, witch hazel, yarrow, belladonna, burdock, cinchona, coltsfoot, dandelion, gelsemium, lettuce, mandrake, sarsaparilla, skullcap, *Veratrum viride,* skunk cabbage, and ipecac. Similar orders for extracts and dried herbs and roots at this time indicated that business was good.

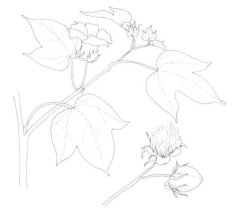

Cotton root

Almanacs Tell the Story

A series of Shaker almanacs was printed and distributed by A. J. White, the Shakers' agent in New York, and those issued after the fire of 1875 told of the great loss suffered. But in an editorial, "A Wonderful Success in Business," White tells how the Shakers got back on their feet in an amazingly short time and continued to produce the medicines "upon which the Shakers had spent much study and labor to bring to perfection."

HERBALISTS TO THE WORLD

The Englishman Hepworth Dixon is quoted in the 1882 almanac as saying:

The writer was struck with the excellence of everything they produced. Their butter was of the very best. Their brooms were prime. The chairs easy, comfortable and durable. Their flannels, of an extra quality. Indeed everything they made was of the very best, and commanded an extra price when offered for sale. Each family had some special industry, by means of which a living was made.

One family made a specialty of medicinal herbs and plants and their reputation for this particular branch has become known throughout the world. Going into one large building the writer found thirty or forty women and children putting up medicine, which they said was being sent to all parts of the world.

They had agencies in England, Belgium, Germany, Italy, Spain, Australia, Constantinople, Greece, India, Africa, and in fact in all parts of the world. They said that they had shipped

enough to London alone within the last three years to make the enormous number of 5,000,000 bottles. What amazed the writer was that such an enormous trade could be created for a medicinal preparation without the usual newspaper puffing and advertising; and what struck him still more forcibly was that this vast amount of medicine was for the cure of one single disease — Dyspepsia. The Shakers claim that modern civilization and modern cooking produce dyspepsia in every country and in every climate. That it is not only a national disease with Americans, but it is a prevailing disease everywhere. That nearly all our bodily troubles have their origin in this one cause, viz: Indigestion.

When asked how such an enormous demand could be created without the usual puffing, they said the remedy possessed merit, and when once used, the party obtaining relief recommended it to others, so that its good name spread from one to another, as the news spreads in India.

Shaker recipes are included on every page of the almanacs for 1882, 1883, and 1884. These covered a galaxy of dishes such as roast mutton, fried chicken, scalloped oysters, and bread puddings. Also suggested were dishes for party fare: okra soup, Spanish cream, lemon cake, and rhubarb pies. They appeared on the same pages with Shaker Family Pills (The Cathartic) and Pain King.

Illustrations portrayed "Mrs. Langtry, said to be the most beautiful lady in England; Arabi Pasha, the Head of the Rebel Army in Egypt; the Khedive of Egypt and William S. O'Brien of Flood and O'Brien, California, the most successful miner in the world."

The "new" Shaker almanacs of 1884 and 1885 gave the history of the Shakers at Mount Lebanon. The issue for 1884 showed photographs for the first time — of the meetinghouse, a group of Shakers, and their dwelling house. In 1885 Dr. White included many more different pictures. The first was of a brother at work crushing the roots for the Shaker Extract or Seigel's Syrup; followed by a view of two brothers in the laboratory boiling the roots for the Shaker Extract; then a picture of Alonzo Hollister, "the famous Shaker chemist," concentrating the Shaker Extract of Roots or Seigel's Syrup in a vacuum pan; and five pictures of the Shaker sisters at work in the medical department filling bottles with the extract, from the enormous vats; corking the bottles, which were held in wooden, slat-bottomed trays; labeling and wrapping the bottles; sealing the bottles; and an ancient sister pasting the labels on the bottles. A final print shows seven brothers packing and shipping the large wooden boxes containing hundreds of bottles of Mother Seigel's Syrup. Dr. White then concludes the 1885 almanac:

We confidently recommend this as the most reliable and trustworthy publication of its kind before the public. No care or expense has been spared in its preparation, and the astronomical calculations are the result of many months' untiring labor, both for us and the scientific men whose services we engaged for this purpose. Most of the so-called Almanacs are simply a rehash of the previous years' figures, and are utterly valueless. The Shaker Family Almanac forms a striking contrast when compared with publications of such a class.

Last Catalogs

During the 1880s seed catalogs were being issued by the Mount Lebanon society and at least seven carried from 13 to 25 herb seeds, "sweet, pot and medicinal." The Shakers offered the seeds of anise, balm, sweet basil, caraway, castor-oil plant, catnip, coriander, dill, fennel, hop, horehound, hyssop, lavender, sweet marjoram, opium poppy, rosemary, rue, saffron, sage, summer savory, winter savory, broad-leaved sorrel, broad-leaved English thyme, tansy, wormwood, and the medicinal white mustard. Those that included herb seeds were published in 1881, 1884, 1885, 1887, and 1888.

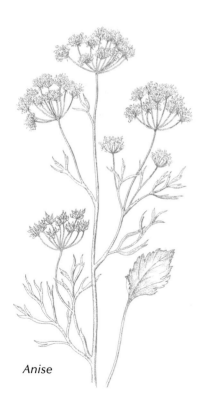

The Shakers have sent to London alone 20,000,000 bottles of their Elixier of Roots to cure Dispepsia and Rheumatism.
FROM THE 1885 ALMANAC

Anise

Waning of the Herb Industry

Despite the advertising, the testimonials, and the known worth of the products, the medicinal herb industry at Mount Lebanon was slipping badly in the 1890s. Henry Clough left for New York City, and a sad letter from his old schoolteacher, Sister Amelia J. Calver, bemoans this fact. In this letter is all the despair of the Shakers as their society began to diminish.

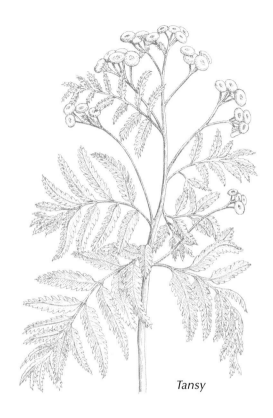

Tansy

April 23, 1890

Dear Brother Henry:

When you read this note you doubtless will be far from home and its many friends. It all seems so strange that I can hardly force myself to realize the truth. . . . It seems hard to us who have hoped and toiled for so many years, to see one generation after another of those reared here who are capable of keeping our home buoyed up to a respectable level, pass out of it and their places filled [by] mendicants, whose only interest is to find an easy corner and care neither for beauty nor order.

I so regret that you disregarded my advice to you last spring. "It is easier to drop out of line of duty, than to take it up." Had you pursued the even tenor of your way, your enemies would have been disarmed, and you triumphant. As it is you and your friends are the suffering party, while that horrid "I told you so", will do its best to crowd us back into the shades of long ago.

But we are used to bearing and suffering, and shall still endeavor to bear up; in fact we shall have to, to save our lives, for the depression we now feel will crush us unless some new line of thought comes to our relief.

We shall try to keep the things in good shape, over which you have toiled, that when you return you will have no need to go the whole ground over again.

But dear brother, you are going to the city. Beware! Homesick feelings will no doubt depress you; new acquaintances may excite you; but do for our sakes keep a steady lookout for the little errors which ruin so many. Don't smoke nor chew; nor taste the social glass. Your nerves your means your happiness; your life will need a safe guard against every thing which your quiet Shaker life has prohibited. Pardon a sister's frankness; but be assured we shall still love and earnestly pray for you, that every blessing of life may be yours. Your sorrow will be our sorrow and your joy our joy and we shall always think of you as our "Lost Boy".

Yours sincerely,
Amelia J. Calver

Henry Clough did return nineteen years later to direct the medicine department once again, according to a February 19, 1909, announcement.

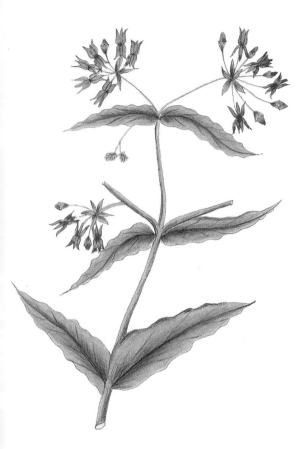

△ Butterfly weed, which the Shakers called pleurisy root, drawn by Canterbury sister Cora Helena Sarle.

It became more difficult, however, to attract converts and increase membership in the society. Keeping the good health of the community therefore became a paramount objective. The study of diuretics to maintain health had been pursued relentlessly by Frederick Evans in earlier days. These methods were now relied upon more than ever and guided many of the Shaker leaders in maintaining the health of the Believers. One sister wrote:

Last note for Mt. Lebanon — Social Life and Vegetarianism, by Martha J. Anderson, Mt. Lebanon 1893. We are increasing our fruit crop every year. Grapes are especially wholesome and are much cheaper and more palatable than drugs. We have not had a fever in the family for 50 years. Judicious water treatment, simple massage and the use of hot herb drinks are our methods of cure in cases of sickness.

Some must always battle with inherited tendencies to disease but if they live strictly moral lives, and adhere to hygienic laws they will live more comfortably. Great good is attained in this direction by fortifying the mind against the ills of the body, and rising superior to them.

Nonetheless, the days when the sisters fifteen strong went to gather thyme and saffron every day for a month, collected sage and stramonium leaves, and cleaned roots all day long for thirty days in October — those days were gone. Gone, too, were the visits recorded so dutifully: "Jan. 13, 1858 Doctor Norwood of New York is here to get some tincture of Hellebore made at our Extract works."

The business became history when Mount Lebanon closed for good in 1947.

CHAPTER 3

Groveland, New York

IN 1826 THE SHAKERS ESTABLISHED a small community on Sodus Bay on Lake Ontario. The land was sold ten years later when a branch from the Erie Canal was projected to pass through it, and the residents moved to Groveland, New York. Then in 1892 this community, which once had about 200 members in two families, was sold, and the Shakers moved to Watervliet, New York.

Although the Shakers apparently did not offer herbs for sale from Groveland, a little book, "Receipts of Materia Medica, written at Groveland, May 1842," contains several herbal remedies. Five of the recipes containing twenty-six different herbs are given here.

Be what you seem to be, and seem to be what you really are; don't carry two faces.

FATHER JAMES WHITTAKER

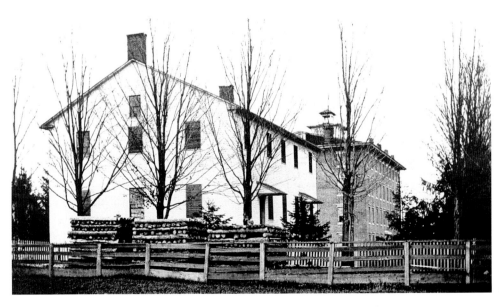

◁ View of the Shaker community at Groveland.

Purifying Tea

- 1 tablespoon Spanish pins [pines]
- 2 tablespoons Bittersweet
- 2 tablespoons Green Ozier bark
- 2 tablespoons Black Birch bark
- 3 tablespoons Black Cohosh
- 2 tablespoons Princes pine
- 2 tablespoons Mountain Lettuce
- 2 tablespoons Sarsaparilla
- ½ tablespoons Saffron. Pulv. & Mix.

1 lb. to be in a gallon of water and boiled down to two quarts. Strain and add three lbs. of sugar and one pint Spirits. This medicine purifies the blood and excites the secretions, in general, it should be taken for a considerable time as much as the stomach will bear. A dose of Billious pills should be taken once or twice a week while taking this syrup.

Indian Consumptive Syrrup

- 4 ounce Wild Turnip
- 1 ounce Skunk Cabbage seed
- 1 ounce White root
- 1 ounce Rum
- 1 ounce Honey

To be put in a stone jug unstopped and boiled in a kettle of water for an hour. Dose ¼ of a wine glass three or four times a day before eating.

Pectoral Syrrup

- 2 tablespoons Wa-a-hoo bark
- 1 tablespoon Boneset
- 1 tablespoon Waterpepper
- 1 tablespoon Princes pine
- 1 tablespoon Bittersweet bark
- 1 tablespoon Black Cohosh

To be boiled in an iron kettle with soft water, when the strength is out, to be strained off then boiled down to the consistency of thin Molasses, to which add one fourth West India Molasses. This should be scalded an hour over a slow fire and it is fit for use. Dose a tablespoon full to be taken three or four times a day before eating. To be used in consumption, Coughs, affections of the liver, spleen, etc.

Cough Drops

- 2 ounces Liquorice root
- 1 ounce Blood root
- 1 ounce Senica Snake root
- 1 ounce Skunk Cabbage
- 1 ounce Elecampane
- 1 ounce Crawley root

Infuse in a quart of soft water until the strength is extracted, strain, then add two ounces of Tint. Lobelia two ounces Tinct. Bloodroot and four ounces Loaf Sugar. Strain and it is fit for use. Dose a teaspoon full thrice or four times a day half an hour before eating.

Syrrup for Pain in the Stomach and Side

- 4 ounces White root
- 4 ounces Skunk Cabbage
- 2 ounces Boneset
- 2 ounces Prickley Ash bark
- ¼ ounce Angelica seed
- ¼ ounce Coriander
- ½ ounce Ginger

To be put in a stone jug unstopped and boild in a kettle of water for an hour. Dose ¼ of a wine glass three or four times a day before eating. From two to three pills should be taken in 24 hours while using this syrup composed of equal parts of Extracts of Butternut and Dandelion worked in White root, Ipecac and ginger of equal parts.

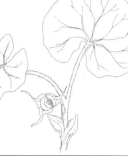

CHAPTER 4

The Hancock or Second Bishopric

Hancock, Massachusetts

Tyringham, Massachusetts

Enfield, Connecticut

THE COMMUNITIES at Hancock, Tyringham, and Enfield were established between 1790 and 1792, just three years after Watervliet and New Lebanon. These societies became known as the Hancock Bishopric. There was complete and close cooperation, love, and respect among the New York and New England families, and constant business intercourse among them.

None of these three societies had a medicinal herb industry to rival those of their fellow Shakers at New Lebanon or Watervliet. Each did, however, build a lucrative seed business during the first half of the nineteenth century. Enfield, in particular, with its relatively mild climate and rich alluvial soil, developed a prosperous seed industry, with sales routes that penetrated deep into the South. Hancock's trade was nearly as vigorous, and Tyringham's seed business was its most profitable industry.

The two Shaker communities in Berkshire County, Massachusetts, command beautiful scenic vistas. They lie in fertile valleys separated from New York by the Taconic Range and from the rest of Massachusetts on the east by what is commonly called the Berkshire Barrier. Tyringham is eighteen miles southeast of Hancock.

Enfield, which was grouped with Hancock and Tyringham as the Hancock Bishopric, is located on the east bank of the Connecticut River just south of the Massachusetts border.

A man can show his religion as much in measuring onions as he can in singing Glory Hallelujah.

ELDER GROVE WRIGHT,
HANCOCK

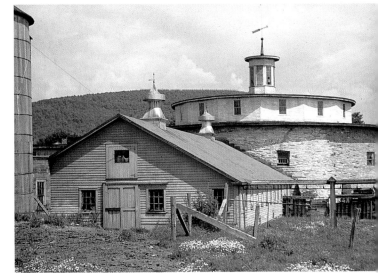

▷ The round stone barn, Church Family, Hancock Shaker Village.

HANCOCK, MASSACHUSETTS

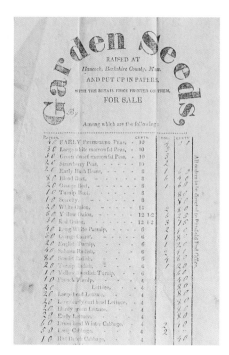

△ Detail of bill for garden seeds dated "Fall of 1821 Spring 1822."

▽ Hancock Shaker brick dwelling and sisters' gift shop (no longer standing).

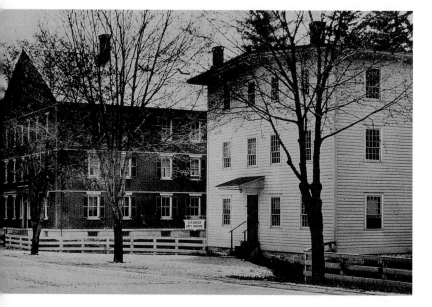

Account books kept by the Hancock Shakers indicate an extremely prosperous seed business. One eighty-page book in particular covers the industry for a period of years starting in 1824, at which time the society had issued its fifth "Catalogue of Garden Seeds." This was a broadside listing fifty-one seeds that stated: "Merchants and others, who wish to purchase seeds, are requested to forward their orders by the 4th of July preceding the time of sale. Directed to John Wright, agent written in Berkshire County, Mass."

The first of the ten broadsides advertising seeds was issued by the Hancock society in 1813 and listed only four herb seeds: parsley, pepper grass, sage, and summer savory. In subsequent catalogs, only burnet, rue, cayenne pepper, and saffron were added.

Before the Civil War the herb and seed business at Hancock was averaging an annual gross of more than $7,000, the herb side of this being largely sage, which was produced in enormous quantities and sold in leaf and ground forms. (Most of the sage was sent to New Lebanon for processing.) In 1864 gross receipts for herbs and seeds had dropped to $2,922.54, and ten years later income from "seeds, brooms and sage" amounted to only $2,525.

Hancock's economy, like that of other Shaker societies, was based on agriculture and horticulture. According to David Lamson, who lived at Hancock during 1847 and 1848, more than 5,000 acres, including several outfarms, were owned and farmed by the six families. Mention is made in a history of Berkshire County of seven herbs cultivated in the gardens of the Hancock Shakers. These are Virginia snakeroot, sweet marjoram, foxglove, gay feather *(Liatris)*, angelica, blue cohosh, and *Thea viridis* (green tea).

On November 25, 1867, a journal that was kept in New Lebanon reported that the West Family at Hancock was about to break up, "removing to the other families of their village. [This family] . . . was on a mountain side much like the Tyringham community, is a very unprofitable and hard place to support a family, the soil is very cold and wet. The buildings, that is, their foundations, difficult to keep in repair, and they have not able abilities to manage a family there." And so as early as 1867 the community at Hancock began to diminish, but it was probably not very noticeable then to the outside world, because the Church and Second Families remained busy and productive. The decline until 1960 was gradual. In that year the remaining Hancock Shakers sold their property to a group of concerned citizens who turned it into Hancock Shaker Village.

Homemade Nostrums

A recipe or formula book kept at Hancock by the Church Family from 1828 to 1846 details the making of homemade nostrums and directions for their use. It claims that they were good for "poor appetite, shortness of breath, pains in all parts of the anatomy, boils, small pox, palpitations, stoppage of water, palsy, diabetes, stones in the bladder, warts and corns, pains of fatality and wounds, not minor, burns and scalds." The botanical material needed to support these concoctions included coriander, blood-root, mandrake root, Culver's root, boneset, elder, marsh rosemary, Canada thistle, spikenard root, white pine bark, red clover heads, sarsaparilla, chamomile, fleabane, hardhack, wormwood, butternut, elecampane, catnip, roots of wild lettuce, sumac bark, avens root, yellow dock, burdock, comfrey, wintergreen, balm of Gilead, smellage, and rhubarb.

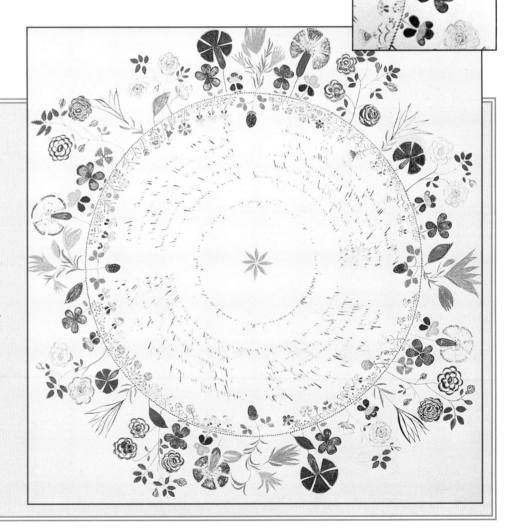

SENSING THE SPIRIT IN NATURE

During the 1840s Hancock, like the other Shaker societies, experienced an outpouring of religious excitement that became known as Mother Ann's Work. The "spirit drawings" were one expression of this enthusiasm. These remarkable drawings were produced after the artist had a vision of the spirit world. They often employed images of herbs and flowers — sometimes familiar, sometimes fantastic — to depict a heavenly landscape.

▷ "A Floral Wreath," with detail.

Tyringham, Massachusetts

In the eighty-three years that the settlement existed at Tyringham, the Believers raised some herbs and gathered many more from the fields and nearby woods for their own use. "Hints and Recipes," a square little manuscript written by Darias Herrick, fills eight numbered pages and includes

▽ Church Family, Tyringham.

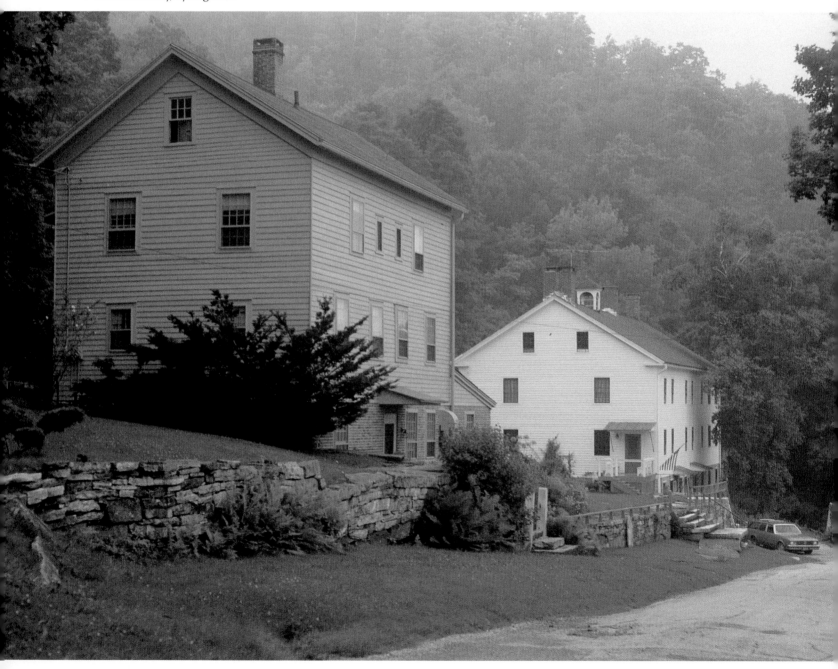

remedies for every ailment: "For The Thrush. To make one pint. A portion of rattle snake Plantain, A small portion of Fox Glove, A little Crawley, some cloves. A good portion of rose Flowers, The same of Balm Flowers, a portion of Camomile. Steep all together, after straining, add 2 table spoonfuls of Sweet Spirits of nitre [native soda, saltpeter], add a small spoonful of balm Giliad. Sweeten very Sweet with honey."

Other formulas were given: "For the Jaundice, To take the Mercury out of the Blood, Pills For to Strengthen the System [containing wild turnip, Peruvian bark, white root, burdock seed, and button snakeroot, among other ingredients]. Syrups for bleeding at the Longues, For the Gravel, the Disentary, the Erisipelas; How to make Egg Ointment and a poltice for swelled feet." There was a "Tincture of opium and Bl. cohosh for the bite of mad dogs; How to Make a Quick Beer; Powders for a cough and loss of Voice," and a dramatic account of a case of lockjaw and its cure. It concerned one Captain C. Gardner of Newport, who "unfortunately jumped upon a scraggy pointed spike which perforated his boot and foot, and he was taken home in most excrutiating torture. The attending Physician could afford him no relief. Providentially, a woman who heard the above came and caused his foot to be put into the warm Lye. The affect was this, in 15 minutes he was released, went to bed and slept well. The application was made for ten succeeding days when the Capt. could walk abroad."

The Tyringham Shakers raised garden seeds in sufficient quantity to print a broadside catalog in 1826, listing twenty-six varieties of seeds, priced from 4 to 12 cents per paper. Another catalog, printed in the 1850s, advises that all orders for seeds are to be directed to Willard Johnson, Agent, South Lee, Post Office.

At this time the Tyringham society was fairly prosperous. There were two settlements, three-fourths of a mile apart, each consisting of two families. The First, or Church, Family had the most buildings in it. The largest building was the five-story seed house used for drying and packaging the flower, herb, and vegetable seeds grown in the large gardens. The seed business was the society's chief source of income, and such was its size that in the seed and herb house a freight elevator ran from the basement to the cupola. A printing press in the same building turned out thousands of herb and seed labels.

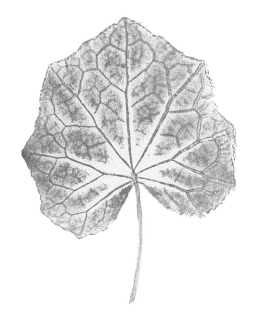

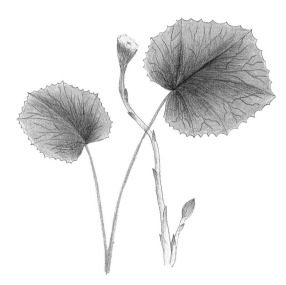

△ Coltsfoot, drawn by Canterbury sister Cora Helena Sarle.

ENFIELD, CONNECTICUT

Happiness is a very common plant, a native of every soil, yet, some skill is required in gathering it; for many poisonous weeds look like it, and deceive the unwary to their ruin.

DANIEL ORCUTT,
ENFIELD, CONNECTICUT

When the society at Enfield, Connecticut, dissolved in 1917, its members went to live at Mount Lebanon and Watervliet, New York. The community had prospered for most of its 125 years, and as Eldresses White and Taylor commented, "Enfield has always been rich in men and women of strong character and historic worth." The community had made its living almost entirely by farming its 3,300 acres of rich land on the east side of the Connecticut River.

The members started a garden seed business as early as any of the other societies and began to sell herbs in 1825 on routes that meandered deep into the south. On their broad sweep of fields the Enfield Shakers also grew tobacco, as did many of their neighbors. This was the large-leaved or "wrapper" tobacco, which commanded a good price from makers of fine cigars.

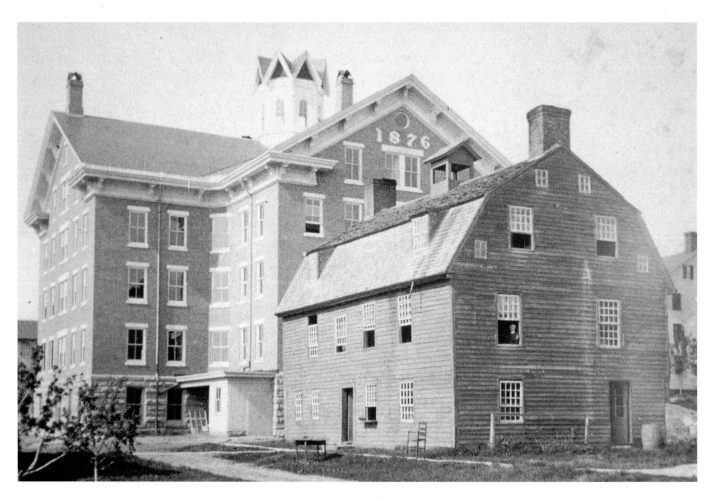

△ Church Family, with dwelling and meetinghouse, Enfield, Connecticut.

Shaker Prescriptions

A book of "Prescriptions Given by Old Dr. Hamilton, family Physician to the Shakers in Enfield, Conn. in 1825 . . ." included a variety of bitters, pills, elixirs, fever powders, cough pills, and a "Spice Cordial" combining myrrh, absinthe, nutmeg, oil of peppermint, and pure water. "Shake them well together," the directions read; "this is a tonic for the patient after he leaves the sick room. Take a small glass 3 times a day."

"Pills for the head" contained "15 grs. of opium and gum and sapo castilo." The directions were: "Mix to a mass with honey and make into pills, one to be taken 4 times a day, dividing the time." A line filling in the bottom of a page reads: "An infallible worm powder is made mostly of skunk cabbage pulverized and Indian hemproot."

Ten catalogs were published by the Enfield Shakers. One listed "Medicinal Plants, Barks, Roots, Seeds and Flowers, with their Therapeutic Qualities and Botanical Names." Also priced were "Pure Vegetable Extracts and Shaker Garden Seeds, Raised, Prepared and Put Up in the Most Careful Manner. . . . First Established in 1802, being the Oldest Seed Establishment in the United States." Seven broadsides were published in the 1850s listing from 46 items at first to as many as 300 items. The Shakers always carried as many as seventeen herb seeds and very often several grass seeds.

A MAN OF PARTS

Enfield seedsman Jefferson White was a talented horti-culturist and a shrewd businessman, but there was another side of him that many Shakers considered even more important. He was one of a number of spiritual "instruments," or mediums, who reported receiving messages from the spirit world during the time of Mother Ann's work. This intense spirituality was especially impressive in a man who had so much interaction with non-Shakers and with the practical matters of the world.

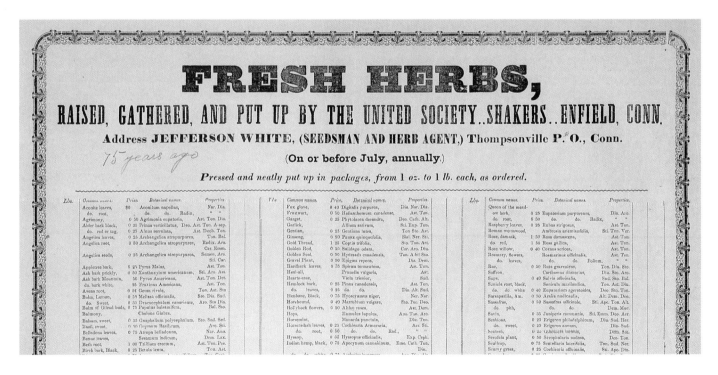

△ Detail of a list of herbs offered by the Enfield, Connecticut, Shakers in the mid-1800s.

Early competition emerged in nearby Wethersfield, Connecticut. James L. Belden's catalog for 1821 carried sixty-one varieties of seeds, among which were mustard, parsley, cayenne, summer savory, coriander, caraway, sweet fennel, dill, saffron, and sage.

Like other Shaker seedsmen and herbalists, Jefferson White made an effort to distinguish Shaker quality from the mediocre products entering the market in the mid-1800s. In the 1854 catalog he wrote:

It is a matter of eminent importance to the interested and benevolent physician, to be able to calculate with certainty, on the effect of any drug or medicine he may administer. This he cannot do, unless he be able to judge of its purity, condition, and carefulness of preparation. Perhaps no class of medicines present so many difficulties, and certainly none which have given such universal dissatisfaction on this point, as vegetable extracts, and some of our best physicians have nearly abandoned their use on this account.

This is not surprising, when we consider the rude and imperfect means generally employed for evaporating, and the want of suitable knowledge and carefulness in the whole process of manufacture. Indeed, it requires much experience and consummate skill, in addition to the most perfect apparatus, to produce extracts that will be uniform and certain in their effects — as much depends on the freshness of the vegetable operated upon, maturity, season of collection and influence of climate.

To remedy the difficulties complained of, and furnish the profession with the article they so earnestly requested of us — pure and reliable extracts — we have directed our attention to this end, and spared no expense to procure the best information and conveniences for the purpose. Our former experience and observations, of thirty years, have been of value, and the possession of large botanic gardens gives us important advantages in the collection and freshness of the vegetables.

Postwar Decline

The Civil War wiped out the southern sales routes and effectively ended the Enfield Shakers' seed business. The herb business, always a much more modest sideline, soon disappeared as well, although garden herbs still flavored the families' meals until well into the 1900s. As in other societies, the numbers of members had dwindled by then, with fewer Shaker hands to do the work of maintaining the farm and gardens. In 1917 the Enfield community closed and the remaining members dispersed to other communities.

The single-hearted should not be impatient with themselves, nor should they be surprised if, with the honestest effort, they sometimes fail to come quite up to the standard they have set for themselves. Soil which has for a length of time been injured by bad tillage, needs care, skill, patience, to bring it to a cropbearing state.

ANNA ERVIN, ENFIELD, CONNECTICUT

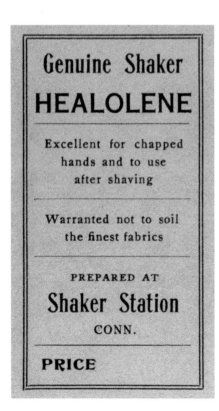

CHAPTER 5

The Harvard or Eastern Bishopric

Harvard, Massachusetts

Shirley, Massachusetts

THE TWO SHAKER COMMUNITIES in eastern Massachusetts developed thriving herb and seed industries. Mother Ann Lee founded these two communities herself, making Harvard her headquarters during a trip she took through New England in 1781, gathering converts.

As with non-Shaker villages, these two communities had to become self-sufficient, providing manufacturing trades and services such as blacksmithing, tanning, shoe making, joinery, and wheel making to meet their own needs and, before long, those of the larger world. As one aspect of this self-sufficiency, the Shakers grew and processed herbs to treat the illnesses within their community. The surplus was offered to their neighbors, and this trade grew into an extremely profitable business in medicinal herbs.

A good name is better than riches.

SIMON T. ATHERTON, HARVARD

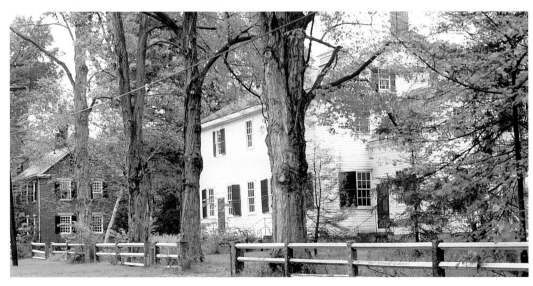

◁ View of Church Family, Harvard Shaker community.

63

HARVARD, MASSACHUSETTS

The Shaker community at Harvard consisted of some 1,800 acres and was located about thirty miles from Boston. High on a hill, it looked due west to Mount Wachusett, also in Worcester County, and north to Mount Monadnock, in southern New Hampshire.

Mother Ann went to Harvard in 1781 to preach the gospel, and for two years it remained the center of her religious mission. The society was formally established in 1791 and eventually reached a population of 200. By the time of the early 1840s it was already prosperous from its farming operations and its nursery business. The herb industry was to flourish also and compare favorably with those of Watervliet and New Lebanon, New York; Canterbury, New Hampshire; and Union Village, Ohio.

An indication of the extent of arboriculture and the nursery business is shown in two journal entries of 1843: "April 28. We take up over five hundred fruit trees to sell," and "May 5. Some of the brethren set out between three and four thousand small apple and pear trees." A catalog issued some years later by Elijah Myrick listed twenty-one varieties of apples and sixteen varieties of cherries.

Herbal Medicine for Home Use

At first the Shakers in Harvard, as in other societies, gathered herbs for the preparation of medicine for home use. A journal kept by the physicians in the society from 1834 to 1843 tells what the medical procedures were and in some cases which herbs were used. It records all the appointments designating nurses and "watchers," those who sat with the very ill twenty-four hours of the day to nurse and observe any change in condition. It was their duty to give constant care.

A Statement of the Changes in the Physicians Order from the Gathering of the Church in 1791 to the present time, 1843.

Sister Sarah Jewett was the first physician. Tabitha Babbit (then a girl) was her assistant. In the autumn of 1810 Salome Barrett succeeded her in the medical dept.

This is the first account of a female physician in the Shaker order.

A vast amount of material was brought in from woods and swamps. As the demand for herbs outside the community increased, fields near the village were cleared and large gardens were planted. But before sufficient quantities could be cultivated, the Shakers made daily excursions for herbs in proper season, the year round. In an entry for January 11, 1824, a journal records searching for herbal material, "mostly for bark."

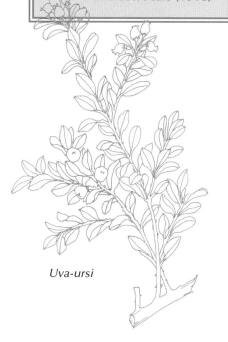

Sept. 1, 2. 1830. Simon T. A., Mary Babbit, Lucy Clark & Selah Winchester to gather herbs.
June 8, 1831. To Dunstable after herbs.
July 15. To south part of Harvard after herbs.
July 22. To Groton after herbs.
Oct. 31. To Shirley after Uva Ursi, or Bearberry.

From Gleanings from Old Shaker Journals by Clara Endicott Sears (1916)

Uva-ursi

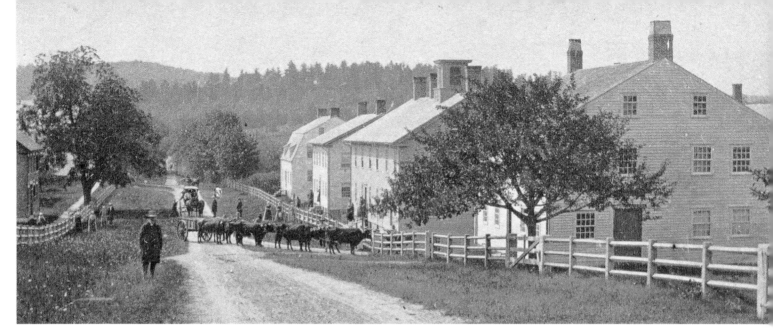

△ Main street, Harvard Shaker community.

Selling Herbs in the World

A journal entry for September 16, 1820, is the earliest known reference to the sale of herbs by the Harvard Shakers. From Joseph Hammond's daybook we learn: "Fair, warm and pleasant but cool. Wrought preparing herbs to go to Boston. September 21. Fair and pleasant but cool. Wrought with Sisters cutting last of things in Garden such as sweet balm, peppermint, spearmint, and various other small parcels of herbs."

The Harvard Shakers ultimately issued ten bound catalogs, the first in 1845 and the last in 1889, and two broadsides, one in the early 1800s and the other sometime later.

Simon T. Atherton was in charge and his first catalog listed 197 medicinal herbs, with eight sweet herbs in canisters, and thirteen extracts. He used the common names and botanical names taken from Eaton's last edition; the price per pound and the properties of each herb were given. This was a practice followed in all but the two broadsides and the last catalog under Atherton's direction, which carried the name of his successor in 1889, John Whiteley. These exceptions listed the common names and prices only.

The 1849 edition was much the same as its predecessors, but the 1851 issue listed 198 herbs, four sweet herbs in canisters, thirteen extracts, and a variety of fruit trees, grapevines, ornamental shrubs, buckthorn hedge plants and seeds, and garden seeds of all kinds, furnished to order. The catalog for 1853 followed the same pattern, listing 200 herbs. In the catalog Atherton wrote:

Medicinal Herbs prepared in bottles require more labor in preparing and extra care and attention in drying, so as to retain all their valuable properties, which necessarily brings them higher [in cost] by the pound than pressed herbs.

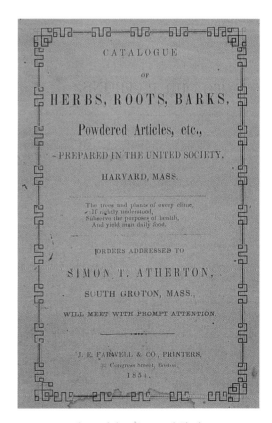

CATALOGUE
OF
HERBS, ROOTS, BARKS,
Powdered Articles, etc.,
PREPARED IN THE UNITED SOCIETY,
HARVARD, MASS.

The trees and plants of every clime,
If rightly understood,
Subserve the purposes of health,
And yield man daily food.

ORDERS ADDRESSED TO
SIMON T. ATHERTON,
SOUTH GROTON, MASS.,
WILL MEET WITH PROMPT ATTENTION.

J. E. FARWELL & CO., PRINTERS,
32 Congress Street, Boston.
1854.

△ 1854 catalog of the Harvard Shakers.

SINGULAR PRAISE

In 1853 Simon Atherton had received an honor from the Massachusetts College of Pharmacy. He used it as a testimonial in the 1854 catalog:

Boston, September 1, 1835
Massachusetts College of Pharmacy.
Resolved: That the thanks of this College be presented to Simon T. Atherton, for superior specimens of Shaker Herbs, presented this College for their Cabinet, and for the exhibition at the meeting of The American Pharmaceutical Association.

A true copy from the records Attest:
(Signed) Henry W. Lincoln, Rec. Sec.

Customers deserving the very best articles prepared in this manner, will have to forward their orders as early in the summer as June, so as to give time for collection in their best condition, and they may rely upon having a superior article, neatly labelled, for $6 per doz. quart bottles, or $10 per doz. two quart bottles by addressing S. T. Atherton.

The catalog of 1857 offered 213 herbs, for which Atherton gave 167 synonyms or alternative common names. As in the 1851 New Lebanon catalog, Atherton urged merchants to consult this list before turning away a customer seeking a plant with an unfamiliar name.

The catalogs of 1860 and 1868 were the same; both listed 212 herbs. In 1873 Atherton offered 213 herbs, but otherwise the catalog did not vary. He issued two broadsides in the 1880s as well, listing 226 herbs, including sweet marjoram, sage, summer savory, and thyme in cans.

△ Details of a broadside issued by the Harvard Shakers in the 1880s.

The Herb House

The original herb house at Harvard had been a small building, and when the Shakers decided they needed more space, foundations were laid for a new one in 1848. Elisha Myrick started a diary in January 1850. In a preface to round up the business of 1849 he wrote:

> This year we cut the timber saw it out at the mill and frame the Herb house ourselves, (the foundation being laid in 1848) get the building so far completed as to be able to occupy the part designed for the herb business Nov. 15th just one year from the day we commenced cutting the timber for the frame. Hire help to cover it [roof it over] and lay two floors and $\frac{1}{2}$ and finish 5 rooms at a cost of about $1800.00 money out.

The building also housed a big woodshed where 300 cords of wood were stored for drying herbs.

Arthur T. West, who lived with the Harvard Shakers as a boy from 1884 to 1889, wrote: "The stone dry-house was where roots were dried by artificial heat. The herb shop was used for stripping, drying by air, and pressing and wrapping the great variety of herbs raised on the broad acres of their estate. There was also the still — no, not what you think, but where rose water was distilled. A very enchanting perfume was made from the real roses."

▽ The herb house at Harvard.

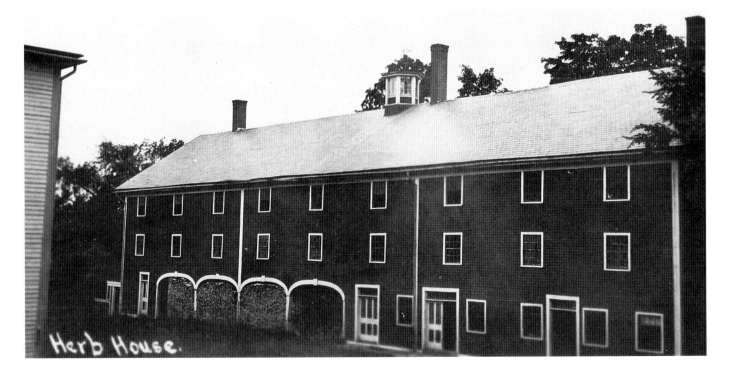

Herb House.

A Year in the Herb Business

Excerpts from Brother Elisha's daybook for the years 1850, 1851, and 1852 describe the organization of the business, the herbs handled, the agents dealt with, and the territory covered. In 1850:

Jan. 3–9. Elisha works at work bench in the Herb House, packing herbs to go to Boston. . . . Sent some dock root to the mill to be cracked. . . . Commence posting accounts for the agents in Boston. . . . The Stoves came down from Fitchburg and were brought from the depot. . . . Elisha puts up the stoves and a lot of herbs for S. W. Fowler and does some writing. After meeting we make 3 herb boxes and Elisha works all night packing and making out bills.

Jan. 14–31. Elisha up at 3 o'clock in the writing and putting up his herbs. . . . Simon brought 2 bushels of Sage from the Depot and Abel 3 bushels of dock root from the Grist mill. . . . Elisha finishes drawing off last year's accounts. Commences in the new books. . . . Elijah brought two tubs of horehound from the depot, and a lot of empty boxes. . . . Elisha puts some

A RECORD-BREAKING YEAR

The daily business of the herb department was the main occupation of Elisha Myrick, who had worked gathering, preparing, and packaging material since he was eleven years old. He described his work of the previous growing season in the preface to the 1850 catalog:

The business this year is carried on by Elisha Myrick, aged 25, and George B. Whitney, aged 22, with the assistance of Isaac Myrick to gather herbs out from home and two sisters to pick over the herbs. . . . We do our pressing and keep our stock of pressed herbs at the Ministry's barn and pick our herbs and do other work at the yellow house. We distilled 165 gallons of peach water and made 134 pounds of ointment, 49 gallons of buckthorn syrup and pressed between February 14, 1849 and February 14, 1850 10,152 pounds of herbs, roots, etc.

The sales for 1849 including all the herbs, and delivered to agent amount to $4,042.31 net. We raise, gather and prepare this year 5,788 pounds of herbs, barks, roots, etc. which is 800 pounds more than was ever collected before.

Elisha Myrick left the Shakers in 1859. His older brother Elijah became trustee after Simon Atherton died in 1888. An excerpt from a Harvard journal appears in the inset.

damper in the stove pipes in the press and counting rooms, puts up an order to go to Worcester and picks over some Buck Bean. . . . Elisha is up at 4 o'clock putting up herbs to go to Boston. After breakfast goes over to the Grist to carry roots to town. . . . Three sisters pick over dry sage in the evening. . . . Elisha chopping dry herbs. Abel brot 4 bushes of Wormwood and 4 Dock Root from the Depot. . . . Elisha at the herb house all day put up 5 bushels sage to be ground. Sent 1 bushel leaf sage to T. Corbett. Sent 4 bushels of Dock to the Grist mill. Had it cracked. Sent 1 bushel of dock to Providence and put up prepared herbs for the agents in Boston, Salem, and Providence. Simon brot 4 bushels of sage in leaf from the Depot. . . . Elisha goes to the North family and gets 104 pounds of Green Horseradish Root cuts it up and puts it into the Oven to dry for E. S. C. Boston. . . . Elisha papers pressed sage in the A.M. A. Blaisdell of Boston here to make a contract for herbs. . . . Elisha papers Spearmint and packs 5 large boxes of herbs for A. Blaisdell & Co. Boston.

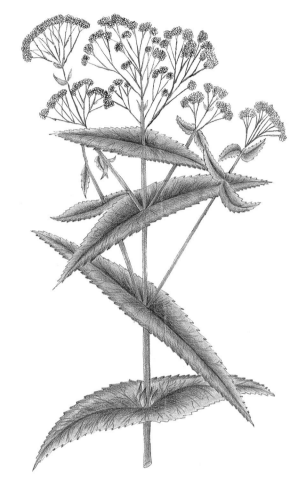

△ Thoroughwort, also known as boneset *(Eupatorium perfoliatum)*, drawn by Canterbury sister Cora Helena Sarle.

The months of February and March were extremely active, filling and labeling cans (sixty-three in one afternoon) and sending off orders to Boston and Worcester. One particular shipment went to Charles Dyer of Providence, containing two barrels of dock root and one of dandelion, all valued at $107.73 net. On February 20 Elisha went to Boston to see about a press and was home the next day and putting up orders. On the 27th he finished putting up 669 boxes of horseradish, which had been dried and ground, as well as three barrels of dandelion root. One day, he wrote, "after meeting in the evening we got some help and put up 18 dozen large cans of thyme till 12 o'clock."

In March orders were received from William Underwood of Boston, among others, for one gross large cans of sage repeated several times during the month. On the 6th "Elijah brot 1,073 pounds of green Horse Radish Root from the depot and dry and ground. . . . March 11th. Put up 4 bushels, 111 pounds of Motherwort and 12 pounds of Bayberry leaves for Chauncey Miller, Watervliet. Put up herbs the remainder of the day to go to Boston." The next day he put up two gross small cans of thyme for Underwood and "the Irishmen put the Horseradish in cans labelled and prepared it to go; 980 cans." Elecampane and pennyroyal were papered and ground to a fine consistency.

Spring meant that, in addition to the regular business of selling, packing, and shipping herbs, the Shakers also had to start growing them.

April 1–14. . . . Build fire in kiln to dry horseradish. . . . Make out bills. In P.M. go to the Corporation Paper Mills after paper. . . . Put up 1 gross small cans Summer Savory for Underwood. Paper some horseradish. . . . Sift 100 pounds Dwarf Elder Root. . . . Work on Herb boxes. Send the Radish Root to the mill to be ground and home again. . . . Put up 560 cans of Horse

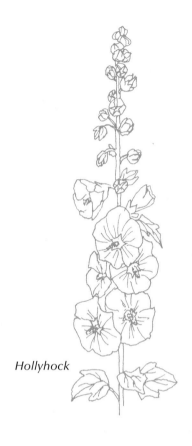

Hollyhock

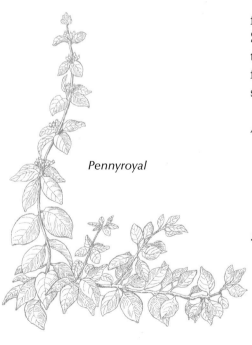

Pennyroyal

Radish with the help of some small boys. . . . FAST. After meeting do some cleaning up back of Herb House. . . . Get some help and put up 48 dozen cans for Underwood, work some in the evening. Wrote a letter to S. W. Bullock. . . . Finished making herb boxes for this year. Made 100. 50 past done, making 150 Total. April 15. Up at 3 o'clock to put up an order to go to Worcester by express. Put up 12 doz. large cans Marjoram and some small orders to go all over the lots. April 17. Prepared the hot beds for use. April 22. We repair the centre part of the double press which was liable to fail. . . . Wrote a letter to S. W. Bullock, N.Y. City ordered up a press. April 30. Took up two waggon loads of sage roots and carried them over to John Blanchard to cultivate for us this year. He is to cut it and bring it to us green and after it is dried he is to have seven cts. per lb.

May 4. Plowed the garden with horses. May 10. Help Mary whitewash the herb house interior. May 11. Sow Hollyhocks and sweet balm seeds. May 13. Sow Jerusalem Oak, Poppy seed and Lavender and do some hoeing and cultivating. May 14. Sow Dock seed, Marshmallow, Pennyroyal seed. Do some plowing, hoeing, etc. May 15. Sowed Horehound seed. . . . To Groton to engage John Boynton to raise Dock Root for 8 cts. per lb. dry and Dandelion Root for 10 cts. per., dry. May 16. Put up 30 doz. cans for Underwood. May 22. Finish the writing desk for use. Put up 150 pounds of Fine Elm in pound papers. May 24. Peel White Oak Bark in the Ox Pasture woods. May 30. Cut 500 pounds of Sarsaparilla Root, 200 pounds of Sage.

Work during the month of June was much the same, but there were fewer entries. The entries for the summer months of July, August, and September were short and to the point and were contained in six pages of the daybook. Most of the herbs the Shakers gathered were catnip, caraway, feverfew, cicuta roots, tansy, wormwood, sweet balm, hardhack leaves, and sumac.

August 6. Commence packing poppy leaves. Cut thyme 5 sheets full. August 21. Seven sister and four brethren go out beyond the depot to pick Wintergreen. Get a small quantity. August 22. Cut the pennyroyal and the thyme. August 24. Cultivate all the gardens. Spread 30 loads of manure. August 31. Cut the savory. Put up some orders [a very large one for Underwood]. Set up the still.

Sept. 2. Put up three kettles of peach leaves. Cut the lavender. Sept. 11. A company of brethren and sister go to Chelmsford to pick Wintergreen. Sept. 26. Pound Savin for Ointment. Cut up a lot of Savory. Sept. 27. Make Savin Ointment at the North House. Put up a barrel of Thyme in cans. Sept. 28. Finish the Ointment. 155 lbs. Sept. 30. Pick the Buckthorn Berries, 1½ bushels. Prepare the juice and put up 16 doz. cans to go to New Bedford.

Oct. 1. Make the buckthorn syrup and put up two hundred cans of herbs. Oct. 3. Go to Leominster in pursuit of herbs. Oct. 5. Put up 730 ounces of peach water and rose water to go to New York. A great number of herbs, etc. sent to Underwood. Oct. 21. Go after chestnuts, put up two gross one half cans of sage for Underwood and prepare a lot of herbs, etc.

Nov. 2. Press yellow dock root all day — 311 pounds prepared and 48 more in the press, making 359 in all. Nov. 5. Put up three barrels of dock root to go to Rhode Island. Nov. 29. Weigh off a lot of herbs bought by a man by the name Vormund Hoyt, of Canada.

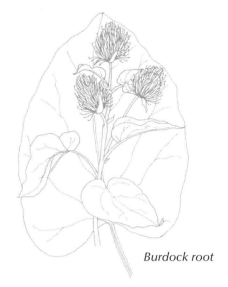

Burdock root

10,767 pounds pressed in 1850	
Sold herbs amount to	$3768.18
Delivered to agent	2305.06
Total amount of sales in 1850	$6073.24 net.

Feb. 26, 1851. Elisha takes up the horseradish root in the dryhouse and carries it to the grist mill and gets it ground, also three barrels of dandelion root. Feb. 26. We work till eleven o'clock in the evening putting up cans of horseradish to go to California.

March 25. Up at two o'clock putting up orders to go to Boston.

May 30. Cut 500 pounds sarsaparilla root and 200 pounds sage.

July 8. Cut horehound and catnip and motherwort. July 18. Cut the canary seed. July 31. Hoe the burdock and henbane for the first time in the west garden; plough the carrot field for dandelions.

Sept. 13. Commence making ketchup in the new furnaces. Cut the marshmallow and sweet marjoram and rue seed. Isaac got a load of life everlasting.

Oct. 24. Put up pumpkin in cans.

Nov. 7. Put up cans of thyme. Nov. 10. Fill 1,000 cans of summer savory. Nov. 28. Put up 200 cans of flour of pumpkin. Pack a lot of orders to go to New York.

Christmas Day. After the solemnities of the day are past I paper a lot of herbs. Dec. 31. This day of the year 1851 closes forever. We have had some hot weather, some cold, some wet, some dry — we have had some joys, some sorrows, some prosperity, and some adversity.

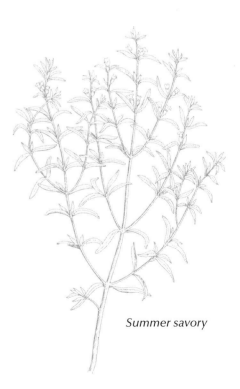

Summer savory

Sold in Worcester and Providence	$ 514.09
Sold to sundry customers	2565.61
Delivered to agents	2573.74
	$5653.44

Elisha Myrick began a new daybook in 1852.

Feb. 16, 1852. Put up ten pounds fine lily root and one hundred pounds ground sage in pound papers. Pack $200. worth of pressed herbs to go to Wilson, Fairbanks & Co. for the California order. Send some herbs to the agents. Feb. 18. Pack four large boxes of prepared herbs to fit out Weeks & Potter, Boston, who have taken the agency.

In one week 1596 pounds of herbs are pressed. In the year brought in $8300.14.

April 2, 1852. The sisters help cut up some herbs to go to New London. April 30. Set out wormwood, marshmallow, and thyme roots.

May 2. Transplant hyssop and feverfew to the west garden. Transplant hore-hound and sage.

Aug. 11. Take up the poppy capsules and work the dandelion root and cut some thorn apple leaves for ointment. Aug. 16. We go with a number of sisters to the intervale to collect a load of hardhack. Gather boneset in the swamp. Isaac gets a load of queen-of-the-meadow.

Sept. 20. Make buckthorn syrup.

March 13, 1853. Pack $7500 worth cans of ground herbs for Underwood. March 14. Pack $7500 worth cans for Davis, Boston. March 16. Pack $200. worth of prepared herbs to go to Wilson, Fairbanks & Co. for the California order. March 23. Finish the hops and commence pressing for an order to go to London, England. March 24. Press 250 pounds and pack 79 different varieties of two pounds each to go to London.

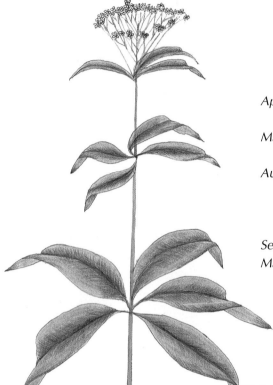

△ Queen of the meadow *(Eupatorium purpureum)*, also known as Joe-Pye weed, drawn by Canterbury sister Cora Helena Sarle.

MUSEUM QUALITY

The Harvard Shakers had made large shipments of botanical material to England. An honor came to Elisha from that country in 1857. It was a scroll with the handsome royal seal, lions rampant supporting *Dieu et Mon Droit* at the top of the parchment, and it read in print and stylish hand lettering:

Royal Gardens Kew

The Director Begs to Convey to Elisha Myrick, Esquire

The best acknowledgements of the Commissioners of her Majesty's Woods and for the undermentioned contribution; Viz:
An interesting set of Extracts of vegetable Pharmaceutical subject, — which together with a large collection of the prepared Herbs in cakes, and deposited in the Museum of Economic Botany.

W. J. HOOKER
DIRECTOR, ROYAL GARDENS, KEW
AUGUST 26, 1857

Business Expands

An account book detailing the work of the "Herb Branch of the Medical Dept" from January 1847 to December 1853 shows that the business had grown sufficiently to warrant the purchase of a new and larger herb press in 1848. This was the press mentioned by a sister from South Union, Kentucky, who visited Harvard in 1869: "They carry on the herb business to a considerable extent; have a remarkably good press, built under the superintendance of an ingenious young man who resided here, but is now a celebrated draughtsman in the city of Washington. This herb business is one of their principal resources, but is now meeting with considerable competition."

The account book lists herbs sold to chemists, doctors, "Thomas Corbett and other Societies," and "July 1, 1850 herbs sold to Indian Doctor. $2.90." The total gross income for seven years as recorded in this one book was $33,706.70. There are many entries for herbs bought from other societies for home use or for resale. Those communities that were mentioned selling herbs to Harvard were Watervliet ("bought from Chauncey Miller: burdock root, rue and lovage root"), Shirley, New Lebanon, and Tyringham. Yellow dock was purchased in large quantities from the Enfield, New Hampshire, society. Thomas Corbett of Canterbury sold herbs to Harvard and also bought considerable amounts from them: "Settled with T. Corbett for short weight on dandelion root."

When Simon Atherton died in 1888 at the age of eighty-five, he was succeeded briefly by John Whiteley, as editor of the catalogs and business manager; then the business passed to trustee Elijah Myrick (Elisha's brother). In the first broadside Myrick printed as successor to Atherton, he wrote:

Medicinal Herbs, Roots and Compounds were first prepared for the market by the United Society, (called Shakers) in Harvard, Mass. From a small beginning prior to 1820, it has grown to an industry of large commercial importance. These natural remedies have supplanted and retired from use the debilitating nostrums and mineral drugs, and instead of aiding the human assassin, moves directly on the enemies' works, and have become the welcome friends in every household. Much of the success in this business is due to the intelligence and strict integrity of the late Simon T. Atherton, who for more than fifty years has maintained the justly deserved reputation of the genuine Shaker Herbs. His motto was "A good name is better than riches." Prime new hops in pound and half pound packages specialty. Call for Shaker Herbs. Also, Rose Water by the Gallon, distilled from Roses. For sale by Wholesale Druggists in Boston and by the Society.

E. Myrick, Trustee,
Successor to the late Simon T. Atherton
P.O. address, Ayer, Mass.

WIDE-RANGING SALESMEN

Year by year the Shakers of Harvard covered more territory. Selling was brisk each fall on Cape Cod, and in Providence and South Providence, Rhode Island. The Worcester route grew rapidly, and more hotels were listed for orders. The Adams House and the Quincy House in Boston were steady customers, sending in large orders for a variety of culinary herbs — especially sage.

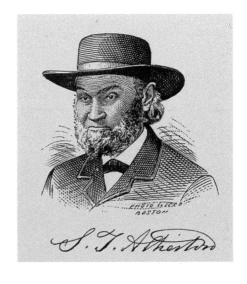

SAGE FOR SAUSAGE

The Shakers at Harvard had a very good account with the Deerfoot Farm Company, makers of sausage. The buyer, W. W. Rogers, had orders filled in November and December 1885, for example, for 289 pounds of kiln-dried sage, "in stem, fine and powdered." In 1886 Mr. Rogers bought 295 pounds; in 1887, 220 pounds; and on January 10, 1888, he purchased for Deerfoot Farms 668 pounds of sage, in stem and ground.

A Sister's Work

"A Journal of Domestic Work of Sisters, Kept by the Deaconesses, from February 1867 to April 1876," describes what the sisters' duties were in their department.

May 29. Cleaning at the Herb house.

June 7. Cut some celandine today, pick it over, the first herb this year. Ellen, the Irish woman came and helped. . . . Elder Grove and Brother John get some butternut bark this afternoon.

July 4. Independence. Have green pease for dinner.

July 5. The Sisters are picking herbs and poppys.

All during the month of July there are daily entries "picking herbs . . . a great deal of picking to do, herbs, pease, beans and currants. We are going our common rounds." The August records are about the same: "Herbs, herbs, herbs, picking over herbs." And finally, "Sept. 30. Finished picking over herbs for this season."

Records for the next year are kept with meticulous care, although not always in the same hand or with equal enthusiasm.

May 22. Clean out the herb house. . . .

July 14. Very warm, begin to pick the peppermint.

July 18. Pick spearmint.

July 21. Picking over wormwood and rue. Herbs, herbs, herbs.

Sept. 1. Picking over Queen-of-the-Meadow.

Sept. 25. We cut coriander seed this week.

Jan. 2, 1869. Papering herbs this week.

Jan. 13. Work in Herb house.

May 7. Clean Herb House.

June 28, 1871. Herbs, herbs, herbs, a plenty of them for all hands.

July 6. Begin to pick over sage.

August 12, 1875. Catnip, catnip, nothing but catnip.

August 13. Very muggy and warm, catnip.

August 21. Catnip. Elder John brought an editer and his wife here. Catnip.

August 30. Horehound.

Sept. 2. Sage, sage, the Eldress came.

Sept. 3. Work on sage. The Ministry Sisters come.

Sept. 8. All hands work on horehound.

Sept. 9. Work on horehound. Elder Henry Blinn from Canterbury come. We see Elder Henry some, he goes at noon. Horehound and rue.

Sept. 23. Finish horehound and rue. Have fresh fish for dinner.

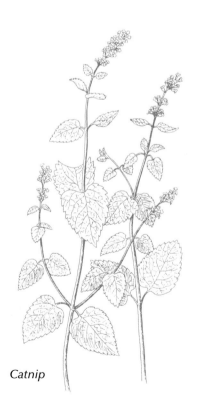

Catnip

Growing Accounts

Orders from many big companies in Boston and in the Providence and Worcester areas are listed in account books from January 1879 through 1888. Deliveries were made in March soon after the devastating blizzard of 1888. S. S. Pierce of Boston placed monthly orders for sage, thyme, marjoram, and sweet savory, five dozens cans at a time, along with gallons of rose water. Park and Tilford of New York City bought about the same amount of sage and thyme and placed orders for 106 pounds of hops at a time, as well as rose water by the hundreds of gallons. A typical order included twenty-seven to thirty-five cans of thyme, sage, marjoram, savory, peppermint, and horehound pulverized or ground fine.

Other companies doing business with the Harvard Shakers over a long period of years were F. W. Hensman and Company of Augusta, Maine, which ordered quantities of lobelia in bulk and pressed; Cheney and Myrick, Boston; Howe and French, and Peek and Velson, New York. In all, 266 accounts were active from 1879 to 1888 and a prodigious amount of material was shipped out.

Decline Begins

The herb business began to decline, however, in the 1890s. A "Home Note from Harvard" in *The Manifesto* of February 1892 described it as being "ably managed," but account books concentrate more on the sale of brooms, and Shakers recorded fewer companies and doctors sending in orders for herbs. Henry S. Norse, writing the history of Harvard, Massachusetts, in 1893, says of the Shakers:

> *Financially the Society is very prosperous and has invested savings. Its resources and support have been largely derived from horticulture farming and the sale of standing wood and timber. Brooms are manufactured to the value of six or seven hundred dollars, yearly and herbs are pressed and packed for the retailers, the sale of which amounts to seven or eight thousand dollars per annum. Eight or ten laborers are permanently employed, besides the members of the community. The chief farm product from which an income is arrived is milk. This is sent to the Boston Market, though the sisters make all the butter used. The variety of herbs, barks, leaves, roots and flowers used for culinary or medicinal purposes, here dried and ground or pressed, packed and labeled, is very large. Many are cultivated or gathered upon the premises, others are bought by the bale. A boiler of ample capacity and a small engine furnish heat and power for the herb-packing department, laundry and dairy, all of which are provided with the most recent scientific and labor saving machinery and economic devices.*

THE WIND OF THE SPIRIT

Writing in the last years of the Shakers at Harvard, Clara Endicott Sears asked one of the Believers: "Eldress where has the fervor gone and all the ardor and enthusiasm, and all the spiritual fire that swayed these men and women? The wind of the Spirit has swept through this place and borne the soul of it away on its wings. Only the outer shell of what was here remains to designate the spot through which it passed,"

And she answered: "But nothing that has gone before is lost. The Spirit has its periods of moving beneath the surface, and after generations pass, it sweeps through the world again and burns the chaff and stubble."

SHIRLEY, MASSACHUSETTS

The earth and all that is therein belongs to God: Man holds them in trust; they are blessings lent, and he will be held to a strict accountability for the use of them.

JOANNA RANDALL,
SHIRLEY

Garden seeds were one of several prosperous industries the Shakers conducted at Shirley, "Harvard's twin sister," for 116 years. Over the years the society acquired some two thousand acres of farmland including several outlying farms; one forty miles away in lower New Hampshire was used to graze stock during the summer. The raising and selling of cattle produced a steady income for many years, but the largest income was from garden seeds.

In July 1795, two years after the community was organized, the Reverend William Bentley of Salem, Massachusetts, visited Shirley. He reported that, although the soil was not good, the cultivation was the best; that there were two fields of thirty acres each planted to rye, and a large field of corn; and that "their flax was in admirable order."

The Shakers enlarged their garden seed business, and they converted fields they had previously mowed for hay to cultivate and plant the seed plants. The production of seeds was first mentioned in a record book kept by Asa Brocklebank, dated August 5, 1805: "We begin to make seed bags." The seeds raised from sale then included fourteen for vegetables and six

▽ Broom shop, North Family, Shirley.

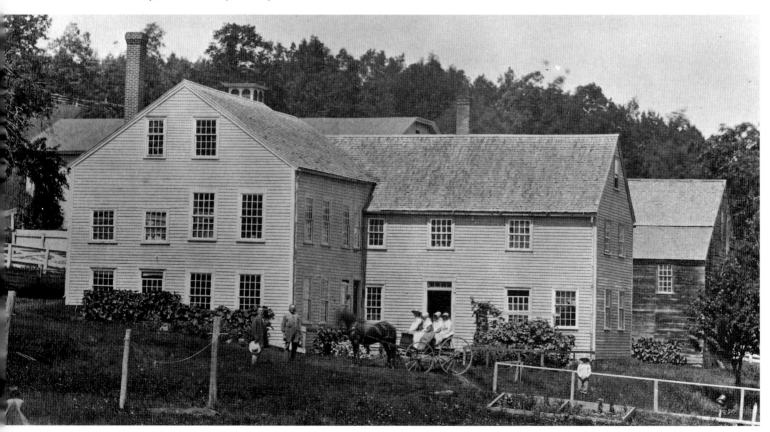

for herbs — caraway, parsley, sage, saffron, lavender, and summer savory. By December 24, 1815, Asa recorded that balm, fennel, and burnet also were being sold.

Another gardener's daybook of 1806 lists sixty-five firms and individuals the Shirley brethren were doing business with for a total income of $1,835.18, "before discount."

Herbs were gathered and raised to be made into medicines for the family's use at Shirley and were carefully collected and processed, but the Shakers' herb business did not comprise an industry as extensive as their garden seed business. A broadside dated in ink from 1810 is probably the earliest catalog to be issued by the Shakers in Shirley. It lists twenty-eight garden seeds, of which six are herbs. Other broadsides were issued in 1826, 1830, and 1855, offering forty-three seeds.

Shirley supplied planed board for herb boxes for Harvard, according to Elisha Myrick's journal, and could be counted on to supply "green herbs." Thus, two hundred pounds of hops were delivered to Harvard in February 1851. The "twin sister" was supportive of Harvard rather than competitive.

> *There was a saying common in that part of the country that when you bought Shaker garden seeds you were sure what you were paying for.*
>
> CLARA ENDICOTT SEARS

SCOLDING WORMS TO DEATH

Asa Brocklebank's journal presents a picture of ceaseless activity and substantial accomplishments. Many farmers of the time believed that worms were harmful to crops, and so they attempted to eradicate them.

Nov. 29, 1805. We stamp bags. 21 vegetables, lavendar, sage, parsley.

Dec. 31. The amount of garden seed sold this year we find to be $1062.

January 1806. Brothers selling in Bolton, Lynn, Groton, Lancaster and Boston.

Feb. 26. Oliver Burt and Joshua go to Boston and stay three days. [This was unusual, as the trips were seldom more than one day.]

May 4–7. Spent raking and hoeing in the new garden and Herb garden. May 16. Oliver goes to Lancester with the widow Burt [his mother]. Plough Vine Ground [vineyards] and sow peppergrass, sage and parsley. May 14. Oliver does what he has a mind to.

June 4. Mother Lucy [Wright] arrives here at half past 2 o'clock. [This remarkable woman had been appointed "to lead in the female line" succeeding Mother Ann and served for twenty-five years at Mount Lebanon.] Oliver kills worms in the garden. Sister Ruth gathers two quarts of worms, but will not kill them and so she scolds them to death.

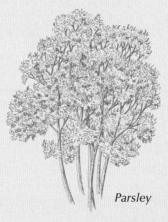

Parsley

A Shaker Nurse's Remedy Book

A handwritten book of formulas is dated Shirley Village, July 12, 1866, and was prepared for the use of the "Nurse-Sister at The Infirmary." It contains seven "Medical prescriptions given by an Indian Spirit Doctor named Pohatton, through James Parker of Shirley Village to G. B. Blanchard." There are remedies for gallstones; for the blood, stomach, and liver; and for a bad back. The ingredients include onion juice, angelica root, bark of the root of prickly ash, bitterwort, seneca, bloodroot, cayenne pepper, brandy, lobelia pods and seeds, burdock leaves, and good pure water.

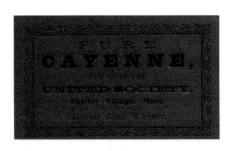

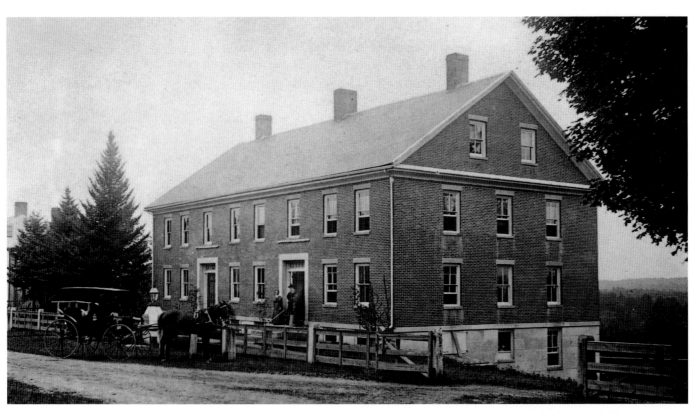

△ Trustees' office, Church Family, Shirley.

CHAPTER 6

The New Hampshire Societies

Canterbury, New Hampshire

Enfield, New Hampshire

LIKE THE MORE SOUTHERLY SHAKER communities, both of the New Hampshire societies began when local farmers responded enthusiastically to missionaries sent throughout New England in the 1780s. The Canterbury Church Family, for example, was established on the farm of Benjamin Whitcher, and he served as an elder for more than thirty years. The Enfield society gathered together on a number of adjoining farms on the western shore of Mascoma Lake.

Both the Canterbury and the Enfield societies closed themselves off from the world for the first few years after their founding. During that period the members worked to clear land, build farms and dwellings, develop industries, and learn to live together as religious communities separate from the world.

Decision, promptness, and perseverance are the prime elements of success in every undertaking in life.

AGNES E. NEWTON,
CANTERBURY

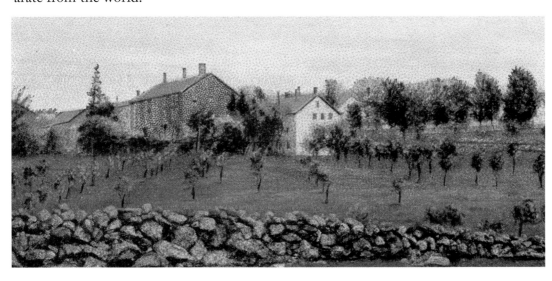

◁ View of the Canterbury Shaker community.

Begin today. No matter how feeble the light, let it shine as best it may. The world may need just that quality of light which you have.

ELDER HENRY C. BLINN,
CANTERBURY

CANTERBURY, NEW HAMPSHIRE

Henry Clay Blinn described his beloved home as being located on gently rising ground, overlooking most of the surrounding country, "high up on the Canterbury hills, twelve miles northwest of the beautiful City of Elms — Concord, the capital of the state." Love for his Shaker home grew from his first sight of it when he went there in 1838 as a boy of fourteen, against the protests of his friends in Providence, Rhode Island. They thought "the wild scheme of going among the mountains of New Hampshire" and with such strange people was not only folly but also extremely dangerous.

His first impression of the village never left his mind. As a talented Shaker teacher, botanist, beekeeper, journalist, printer, and dentist, this dedicated elder would return from the many journeys that were a part of the ministry's life and always thrill with pride and expectation as he had on that youthful trip in 1838.

Writing about the occasion later he said: "On reaching this last elevated spot, the whole of the Church Family was presented to view and the presentation was a beautiful picture on the mind. At that date, the white and yellow houses with bright red roofs, heightened the beauty of the village very much and to my mind, after a long and tedious journey, it seemed to be the prettiest place I had ever seen."

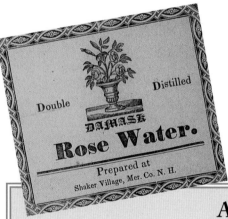

A YOUNG SHAKER BOTANIST

William Tripure the Botanist who has the personal charge of the Botanic Garden, and who at the same time practices physics in the Shaker families, the individuals of which seldom need medicine of any kind, was taken by the Shaker when very young, a poor boy from Elliot in the state of Maine. Probably there is not the second individual in the United States of his age who had so extensive a practical knowledge of botany as this young man. There is not a plant in the herbiary that he cannot give both its common and its botanical name with a description of its peculiar qualities.

This young man takes upon himself a large share of the personal labor of the Botanic garden; he excused himself for the few weeds that had recently got under way in it by saying, that as they were short-handed on the farm he had been at work haying a greater part of the time for four weeks.

The Botanist is making the experiment on his garden of the efficacy of the soil manure. He had planted side by side, three hills of medicinal beans. One hill he manured with peat and a solution of potash — another with vault manure — and the third with oil; the second hill was larger and more vigorous than that manured with peat; and the hill manured with oil was three times as large as either of the others.

FROM *THE FARMER'S MONTHLY VISITOR*,
AUGUST 31, 1840

Talented Members

Among the Canterbury Shakers lived a number of talented members whose combined abilities in healing, herb growing, botany, and business made their community's herb industry flourish in just a few decades.

Thomas Corbett

Thomas Corbett was not a doctor, but took up the study of medicine in 1813 when he was thirty-three years old at the request of the leaders in his community. Brother Thomas became known as a good physician outside the Shaker boundaries, and built up a large and profitable business in pressed herbs, pills, and syrups. Corbett's Shaker Vegetable Family Pills, "that medicine which goes slowly and without irritation along the intestinal canal," was endorsed by the celebrated professor of surgery of Dartmouth College, Dr. Dixi Crosby, who helped Corbett work out the sarsaparilla formula. Corbett's Wild Cherry Pectoral Syrup was also endorsed by several distinguished doctors and was said to have been given their highest commendations.

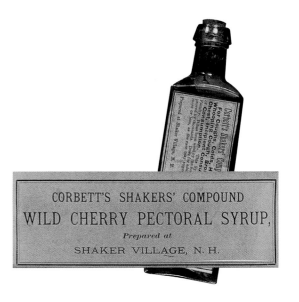

David Parker

David Parker, in his day, was doubtless one of the most widely known of all the Canterbury Shakers. He was remarkable for his industry, thrift, and shrewdness, but combined these with absolute honesty, which stamped him with the reputation of being perfectly reliable in every business transaction. He was admitted to the society at Canterbury in 1817, when he was ten years old.

▽ Elder Henry Blinn, shown here with his beehives in an orchard in full bloom.

Henry Blinn

Parker was seventeen years older than Henry Blinn and had been at the Canterbury community twenty-one years before young Henry was admitted in 1838. Despite the difference in years the men were congenial, and Brother Henry was placed under the watchful eye of the experienced trustee. This early training proved to be enormously valuable to Henry Blinn, who became a botanist, a printer, an editor, an author, a beekeeper, a stonecutter, a tailor, a musician, and a cabinetmaker. In addition to his other abilities, Brother Henry was a devoted and inspiring teacher, and he taught at the Shaker school from 1842 until 1852. That year, at the young age of twenty-eight, he was appointed elder and served until 1880. His wide range of activities and achievements shows the richness of life possible for a Shaker.

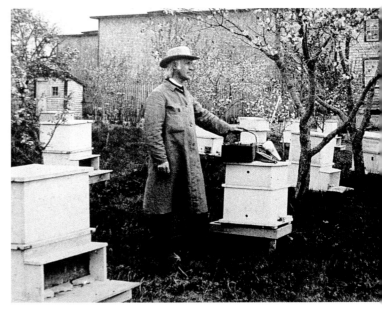

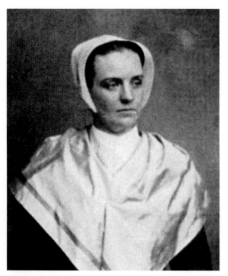

△ Sister Cora Helena Sarle.

Cora Helena Sarle

Elder Henry served as a mentor to a number of young members, including Sister Cora Helena Sarle. At the age of nineteen this talented young woman was in frail health. To get her out in the fresh air, Elder Henry asked her to draw the local weeds and wildflowers as a teaching aid to help Shaker children identify native plants. Over several years she filled two notebooks with her detailed, delicate drawings, and grew strong and sturdy in the process. Elder Henry added descriptive comments to most of the illustrations.

In addition to her drawing talent, Sister Helena was renowned for her beautiful soprano voice and for her ability to bake pies and breads. She remained in the Canterbury community until her death in 1956.

A Farmer's View of the Shakers

Isaac Hill, writing in his paper *The Farmer's Monthly Visitor*, gave a full account of the Shakers' botanical medicine industry in 1840:

▽ A page from Sister Helena's journal.

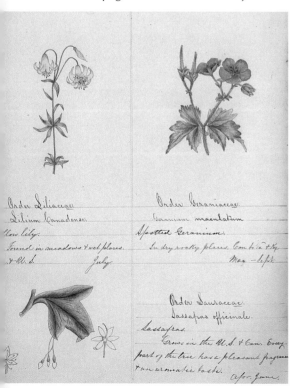

> The Botanic garden and Herbiary at the Shakers' first family contains probably a greater variety of the useful medicinal plants than any other establishment of the kind in New England. This garden was commenced by Thomas Corbett, one of the family and a self taught botanist and physician, twenty-four year old; it has been enlarged by the introduction of new species and new varieties until it covers a full acre and a half. We have before us a catalogue of Medicinal Plants and Vegetable Medicines prepared in the United Society of Canterbury, N.H. "printed at Shaker Village" (for they print here as well as perform almost every other mechanical business) consisting of about two hundred varieties. . . .
>
> The vegetable preparations have grown annually into an establishment probably more extensive than any other in the United States. The vegetables were introduced in the shape of dried leaves pressed into a solid cake weighing a specific quantity, in shape like a brick. When these articles of different kinds, such as chamomile, coltsfoot, elecampane, goldthread, horehound, johnswort, rose flowers, saffron, sage, summer savory, and the like, were first

> *One can always find someone whom he can serve by a kind deed, a timely word or a sympathizing prayer, and in so doing he finds that humility leads to honor, and that service is the sure door to true greatness.*
>
> CORA HELENA SARLE, CANTERBURY

introduced and left at the apothecary store in Boston, they were the food of merriment to some of the regular physicians. Gradually, however, Dr. Corbett has succeeded in their introduction until the prejudice of the doctors has been so far conquered that many of the faculty are constantly applying for them.

The medical establishment at the Shakers is not confined to articles raised by themselves — they purchase all the varieties of vegetable articles of extensive use in the materia medica. As a single item of purchase at one time was mentioned six tons of the ulmus fulva or bark of slippery elm, which was procured from the northern part of Vermont and Canada. This article, like many other barks and roots, is pulverized into fine flour and pressed into pound cakes; it is a most valuable medicine to be used in inflammation of the mucus membrane, in catarrhs, influenza, pleurisy, dysentery, strangury, and inflammation of the stomach and bowels.

Not only as medicine, but as articles of extensive family use in cooking, are the preparations of vegetables invented by the Shakers, two of which are of great value to the inhabitants of cities; they are sage and summer savory, two articles of vegetable growth which impart the finest flavor to various items of cookery. They are preserved and pressed into that compact form that they may be carried anywhere and used with as much convenience as a compressed hand or roll of manufactured tobacco.

In all these productions and preparations, as in almost every other enterprise they undertake, the Shakers find their account to be a constant gain. If others undertake to imitate their inventions and improvements, by the time their articles are finished, they will find the United Brethren in advance of them in some other improvement which always makes theirs to be preferred.

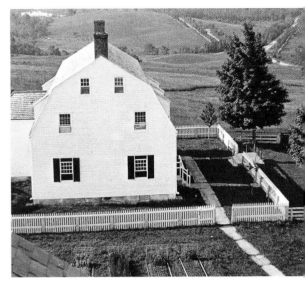

△ View of the Canterbury Shaker meetinghouse and gardens.

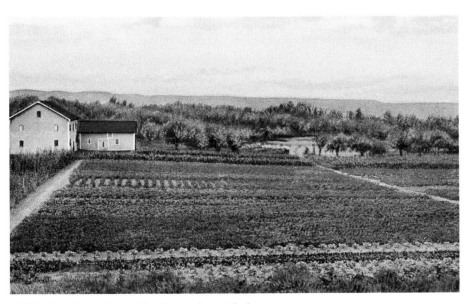

△ The family garden of the Canterbury Shakers.

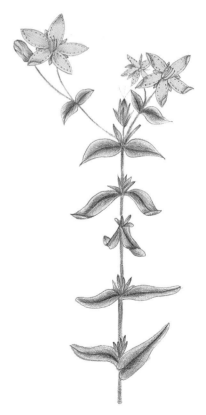

△ St.-John's-wort, drawn by Sister Helena Sarle.

Catalogs

The first medicinal herb catalog prepared in the Canterbury society was printed in 1835. This catalog covered 180 herbs, with common and botanical names and the price per pound, and twelve extracts: butternut, cicuta, clover head, cow parsnip, dandelion, garget or poke, henbane, garden lettuce, nightshade, poppy, thorn apple, and thoroughwort. Any other kinds not mentioned could be made to order. Oils made from cedar, fir, goldenrod, snakeroot, wormwood, and wormseed were listed.

Three compound syrups were offered: Syrup of Liverwort, "a safe and valuable medicine for coughs, spitting of blood and consumption"; Syrup of Black Cohosh, "one of the most powerful deobstruents, and alternatives in the vegetable kingdom; and as such has proved an effectual remedy in rheumatism, gout, chronic lameness; and in scrofulous, glandular and eruptive diseases"; and Syrup of Sarsaparilla, "taken in doses of an ounce, four or five times a day, will fulfill every indication that the boasted panaceas and catholicons can perform; is free from the mercurial poison such nostrums contain; and is much more safe and efficient as a medicine for cleansing and purifying the blood."

Other medicines listed in this 1835 catalog are similar to those in the early catalogs isssued by the Watervliet and New Lebanon societies.

"We recognize Vegetable Antidyseptic [Antidyspeptic] Restorative Wine Bitters," the text proclaimed, a "superior tonic" guaranteed "to restore the appetite, tone up the stomach, dispel torpid feelings and headache and warm the system." Vegetable Bilious Pills, Digestive or Stomach Pills, and Vegetable Rheumatic Pills were listed with familiar ingredients, much the same as those offered by other societies. The Rheumatic Pills were endorsed by six doctors, who stated: "This may certify that the subscribers have examined by request the formula for the Vegetable Rheumatic Pills made by Doctor Thomas Corbett of the United Society of Shakers at Canterbury, New Hampshire, and having compared it with that for the celebrated Dean's Rheumatic Pills, are of opinion, that the substitution of 'Extracts' in the former, for the vegetables in substance in the latter, with some alterations, gives to his formula a decided preference as a mild and efficient cathartic over that of Dean's."

Corbett's Syrup of Sarsaparilla

The Shakers' 1848 catalog carried a detailed description of Corbett's Compound Concentrated Syrup of Sarsaparilla, along with four pages of signed testimonials from physicians and agents. David Parker, trustee for the community, claimed that Corbett's Syrup of Sarsaparilla was composed

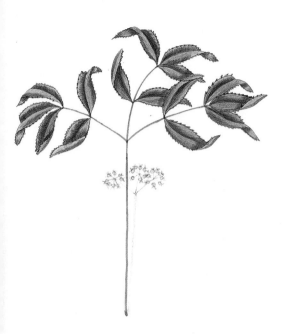

△ Sarsaparilla *(Aralia nudicaulis)*, drawn by Sister Helena Sarle.

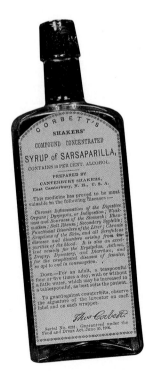

entirely of vegetables and herbs. One ounce of pure iodide of potassium was added to every twelve bottles "to insure a pure article." The society stated that the formula was a combination of the roots of sarsaparilla, dandelion, yellow dock, mandrake, black cohosh, garget, and Indian hemp, along with the berries of juniper and cubeb. Parker added that "this medicine had proved to be most valuable in the following diseases: chronic inflammation of the digestive organs, dyspepsia of indigestion, jaundice, weakness and sourness of the stomach, rheumatism, salt rheum, secondary syphilis, functional disorders of the liver, chronic eruptions of the skin, and all scrofulous diseases. Also it is found to be an invaluable remedy for the erysipelas, and the distressing disorder of asthma. It has proved highly beneficial in some cases of dropsy, dysentery, and diarrhea."

The following account from the *Granite Monthly*, for September 1885, gives the best of many descriptions of the origin and ingredients of this medicine:

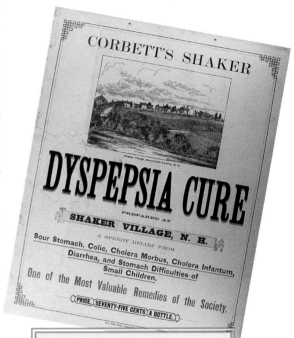

> Some fifty years ago Dr. Dixi Crosby, the celebrated physician of Hanover (New Hampshire), gave his counsel and advice to the Shakers, Dr. Thomas Corbett and David Parker, to aid them in the preparation of a curative compound of herbs and roots, which should meet the wants of the medical fraternity. The learned doctor wanted his prescription honestly and conscientiously mixed; and, reposing confidence in the fidelity of the Shaker community, he and his friend Dr. Valentine Mott gave the new medicine the benefit of their approval, and widely advertised its merits. . . .

> From the most euphonious of its constituent parts, it was called "sarsaparilla," and became so famed for its curative properties, that great fortunes have been made in manufacturing imitation or bogus articles of the same name. The medicine was designed for impurities of the blood, general and nervous debility, and wasting diseases and, for the half century during which it has been prepared for the public, it has been an inestimable boon to the sick and suffering.

> To fully appreciate the care given to the preparation of this remedy, one should visit the Shaker community in Canterbury, the home of Dr. Thomas Corbett and David Parker,   both long since gone to their final reward, — and see their successors in the field and in the laboratory, working to compound the sarsaparilla. A little north of the kitchen garden of the First Family, and east of the great barn, near where the saintly Elder Henry [Blinn] caresses his pet bees, and jovial Friend George attends to the grape, the pear, and the apple, the brothers of the family cultivate the curative herbs in a garden especially tilled by them. At the proper season the plants are gathered into storehouses, the roots and berries subjected to chemical changes by skillful hands, dirt and impurities are absolutely banished, and in time Shaker Sarsaparilla is ready for the market.

SELLING SARSAPARILLA

According to the record, the amount of sarsaparilla sold from Canterbury is impressive:

1849   551 bottles sold.

1850   668 dozen bottles and 10 jugs sold.

1853   Eleven barrels sold.

1857   303 dozen bottles sold.

1859   154 dozen bottles and 6½ dozen jugs sold.

1861   400 dozen bottles and 20 gallons in jugs.

1879   154 dozen bottles and 6½ gallons in jugs.

1894   100 dozen bottles sold.

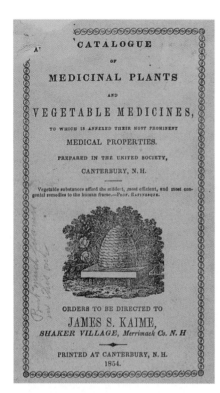

△ The 1854 catalog issued by the Canterbury Shakers.

A Variety of Products

The 1835 catalog listed a remarkable variety of medicinal products. Among these were:

Cephalic Pills; Vegetable Cough Pills; Bitter Root, highly valued by the Southern Indians; Compound Emetic of Lobelia; Flour of Slipper Elm; A Chemical Liniment for bruises, sprains, rheumatism, pain in the neck, chilblains, etc.; Nitrous Salts, a new and valuable medicine for physic in fevers, influenzas and colds and also in St. Anthony's fire and most kinds of eruptive diseases. In cases where the food lays hard on the stomach, it is an infallible remedy; and Beth Root [trillium] one of the mildest but most efficient remedies in Haemoptysis as well as all kinds of hemorrhage.

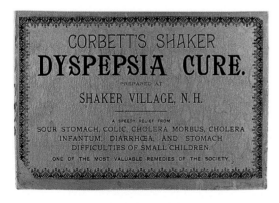

△ In packing boxes like this the Canterbury Shakers shipped their products all over the world.

SOLICITING HERBS FROM THE WORLD

In 1853, David Parker circulated a handbill soliciting the gathering of herbs by people outside the community.

WANTED

The following Roots and Herbs are wanted, delivered at Shaker Village, Merrimac Co. N.H. for which a fair compensation will be given, if the following directions are observed.

All herbs must be well cured by being dried in the shade that they may retain a bright appearance, and must be freed from all other articles, as dirt, grass, etc. and those having large stalks must be stripped therefrom. They should be gathered in time of blossoming or soon after.

Roots must be cleansed from dirt, and if large, split and well dried. None will be received unless the above directions are strictly regarded.

Roots should be gathered in the fall or very early in the spring. June is the best time for peeling barks.

1853. David Parker.

Avans Root	Dragon's Claw	Scabish
Alder Bark, Black	Crawley root	Spearmint
Bittersweet	Dwarf Elder Root	Snakehead
Blackberries	Harvest Lice	Stonebrake (Purple
Blue Flag Root	Horsemint	Thoroughwort)
Bugle, Sweet	Horseradish Leaves	Sumach Leaves
Burdock Leaves	Lobelia, Herb and Seed	Sweet Flag Root
Root	Marigold Flowers	Thoroughwort
Seed	Motherwort	Vervain
Catmint	Peppermint	Witch Hazel Leaves
Coltsfoot	Rose Flowers, red	Yarrow
Dragon Root	and white (Separate)	

A broadside printed a few years later listed 200 herbs with common and botanical names, but the next bound catalog was not issued until 1847. The back cover listed the Reimproved Rocking Trusses, "Single, Double, and Umbilical adapted to all ages and sexes, for the relief and permanent cure of Hernia, or Rupture; invented, manufactured, applied and sold in the United Society of Shakers, in Canterbury, N.H. All orders to be addressed to Thomas Corbett." The ointments offered were bone or Kittredge, savin, and thorn apple. Sweet marjoram, sage, summer savory, and thyme were sold in canisters, small and large. Without giving specific ingredients, five syrup compounds by the gallon bottle were listed. They were called black cohosh, liverwort, poppy, sarsaparilla, and wild cherry pectoral.

The Shakers of Canterbury published their last catalog of medicinal plants and vegetable medicines in 1854, offering 242 herbs with common and botanical names and prices, and listing thirty-six properties. They also offered the same extracts, oils, ointments, syrups, and sundries for sale.

△ Bittersweet *(Solanum dulcamara),* drawn by Sister Helena Sarle.

A Shaker Cookbook

In addition to their catalogs, the Shakers issued a little booklet of thirty-four pages, called *Mary Whitcher's Shaker House-Keeper,* to sell Shaker medicines. Originally published in Boston in 1882, this is the earliest cookbook in Shaker culinary literature. Sister Mary had been a member of the Canterbury community since early childhood; she also served as kitchen deaconess, trustee, and eldress.

Corbett's Syrup of Sarsaparilla was described as "The Most Economical Medicine," the best for "Mothers When Worn Out," a restorative for "Good Appetite and Rich Blood," and was endorsed by doctors, druggists, and chemists. Menus and recipes in one column were side by side on each page with testimonials and "kind words" as to what Corbett's would do. In a column beside "Brown Bread No. 3 and Graham Gems" was a note of gratitude: "[Mary Whitcher] has done more to adapt the Sarsaparilla to the wants of mother and children, than any other person."

But in spite of all the advertising and testimonials, the last of Corbett's sarsaparilla was made in the syrup house at Canterbury in 1895. Competition with commercial firms had become increasingly stiff, and since the trustees were counseled not to sell inferior articles, it was impossible to maintain their high standards and realize a profit.

Enfield, New Hampshire

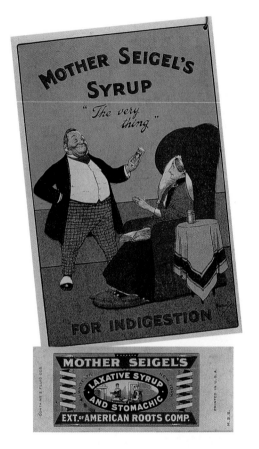

Enfield is situated near the western border of New Hampshire, thirteen miles southeast of Hanover — home of Dartmouth College. Although not as close to each other geographically as were the "twin villages" of Harvard and Shirley, these two, Enfield and Canterbury, on opposite sides of the state, were close in spirit.

"Shaker Hill," the rich farmland on the west shore of Mascoma Lake, belonged to James Jewett and eventually became the site of the society when it was formed in 1793. As more farmers joined and gave their land to the society it increased to about 3,000 acres, productive uplands of the Connecticut River further enriched by acres of alluvial mowing grounds. A lake on a mountain 1,500 feet above the village supplied water.

Isaac Hill reported in the September 20, 1839, issue of *The Farmer's Monthly Visitor* that the garden of the Center Family covered five acres of ground on the margin of the "Mascomy pond." He wrote:

Of the garden one half an acre was sage, a portion of which had been forced in early hot beds. The Shakers also raise large quantities of summer savory. The preparation of sage and summer savory is by drying and pressing into a solid mass. The profits of these and other botanical preparations are best understood by those who are well acquainted with the best methods of raising and preparing them.

Five hands, two men and three boys, are sufficient for the labor of these five acres of garden, which yields annually in cash its thousand, if not its thousands of dollars.

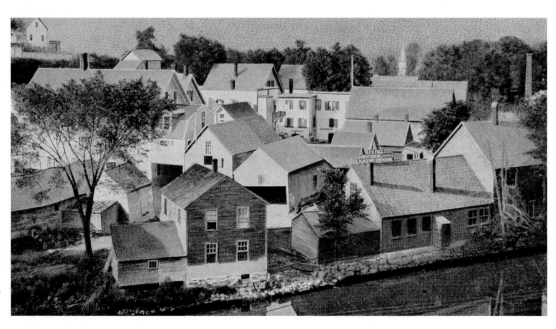

▷ Church Family, Enfield, New Hampshire.

Dandelion and Valerian

Extract of Dandelion was made in large quantities at Enfield, as it was in the medical departments of other Shaker communities, to act upon "the derangement of hepatic apparatus, Liver and Gall and of the digestive organs generally. In Congestion and Chronic Inflammation of the Liver and Spleen; in cases of suspended or deficient biliary secretion, etc., if employed with due regard to the degree of excitement, our own experience is decidedly in its favor. Nothing further need be said, its use is so common and generally understood."

Among other preparations manufactured at Enfield were a gargle for the throat and tongue; pure Jamaica ginger, which was highly recommended for dyspepsia and indigestion, and as a tonic for debilitated systems, "which if taken in season" would cure colds and coughs and was the best-known remedy for summer complaint, toothache, earache, cramp, and cholera; Mother Seigel's Curative Syrup for Dyspepsia; and Brown's Extract of English Valerian.

Valeriana officinalis was the botanical name of the principal ingredient of Brown's Extract. The Shaker catalog called this extract "the best remedy yet discovered for the cure of Nervousness, Lowness of Spirits, Debility, Hypochondria, Neuralgia, Hysteria, Restlessness, Tic Douloureux, Sick Headache, and every other disease arising from mental affection and nervous exhaustion. One trial will prove its great superiority over all other remedies now in use. It is also an invaluable remedy for outward application, in all cases of Cuts, Bruises, Sores, Sprains, Scalds, Burns, Lameness, Skin Diseases, and every affection requiring external treatment."

The Enfield Shakers printed advertising circulars and broadsides and two pamphlets of several pages each containing facts about Brown's Extract in 1879 and 1880.

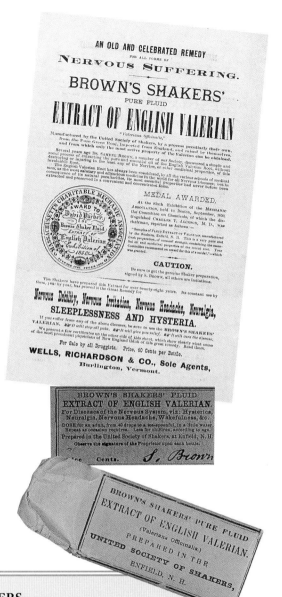

RECOMMENDED BY FORTY-NINERS

The Enfield Shakers manufactured a list of medicines "composed of native vegetables," as stated on the labels. They prepared a Family Cough Syrup, and a big seller called Arnikate of Tannin, which was a specific for all choleric diseases. This was "first recommended to a Company going to California, in 1849, by whom its virtues have been fully tested and is now put up by their advice expressly for that numerous portion of our countrymen who are going to the infected region for gold."

The Shakers claimed that their Vegetable Pills were an almost sure preventive of epidemic complaints, such as cholera morbus, bilious colic, and bilious and typhus fever. The pills were also "a safe and powerful cathartic," the label read. An Alterative Syrup, "A Compound Concentrated Decoction of Rumex highly recommended as a natural efficient and safe alterative to the system affected with scrofulous, cancerous and other accidental or hereditary diseases," was in general demand.

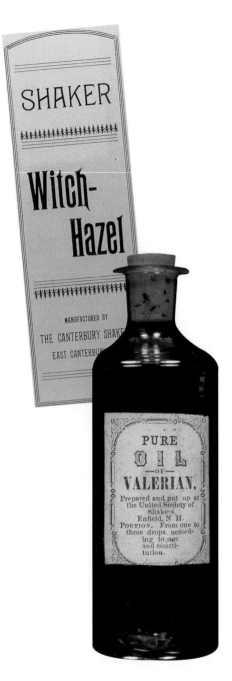

A Catalog of Medicinals

The medical department of this community also published a seven-page catalog of medicinal plants and vegetable medicines, with their most prominent medical properties. Although it was not dated, it was probably an earlier issue than the pamphlets published in 1879 and 1880 because it listed valerian as an available root for medicinal purposes but did not list the manufactured product, presumably because it predated the medicine.

In selling the extract in their printed material the Shakers gave this information about valerian:

This highly valuable article is a preparation manufactured by the United Society of Shakers, at Enfield, N.H. It is simply an extract from the pure green roots of the Valerian plant; and owing to their favorable position for obtaining the fresh, green roots of the Valerian plant at the proper season for digging when they are strongest, they claim greater efficacy for their preparation than is secured by that made in the usual way from dry roots of uncertain age and strength.

For years the Enfield Shakers enjoyed a well-earned prosperity, their farm and garden operation accounting for a large part of it. In 1874 they were doing a business of $30,000 in the sale of seeds and $4,000 in distilled valerian. Boston was their best marketplace.

Sister Frances Carr, a member of the Sabbathday Lake Society in Maine, wrote in *The Shaker Quarterly* for the summer of 1963: "Brown's Fluid Extract of English Valerian compounded at Enfield, New Hampshire, by Br. Samuel Brown of that Society, remained in demand as late as 1897, though he died in 1856. From his youth and for many years, he worked closely with Br. Ezekiel Evans, who was charged with raising and preparing herbs for the market. Their work contributed considerably to the advance of the herb industry at Enfield."

After 130 years the Enfield community, which at one time counted close to 250 members, closed its doors in 1923, and the remaining seven Shakers moved to Canterbury.

CHAPTER 7

The Maine Societies

Alfred, Maine

Sabbathday Lake, Maine

THE LAST OF THE SHAKER SOCIETIES to be settled in the Northeast, Alfred and Sabbathday Lake were established in 1793 and 1794, respectively. In 1781 an Alfred man, John Cotton, encountered ardent Shakers in Enfield, New Hampshire, and brought the news of this new faith back home, where he persuaded friends and neighbors to convert. Shaker missionaries then visited from New Lebanon and Hancock and found many receptive hearts throughout the area. A few Maine Shakers visited Mother Ann and the Elders at Harvard, Massachusetts, and then a larger group made the long and difficult journey by ship down the Atlantic coast and up the Hudson River to see Mother Ann at Watervliet. After their return, Father James Whittaker traveled to Maine to visit the eager communities there, the most active of which were Alfred, Gorham, and "Sabbathday Pond."

During this period Maine was still part of Massachusetts; it did not become a state until 1820. Thus Massachusetts had seven Shaker societies within its borders at one time.

Of the two Shaker societies in Maine, Sabbathday Lake had a much more vigorous herb industry. The community still thrives and the herb industry is enjoying a tremendous revival today.

What might at first seem to be mere labor becomes, in fact, the occasion for sharing both socially and spiritually.

FRANCES CARR,
SABBATHDAY LAKE

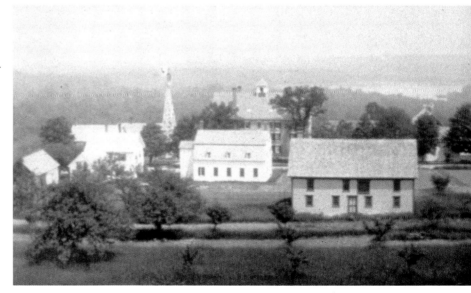

▷ An early 20th-century view of the Church Family at Sabbathday Lake.

ALFRED, MAINE

According to Sister R. Mildred Barker, formerly a member of the Alfred community, writing in *The Shaker Quarterly:*

> *The herb and medicine business does not seem to have gained the prominence in Alfred that it did in most Societies, though their use within the family itself was prevalent. During the latter half of the [nineteenth] century, Elder John Vance, who had studied medicine to some degree, provided the family with a most capable physician during most illnesses. There were, however, some herbs gathered and sold to Harvard and some of the other Societies where the herb industry prevailed to a larger extent.*

Alfred is about thirty miles southwest of Portland. The Alfred Shakers' 1,200 acres were situated between sizable hills and included a large pond that provided them with important waterpower. Charles Nordhoff reported in 1875 that the land was not very fertile or easily cultivated, and when an outlying tract of timberland was sold for $28,000 the Shakers "were glad to be rid of it."

The raising of garden seeds was a much larger business; the Shakers started growing them in Alfred as early as 1835. A broadside dated 1850 lists forty-seven seeds, including ten herbs: summer savory, sage, lemon balm, sweet balm, rue, parsley, saffron, English sorrel, marigold, and hyssop.

The herb business became sufficiently successful for the trustees to issue a broadside listing eighty-two medicinal herbs, including rose flowers, belladonna, poppy flowers, raspberry leaves, Roman wormwood, and sumac berries. Although this business did not compare in size with that at Sabbathday Lake, where almost twice as many herbs were offered for sale, it was still a good source of income.

A Visiting Farmer's Praise

Editor Isaac Hill furnished an account of Alfred in *The Farmer's Monthly Visitor* for July 31, 1840. Although this description focuses on the seed and vegetable business, it gives an idea of the degree to which outsiders admired the Shakers' agricultural expertise.

> *Their garden for the production of vegetables and seeds was what we always expect to see when we visit a Shaker family in the summer season; they had recently erected an extensive seed house, in the lower story of which were preparation rooms for labelling and packing seeds, and in the two upper stories ample space was given for drying, curing, thrashing and cleaning the seeds as they are collected from the field.*

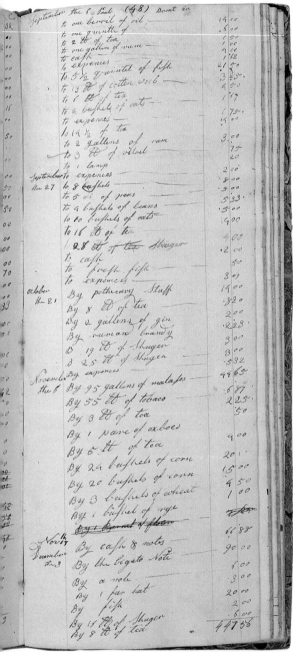

△ An excerpt from the Alfred Shakers' Daybook, 1815, mentioning a "pothecary."

The persevering attention which the several Societies of Shakers have paid to the production of Garden Seeds for many years, commends them to the public patronage. They have steadily pursued this business for more than half a century; and they are not a people to relax in any laudable effort which is likely to be crowned with success. Others following their example have gone extensively into the production of garden seeds; but the growth of the country still affords the consumption which induces the Shakers to continue this as a profitable business. Of them useful lessons may always be taken in everything connected with domestic economy and in the productions of the earth. If they raise garden seeds, they know how to preserve the pure varieties of onions, beets, carrots, cabbages, melons, squashes, etc., not suffering them to intermix by growing in the near contact; and they are in advance of most other horticulturists in a more sure and better method of curing and preserving seeds.

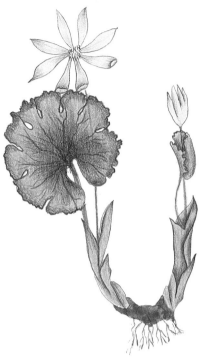

△ Bloodroot, drawn by Canterbury sister Cora Helena Sarle.

SABBATHDAY LAKE, MAINE

In 1794 this Maine community, the last of the eastern societies to be founded, was organized into full gospel order. It was called New Gloucester, then West Gloucester; it is now known as Sabbathday Lake. The society owned 2,000 acres of land when Charles Nordhoff wrote about it in 1875, and according to him its income was derived from the raising and selling of garden seeds and the making of brooms, quantities of woodenware, and old-fashioned spinning wheels. He said: "Its most profitable industry is the manufacture of oak staves for molasses hogsheads, which are exported to the West Indies. . . . They made last year also a thousand dollars worth of pickles; and the women make fancy articles in their spare time."

During her tour of the eastern Shaker societies, Eldress Betsy Smith from Pleasant Hill wrote in her journal in July 1869:

First Order, New Gloucester, their dwellings have the neatness of a flower bed. . . . There are about 60 persons in this Society composed of two families, the Church and the gathering order, Poland Hill, and they are a little band of very clever, social good folk. They have a very nice terraced garden on the hillside just west of the road and buildings that looked lively and thrifty where they raise herbs and vegetables for sale. . . .

▽ The Sabbathday Lake Church Family, showing flower garden.

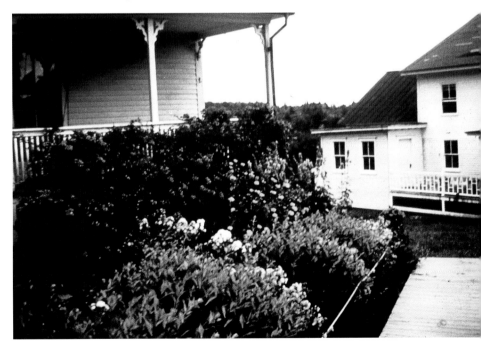

Growing and Selling Medicinal Herbs

At first the Sabbathday Lake Shakers grew and processed medicinal herbs as those in other Shaker communities did, only for the benefit of their own families. When they grew a surplus, they sent the excess to market. They soon issued "A Catalogue of Medicinal Plants Prepared in the United Society of Shakers, New Gloucester, Cumberland County Maine," with prices per paper, in 1840. In broadside form eighty-three herbs were offered.

James Holmes (1771–1856) founded the seed business and printed the labels and packets needed for the herb and seed industries. He was a deacon in the society and also the author of three little books, which he printed in the garden seed house. The first one of eighty-one pages printed in 1850 gives instructions for the treatment of hydrophobia; recommends camphor to destroy lice on cattle; gives a cure for piles; and recommends human urine in a bucket of water as a simple cure for "Cough in Horses," and heather root for treatment of whooping cough in children.

This collection of useful hints for farmers and many valuable recipes,

▽ The 1794 Meeting House at Sabbathday Lake, with bee balm in the foreground.

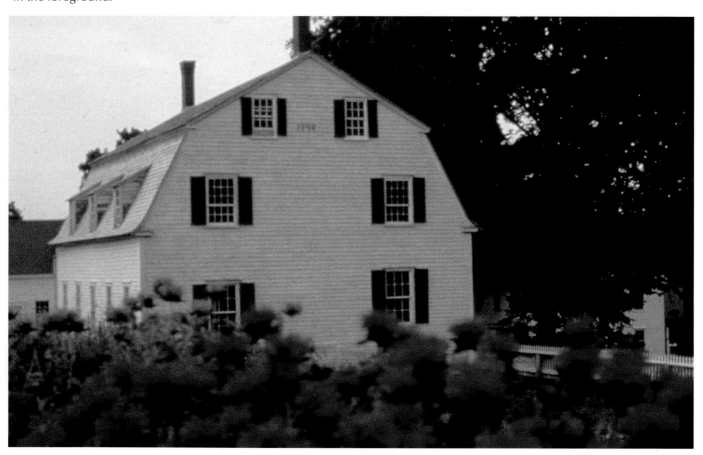

collected and compiled by James Holmes, appeared with this preface: "The compiler of this little work in his leisure moments, has collected the following recipes, maxims and useful hints in farming and other matter of economy, considering them worth preserving and believing they might be useful and of great benefit to those who may wish to avail themselves of every improvement, and the best methods of performing business." The garden seed house, where these little books were produced, was razed around 1920 and all the contents destroyed.

During the summer of 1993, however, Brother Arnold Hadd, community printer and a trustee of the Sabbathday Lake Shakers, printed a small booklet on James Holmes with the help of John Cutrone, entitled *Collected and Compiled by J. H. (The story, in Many Voices, of Deacon James Holmes, first printer of the Sabbathday Lake Shakers).*

Sage was the culinary herb grown in the largest commercial quantities, and from all accounts it was a large crop. There are several entries in Elder Otis Sawyer's journal bearing on this:

March 6, 1873. Brother William Dumont went to the depot in the afternoon with four barrels of Sage for Thompson and Leighton of Portland.
March 25, 1874. Brother William Dumont ground and put up a barrel of Dockroot for Brother Samuel. March 31. Brother William Dumont went to the depot with 5 barrels of herbs. Brought back 10 bushels of corn.
January 16, 1878. Herbert West took five barrels of sage to the depot to be shipped to Portland. January 18. Herbert West took another five barrels of sage to the depot to be shipped to Portland.

The society issued only one bound herb catalog, in 1864, listing 155 herbs, barks, roots, and powdered articles. Herbs were ground and pulverized and sweet marjoram, sage, summer savory, and thyme were sold in canisters, in two sizes, for $1 or $2 per dozen. Also offered were grapevines, plants, garden seeds, horseradish in jars, applesauce, peach water and rose water by the gallon or bottle, and sieves and brooms.

The Shaker Tamar Laxative

Many Shaker communities specialized in creating one product in the medicinal herb department, which provided a source of income larger than all of the other medicines they made. At Mount Lebanon, Seven Barks and Veratrum Viride were in this category. At Canterbury it was Corbett's Syrup of Sarsaparilla, and at Enfield, New Hampshire, it was Brown's Pure Extract of English Valerian. At Sabbathday Lake it was the Shaker Tamar Laxative, a fruit compound. How this came to be manufactured by the community is told in the *Church Record:*

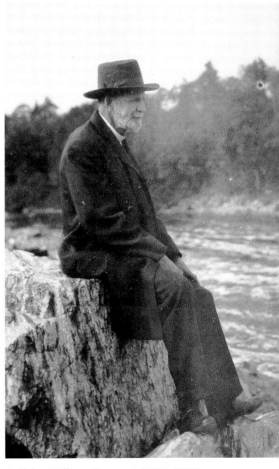

△ Elder William Dumont (1851–1930).

SHAKER TAMAR LAXATIVE

Take Cassia Fistula, crushed, 400 lbs; Tamarinds 135 lbs; Prunes, 100 lbs; Digest each in warm water and strain through sieve or fine cloth. Then mix the strained liquid and evaporate in vacuo to a thick extract. Then take of this compound, Fruit extract, 579 oz; Fruit of Cassia Obovata, 192 oz, Glycerine, 24 oz; Sugar, 80 oz; Powdered Hyoscyamin, 1½ oz. Mix thoroughly and make into Tablets of 53 grains each which are then to be covered with Gelatin.

According to Sister Frances Carr, after the compound was cut into lozenges, each one was placed by hand onto a specially prepared drying board that was studded with wire pins. On these the lozenges remained until the coating was thoroughly dried and they could be packed. Each box, when ready for sale, had both the compound's formula and the directions for its use printed on the bottom.

The formula does not include wintergreen, but a church journal with a March 13, 1884, entry states: "Laxative rolled into sheets today. Two pounds of glycerine and two ounces oil of wintergreen put into full batch."

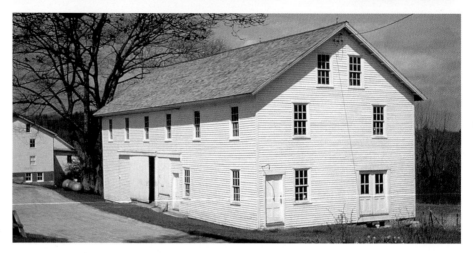

△ The 1821 herb house. Processing and packaging took up the second floor. The double doors open into the former shipping room. The top floor is still a drying attic for herbs.

October 5, 1881. Brother Benjamin came to offer the Church a chance to prepare and put up a new medicine compounded and invented by A. J. White of New York who gives preparations to the amount of twelve hundred dollars and New Lebanon gives two hundred. The Church gladly and gratefully accept the offer. Brother Benjamin went around to the Laundry, the Herb House and other places to see where the business could be carried on and decided that the large Herb room in the chamber of Middle Wood House was a very appropriate place. The medicine is to be made in the shape of Lozenge and to be called "The Shaker Tamar Laxative." A meeting of the principal part of the family was called and decided in favor of prosecuting the business.

October 8, Saturday. Brother Hewett went to New York to meet Brother Benjamin Gates to learn more about the preparation of medicine.

October 24. Monday. Brother Hewett is making preparation for the manufacture of the Shaker Tamar Laxative. He has purchased a kneader to work the stuff through.

October 28. Friday. Brother Hewitt went to Lewiston. He is having a machine made to cut out the Losenges.

November 24. . . . The New Medicine started this afternoon. Brother Hewitt and Sisters mixed one batch of The Shaker Tamar Laxative and cut a few tablets. That it may prove a profitable business is the prayer of every person in the Church.

December 29, Elder William and Sisters are making the Tamar Tablets with a hope to make sales and render the medicine Popular.

January 16, 1882. Monday. The first order for Shaker Tamar Lozenges came Thursday, January 12, from Dr. Russell of Minot; 4 boxes. Tall oaks from little acorns grow.

March 22. A large lot of Tamar now packed for parties in Boston, New York City, Philadelphia, Chicago and Troy, New York.

And so a medicine was manufactured that from the very first and for thirty years was an outstanding success. The last batch was made in 1911. A four-page leaflet of testimonials, directions on its use, and the admonition "The West Gloucester Society are the only Shakers who make the Shaker Tamar Laxative, and all others bearing the name of Shaker are not genuine" was distributed under the name of Brother William Dumont, the trustee in charge of its manufacture.

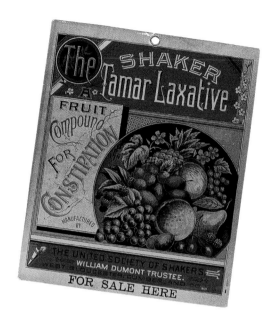

The Revival of the Herb Industry at Sabbathday Lake

In the same way that the herb industries at other communities declined at the turn of the century, so did the business at Sabbathday Lake, but it did not die. The medicinal herb department at Sabbathday Lake was closed in 1911. As the century progressed, the community's herb house, built in 1824, became the only Shaker herb house still standing in any of the communities, but it was not used for herb processing. On a very small scale, a couple of the sisters continued to sell sage, savory, and candied sweet flag root in the village store. Yet according to community member Sister Frances Carr, from the time the herb department closed until the 1950s, "very little herb activity was carried on here."

By the mid-twentieth century Shakerism seemed to most people to be like a garden in winter — a few remaining traces of former glory but lifeless nonetheless. To a perceptive few, however, the remnant of the Shakers still held promise. Writing in 1956, John S. Williams characterized Believers of the time this way: "Strength still exists, and the few remaining members (some 35) follow the precepts with a dignity that makes their friendship a vital experience. The curtains have not closed." Mr. Williams proved to be correct, for at Sabbathday Lake a quiet "opening" was about to occur.

Under the guidance of Theodore Johnson (Brother Ted), who moved to Sabbathday Lake in 1960, the society began a more vigorous outreach to the world. The most important aspect of this outreach was spiritual: the presentation of Shakerism as a viable spiritual way of life for today. The meetinghouse was once again opened in the warm weather for public meetings on Sundays, and pamphlets and articles began to appear explaining Shaker theology in modern, easy-to-understand terms.

On the scholarly level, the launch of *The Shaker Quarterly* in 1961 seemed a fulfillment of the hope of Canterbury Elder Henry Blinn, when he regretfully ended *The Manifesto* in 1899, that a "wave of enthusiasm" would someday revive Shaker publication. Thus it is not surprising that before the 1960s were over, the Sabbathday Lake Shakers had revived a few of the traditional Shaker industries, one of which was the herb industry.

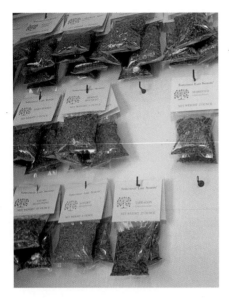

△ Sabbathday Lake culinary herbs are packaged in smaller quantities in poly bags for "occasional cooks" and one-time users.

▽ View of present-day Sabbathday Lake herb gardens taken from the meetinghouse, with the orchard visible in the background.

The survival of the herb house, a visible reminder of what once was, and the fact that "people were beginning to discover both the beneficial aspects of herbs as well as the pleasure they brought to one's culinary sense" caused Brother Ted to feel that "this was the time to re-establish the herbal industry once so much a part of nearly every Shaker community's existence."

Wild Mint and Pipsissewa

In 1964 the first small efforts were made. Some mint was transplanted from the shores of the lake to a small garden in the village. Gradually the Shakers added other plants to this garden. Once again, Sister Frances chronicles what was happening: "We began looking for and discovered many herbs growing wild on the property. No doubt they were left over from the once thriving industry which once encompassed acres here at Shaker Village. We still find such things as Pipsissewa in the old granite quarry and other relative rarities in the fields and woods."

By 1969, Brother Ted had the firm intention to grow enough herbs so that they could be sold in the Shaker store. "The first tangible results" of his efforts appeared on August 10, 1971, when tarragon vinegar went on sale in the village shop. Immediately following this success, dried thyme, rosemary, sage, savory, basil, spearmint, peppermint, marjoram, oregano, dill seed, and Shaker Herb Tea were offered for sale in small glass bottles.

The final two pages of the Winter 1971 issue of *The Shaker Quarterly* listed eighteen culinary herbs and eleven herbal teas for sale. The price for the one-ounce glass jars was $.50 each; the herbal teas sold for $1 a jar. At

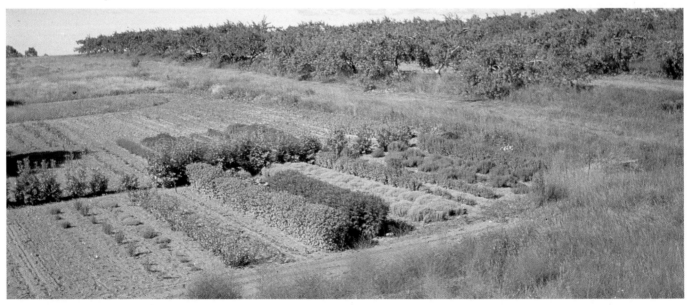

that time the community also offered Shaker Rose Water in both four- and eight-ounce sizes. They cost $.95 and $1.75, respectively. It is interesting that after the list of herbs and rose water a long list of non-Shaker publications appeared. Books on herbs, herb growing and gathering, herbs in the kitchen, herbs and health, and dyes and dyeing could be ordered. By 1971, in anticipation of an ever greater demand, fifty-seven distinct varieties of herbs were grown at Sabbathday Lake.

Mail Order

That fall the Shakers began a mail-order business, replacing the small glass bottles with specially made tins that were exact reproductions of the tins used by the community in the 1860s. The labels were printed by Brother David Serrette on a press belonging to the community.

The response was tremendous:

The processing and packaging of herbs and herbal teas had occupied many of us off and on all fall long. On the 27th [of October, 1973], we found the busiest production line we had yet had. Sisters Elizabeth, Elsie, Frances, Marie, and Mildred, along with Brother Ted and David spent much of the day working very hard indeed over our revived industry. Although the processing is without doubt hard work, it also affords the opportunity for close family fellowship. What might at first seem to be mere labor becomes, in fact, the occasion for sharing both socially and spiritually.

Activity continued at a hectic pace in 1974 from April, when "the first ploughing for the vegetable and herb gardens began on the 23rd," until June 4, when "everyone who was available joined forces in packing herbs." Ironically, none of this herb activity took place in the 1824 herb house. The sisters' shop and laundry served the purpose in a far better manner. The building's attic was used for drying herbs, and the ironing room below for preparing and packaging.

Naturally this revival of the Shaker herb industry did not go unnoticed by the press, especially since 1974 was the 200th anniversary of the arrival of the Shakers in America. Various newspaper and magazine articles provide yet more glimpses at the industry. For the July 1974 issue of *Down East* Marius B. Peladeau wrote an essay titled "Anyone for St. Johnswort?" detailing the revived herb industry at Sabbathday Lake. Included are five photographs of the Shakers working at various tasks, from gathering herbs to packing. In addition there is a photo of the herb house and one showing a pyramid of tins.

In 1974 the society offered seventeen culinary herbs and twenty-eight teas. That Christmas the Shakers shipped 1,100 tins to Bloomingdale's department store in New York City.

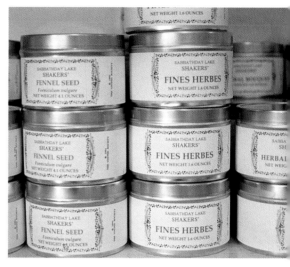

△ Herbal teas and culinary herbs are still packaged in tins, a practice that replaced paper-covered herb bricks in the 1860s.

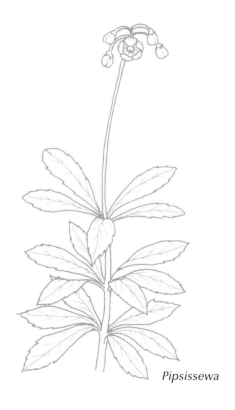

Pipsissewa

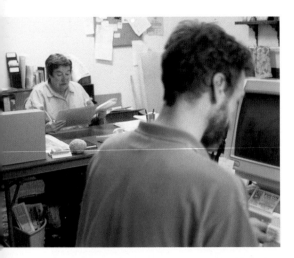

△ Sister Frances Carr (left) and Brother Arnold Hadd (right) working in the office in the 1883 Dwelling House.

Shaker Cooking

In addition to the growing and selling of herbal products, the Shakers have used another means to present their herbs to the world — Shaker cooking. By the 1980s, Sister Frances and Brother Ted began presenting programs on community life at Sabbathday Lake that included examples of Shaker food preparation. The culmination of these efforts was the publication of *Shaker Your Plate: Of Shaker Cooks and Cooking* by Sister Frances in 1985. Now in its fifth printing, this book has more than 150 pages on all aspects of Shaker cooking at Sabbathday Lake. Almost all of the recipes call for herbs, and an entire section is given to a description of the revived herb industry and how to use herbs effectively in cooking. This book, however, was not Sister Frances's first work on Shaker herbs. In 1963, in anticipation of the revival of the herb industry, she wrote a five-page article, "The Shakers as Herb Growers," for the summer issue of *The Shaker Quarterly*.

The Herb Business Today

Today the herb industry still continues as a vital part of the Shaker community, although it is carried on by other hands. Brother Ted died in 1986 and Sister Mildred in 1990, and Brother Steven is no longer a Shaker. Various members of the present community work in the herb department, still housed in the sisters' shop. Outside labor is also used.

The 1997 catalog, printed on the Shaker press by Brother Arnold Hadd, lists twenty-five culinary herbs and fourteen herbal teas. These are packed in slipcovered tins with colorful labels and are also available in plastic bags. Among the culinary herbs, nine are "superior blends" developed by the Sabbathday Lake Shakers themselves. According to the catalog, "These mixtures have been time tested by the Shaker Sisters in our own kitchen to the applause of the Community and our guests." In addition to these herbal products the Shakers also sell four-ounce bottles of rose water and an aromatic potpourri using a community recipe from 1858.

Visitors to the Sabbathday Lake Shakers can see the large herb gardens and the stacks of tins used in the industry. If they are fortunate, they can also enjoy deliciously herb-flavored food from the kitchen in the dwelling. The quiet voice of the Shakers thus can still be heard in a fully revived herb industry.

PRINTING AND PUBLISHING

The Shaker press and Shaker publications dealing with herbs were also an important part of the herb industry at Sabbathday Lake. Today the printing business is carried on by Brother Arnold Hadd, a trustee for the community. In addition to the labels for the herb tins, the press has produced labels for rosewater bottles and fir balsam pillows, posters, placards, greeting cards, and many other items. These include a flyer entitled *Shaker Culinary Herbs, Suggested Uses* in 1982 and the more recent *Shaker Herbal Teas*, a seven-page booklet prepared by the herb department discussing the uses of forty herbal teas.

CHAPTER 8

The Western and Southern Societies

Union Village and North Union, Ohio

Pleasant Hill and South Union, Kentucky

THREE MEMBERS FROM the New Lebanon society, John Meacham, Benjamin S. Youngs, and Issachar Bates, set out for the West, traveling mostly on foot to see for themselves the religious fervor then sweeping over the southwestern part of Kentucky. This journey of more than a thousand miles was begun on the first day of January 1805, and the missionaries arrived in Kentucky about the first of March, weary but exalted, having experienced great hardship and many indignities.

The arduous journey resulted in the eventual founding of six Shaker societies in the west by 1826 — two in Kentucky and four in Ohio. Union Village, Ohio, and Watervliet (Dayton), Ohio, were founded in 1812 and 1813; Pleasant Hill, Kentucky, 1814; South Union, Kentucky, 1811; North Union (Cleveland), Ohio, 1826; and White Water, Ohio, 1824. (A community at Busro, Indiana, was organized in 1810, but lasted a few years only; its members moved to Union Village, Ohio, in 1812.)

The Shakers followed the same pattern for organizing the western villages as others had in the eleven eastern societies. Each community bought land, continuously, amassing from one to six thousand acres to pasture their fine herds of cattle and sheep, graze horses, and grow their diverse crops. At first, the settlers had to build dwelling houses, huge barns, large sheds for many different uses, and mills and shops. Then they established industries to manufacture goods first to provide for the needs of the members of the families and then to sell materials in the general markets to produce necessary cash income.

When we sow words and deeds of kindness,

We will rejoice in the time of our harvest.

LARZ ERICKSON, PLEASANT HILL

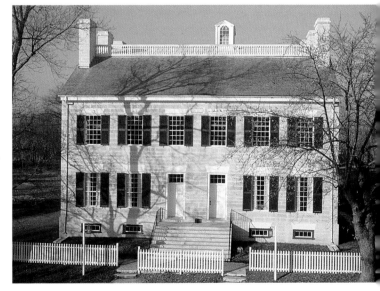

△ Centre House at Pleasant Hill.

101

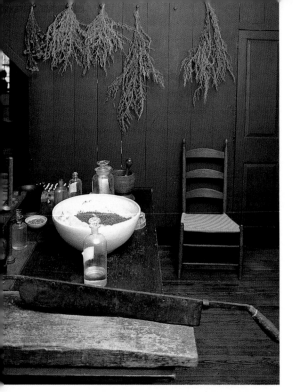

△ Herb drying room at Pleasant Hill.

Although herbs were first gathered in their natural habitat, all of the western societies soon raised herbs for the use of their families, as was the custom of the day on the frontier. Each community had herb gardens, with drying houses. In most of these societies the Shakers sold the surplus of herbs or medicines to the outside world. In some cases this practice became a good business. In others it was more of a thrifty procedure to avoid waste.

UNION VILLAGE, OHIO

Union Village, situated between Cincinnati and Dayton, three miles west of Lebanon, had as its spiritual name "Wisdom's Paradise." It was the largest in size and population of the western communities and for a short while it was as large as New Lebanon. Six families, comprising 600 members, lived there when it was at its height. It prospered for ninety-eight years, until, after a period of decline, it was sold in 1910.

O. C. Hampton, who joined the community in 1822, frequently audited diaries and in 1849 compiled a summary, not always in chronological order, from several covering the life of the society.

We were at this time [1849] still running many of our former branches of business such as the tanyard, selling, preparing of herbs, roots, extracts and oils. The woolen factory operated in 1819 as did a fine garden of sage and sassafras. In 1834 among the other methods of making a living at this time and for many years previous was the distilling of oils and fragrant waters which paid as well as almost any other resort, considering the small expense of procuring raw material. And sometimes in the distilling, we would occasionally double distill a barrel of Whiskey for the sake of the Alcohol for medical purposes.

DRAWING ON NATIVE AMERICAN PLANT LORE

In order to cultivate herbs successfully, the western Shakers accumulated and relied upon Native American plant knowledge. Thus Peter Boyd, one of the Shakers of Union Village, notes on February 26, 1845, that the Indians had brought gifts of herbs and roots. He also tells of Issachar Bates and Richard McNemar visiting the Shawnee tribe. At Union Village, as was the case at New Lebanon, the Shakers used herbal material provided by Indians.

▷ North Family dwelling, Union Village Shaker community.

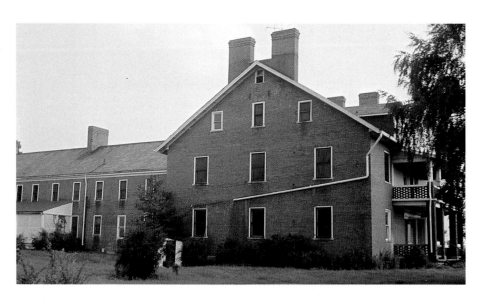

A Sister's Work

Another journal titled *A Register of Work performed by Second Family Sisters, Together with the Most Important passing Events, Recorded by Amy Slaters* is full of minutiae, all of it forming the picture of a busy family. From January 10, 1848, with few dates given until May, the entries cover many industries and household chores. The entries for 1848 and 1849 are concerned with the dates when strawberries, new potatoes, green apples, and eggs for breakfast were offered to the family. In addition, the diarist records the sisters' work picking and processing herbs.

> *July 22nd. Rained again today, picked the saffron. [She also picked saffron on the 24th and 26th.] July 27th. Rhoda Evens here today to pick the saffron. [Also picked saffron on the 31st.]*
>
> *August 2nd. Amelia went with her brother [left the community], picked the saffron. August 5th. The brethren gathered boneset, the sisters commenced stripping it off the stems. August 6th. Continued stripping boneset, picked the saffron. August 25th. Stripped boneset.*
>
> *September 1st. Gathered elder berries to make wine. September 2nd. Brother Abner come here to show about the wine. September 3rd. Gather more elder berries.*
>
> *October [no date]. Stewed and dried pumpkins. Gathered husks for mattresses.*

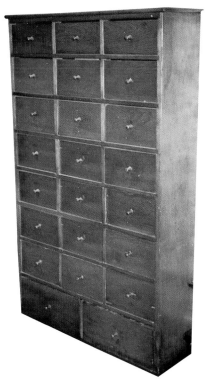

△ Apothecary chest at the Shaker community at Watervliet, Ohio.

Catalogs

The Shakers' herb business had expanded sufficiently so that in the 1840s they had issued a four-page catalog listing 170 medicinal herbs and eighteen extracts. In 1847 the catalog doubled in size, and they offered 156 herbs, twenty-five extracts, nine essential oils, and four culinary herbs: pulverized sage, summer savory, sweet marjoram, and thyme. Seven fragrant waters were also listed in their eight-page catalog. Thirty-four properties with abbreviations were explained, and there was a lengthy testimonial from R. D. Mussey, Professor of Surgery at the Medical College in Cincinnati:

> *I have the pleasure in saying that I have used the extracts of Sarsaparilla, Hybrid Colocynth, and the Belladonna prepared at Union Village by A. Babbit & Co. and that I have never found better articles of the kind. From the fidelity with which these articles are prepared, I can have no doubt that other medicines prepared and vended by them are of prime quality, and may be fully relied on.*

SELLING SHAKER WINE

Winemaking at Union Village was of sufficient volume to sell to the world and to print an illustrated eleven-page booklet on the subject.

Shaker Community Wines. A treatise on Pure Wines and its Beneficial Uses. *Shaker Community Wine Growers, William G. Ayer, Assistant Trustee, Union Village, Ohio, Vineyards on the Shore of Lake Erie. Established 1805. Shaker wines are medicinal wines. They are for medicinal purposes. . . . Above all things they are not incentives to drunkenness.*

Six preparations were advertised on the back cover of the catalog: "Fluid Extract of Sarsaparilla and these simples which for their important therapeutic qualities deserve to be more extensively known and used, Bugle, Button Snake Root, Golden Seal, Indian Hemp, and Pleurisy Root." The diseases for which these preparations were recommended were the same as those set forth by the eastern Shakers, as were the doses and properties.

A three-page catalog was printed the next year listing 206 herbs, eighteen extracts, seven essential oils, and twenty-six powdered herbs, roots, and barks. (As was the case in all Union Village catalogs, the botanical names were taken from *Eaton's Manual of Botany*, *Griffith's Medical Botany*, and *Raffinesque's Medical Flora*. Common names were such as were in use in the cities of Cincinnati, St. Louis, Louisville, and New Orleans.) Prices were given per pound and a 25 percent discount was allowed regular retail customers.

▽ Center Family dwelling at Union Village.

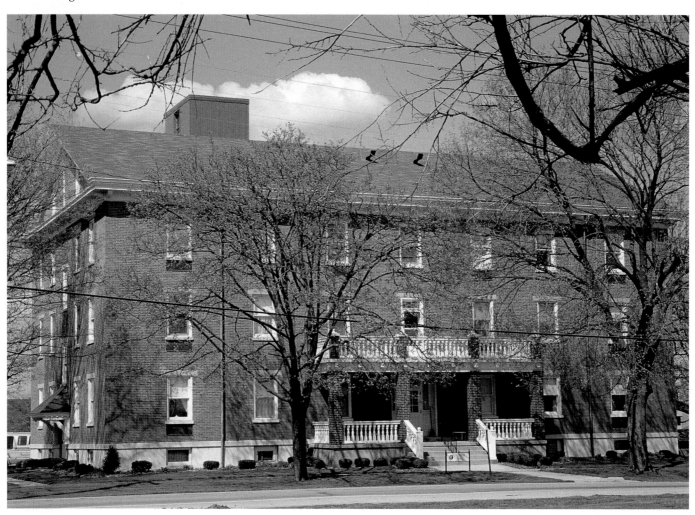

In 1850 a twelve-page "Annual Wholesale Catalogue" was offered by Peter Boyd, listing:

252 *drug plants: leaves, roots, seeds, bark, flowers, and berries.*
 46 *extracts*
  8 *inspissated juices*
 15 *essential oils*
  4 *pulverized sweet herbs: sage, summer savory, sweet marjoram, and thyme.*

MEDICINAL WATERMELON

According to their 1847 catalog, the Union Village Shakers had developed an unusual hybrid plant: a cross between the colocynth and a watermelon. It yielded a bitter fruit that had the medical virtues of colocynth and was an important addition to the medical plants grown at the village. A note explained colocynth:

Both the Simple and Compound Extracts of Colocynth, are prepared from the Hybrid Colocynth, which was originated at Union Village, Ohio, in 1842. This Hybrid was produced by planting seeds of the genuine colocynth, and at the proper time the flowers of the colocynth plant were fecundated with pollen from those of the watermelon. Hence we have given the plant thus derived, the Botanical name of Cucumis colocynthis hybridum. But we propose to call it the American Colocynth, and give it the Botanical name Colocynthis Americana. The following reasons for this are respectfully submitted. It is now reduced to a certainty that the Colocynth does not belong to the genus Cucumis where botanists have placed it. It has no resemblance to the cucumber; but both the plant and its fruit have a striking similarity to the Watermelon; and the fact that it freely mixes with the latter plant demonstrates that it belongs to the same genus. It ought therefore to be put in the genus Cucurbitas.
In all the editions of the United States Dispensatory previous to that of 1845 (sixth edition)

the Colocynth is called the "bitter cucumber," and said to bear considerable resemblance to the cucumber of our gardens. This mistake was pointed out by the writer to the learned and much respected author of the Dispensatory previous to issuing the sixth edition. Consequently the description was altered and the plant described as resembling the watermelon and the following note appended by the author:
"In a letter from R. W. Pelham, of the Shakers' Village near Lebanon Ohio, the author was informed that a hybrid plant between the colocynth and the watermelon had been successfully cultivated in that place, and yielded a bitter fruit having the medical virtues of Colocynth. With the letter I received some seeds of the plant, and a portion of the extract prepared from the pulp of the fruit. This was found upon trial to be actively cathartic. The seeds planted in the garden of the author, produced vigorous plants, which perfected their fruit. The plant appeared intermediate between the colocynth and the watermelon. The fruit was globular, about four inches in diameter, green like the watermelon externally, having the same odor when cut, but of an extremely bitter taste."

The author of this "note" was R. D. Mussey, Professor of Surgery, Medical College of Ohio at Cincinnati, writing in 1846.

TRIAL BY FIRE

From a note in Brother Oliver
Hampton's diary we learn of
a fire on March 4, 1865,
which destroyed the Old
North House and its contents
— the tin shop, broom shop,
carpenter shop, and sarsaparilla laboratory. By 1897,
according to an anonymous
editor, the entire community
numbered only thirty-two
members, but the members
still cultivated gardens and
orchards.

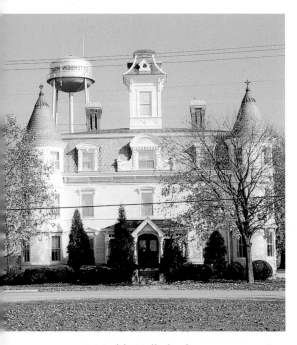

△ Marble Hall, the former trustees'
office, Center Family, Union Village.

Extracts and Essential Oils

Extracts and essential oils produced from herbs raised at Union Village were given and are listed here in full for the purposes of comparing them with similar products offered in the eastern Shaker catalogs.

The extracts were belladonna, bittersweet, boneset, butternut, cicuta, cowparsnip, colocynth (simple and compound), dandelion, yellow dock, foxglove, garget or poke, henbane, horehound, lettuce (garden and wild), mayapple, garden nightshade, poplar bark, poppy, snakehead or balmony, thorn apple, tomato, white ash bark, wood sorrel, and wormwood.

The essential oils offered were fennel, fleabane, pennyroyal, peppermint, spearmint, summer savory, tansy, wormseed, and wormwood. The catalog also included seven double-distilled and fragrant waters — rose, wild cherry, peppermint, elder flower, peach, sassafras, and spearmint — along with thirty-one roots, herbs, and barks "in a powdered state." The price per pound was given for all of the items, as well as both the common and botanical names. Thirty-four properties with abbreviations were explained.

The catalog also stated that other kinds of extracts would be made to order and said: "Of the above, though placed under the general head of EXTRACTS, the following are always INSPISSATED JUICES: Belladonna, Cicuta, Poke, Henbane, Lettuce, Thornapple and Tomato. As mere Extracts of the Narcotic plants are nonoffi[cial] preparations, we never make them; but follow carefully, the directions of the United States Dispensatory. The prices however, of these articles, are set down at the common rate of extracts, though it is customary to charge double for Inspissated Juices. Hence it will be seen that our articles of this class are very low." The prices for one-pound amounts ranged from $1 to $2.50, except for foxglove, which was $3.

The Union Village catalogs not only listed botanical products and medicines but also guaranteed them, as in the 1850 edition:

To Our Patrons
The articles contained in the following catalogue are prepared and put up with the greatest care and fidelity. The various Herbs, Roots, and Barks, are gathered in the season proper to each; the stalky and coarser part being rejected; they are then uniformly dried under shelter, after which they are neatly prepared and papered in assorted packages for the convenience of the purchasers.

Our Extracts are prepared by experienced persons; they are vaporized by steam, and great care is used that they are not burned, or otherwise injured. Our Inspissated Juices are of superior quality and excellence.

We pledge ourselves that our preparations shall be inferior to none offered in market, and that they shall be such as will meet the approbation of dealers and practitioners generally, to whom we confidently recommend them.

Orders for such Native Plants as are not in the Catalogue will receive due attention.

The back cover was devoted to Compound Fluid Extract of Sarsaparilla, testimonials by Dr. Mussey, Dr. Andrew Campbell of Middletown, Ohio, and a resolution from the Lebanon, Ohio, Medical Society:

That this Society have entire confidence in the purity of the Pharmaceutical preparations of the Shakers at Union Village, Ohio, and that we heartily recommend these preparations to the profession; especially the extracts of the Narcotic Plants and of Sarsaparilla.

The final paragraph states:

We wish the public to understand that, as we never on any occasion obtain any patents for our medicines, or sell any receipts, or sell any medicine of which the materials are secret; any publication purporting to have obtain receipts of us, is a fraudulent attempt to obtain money on our credit.

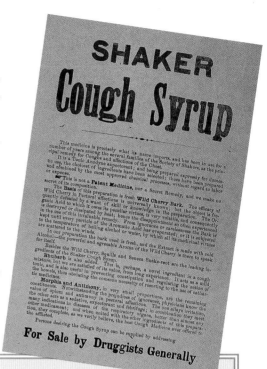

PLANT MEDICINES

Several broadsides were printed during the 1850s, including one for Shaker Cough Syrup and another for the Extract of Sarsaparilla. The basis of the cough syrup was fresh wild cherry bark, squill, and seneca snakeroot, to which was added rhubarb and, in very small proportions, morphine and antimony. A paragraph states:

Notwithstanding the prejudices of ignorance, physicians know the value of opium and antimony in pectoral affections. The one allays irritation, the other acts as a sedative, expectorant and febrifuge; in combination they meet many indications in diseases of the respiratory organs, better than almost any other medicament; and when united with the other ingredients of this preparation, they complete, as we verily believe, the best Cough Medicine ever offered to the Afflicted.

The broadside advertising sarsaparilla claimed the medicine could be successful in cases of chronic rheumatism, scrofulous affections, obstinate skin diseases, and derangement of the liver, internal organs, and nervous system. It pointed out:

It is a fact well known, that the general character of the Extract of Sarsaparilla, now in market, is deficient in quality. The truth is, a perfect article costs more than can be afforded for the price at which it is generally sold; therefore, we would say to the public, and will appeal to the medical profession for the truth of the statement, that wherever a quart bottle of "said to be" Sarsaparilla Extract is offered for one Dollar, it is utterly deficient in quality, and can not be a true and legitimate article.

In 1850 the Shakers issued a four-page illustrated leaflet advertising Extract of Sarsaparilla, signed S. D. Howe and Co., Cincinnati. It shows a Shaker brother on the back cover, holding a sarsaparilla bottle. A testimonial signed D. M. Bennett states that this is the same recipe as that used by the Shakers in New York and New Hampshire. Bennett, formerly a physician to the New Lebanon Shakers, seceded in 1846, and it can be assumed that he furnished Dr. Howe with the formula for Howe's Shaker Sarsaparilla.

CLOSING THE DEAL

William Glowny: Respected Friend. We have to state that we sell our Sarsaparilla syrup for $8.00 per gallon, always cash. If you wish a supply we can send it to the City almost any week by our own market waggon which stands at 5th Street Market on Fridays in each week. The name of the person with whom you can make the payment is Moses Miller. You can furnish him with a vessel of suitable size to contain what you wish free of charge to us and it will be sent down the next week. Your Friend, etc. P.S. Send for but little at this time as we are scarce of the article.

ACCOUNT BOOK
OF PETER BOYD, 1851–52

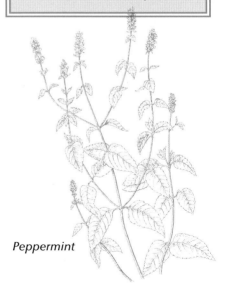

Peppermint

A Brother's Work

Peter Boyd wrote journals, diaries, and letters from 1833, the year the medicine garden came into importance, until the late 1850s. These records give a good idea of the meticulous care he took building up and maintaining the industry. In 1833 he wrote:

January. Have had a frame built, a cold frame, a hot house frame. It is well ventilated and elevated, banked with sod and leaves to the waist height. Seed will begin to do well when planted here in February and March. It being well protected.

In June of the next year he says: "I will build and frame a hot house to enter and work within."

Some material in Peter Boyd's diaries is cut out, but enough remains to follow his numerous activities.

January 16, 1844. David Parkhurst and Peter Boyd start to Cincinnati and sell a two horse waggon loaded with sage and brooms. . . . January 25th. Peter Boyd starts to Cincinnati with brooms, sage and other herbs. . . .
February 19, 1844. Peter Boyd went to Dayton after flax, bought 419 pounds.
April 10th, 1844 David Parkhurst and Peter Boyd start to Kentucky after squaw root weather is warm.
April 13th. Got home, planted corn.
April 14th. The apple trees are in full bloom at this time.
*   15th. Ministry start to the East on their visit.*
April 29th. We begin to plant the peppermint south east of the apple orchard. I seed red clover in bloom last Saturday in the dooryard. The grass and trees are very forward.
April 30th. We finish planting the peppermint.
May 1st. Richard Pelham and Peter Boyd start to Watervliet, or in the neighborhood of Dayton after roots with two colts and the light waggon.

On May 4 they returned with a load of roots and on May 8 Peter was off again to sell herbs and brooms and to buy a casting "for grinding herbs."

On February 6, 1845, Brother Peter recorded that he sold brooms, herbs, and extracts in Cincinnati in weather very warm for the season. A few days later he was called to a momentous new position of leadership: He "was notified by Elder John [Rankin] of his intended removal to the Meetinghouse to take part in the Ministry." Rankin also informed Richard W. Pelham that he must move into the office to take Peter Boyd's place there.

Correspondence with Customers

Despite his increase in responsibilities, Peter Boyd remained active in the herb and medicine businesses. His account books and letters for 1851 and 1852 tell the story:

To G. H. Reynolds, Cincinnati. We should be thankful to obtain your check and will be pleased to supply you with more items on our most liberal terms. We have made considerable additions to our gardens and other conveniences for pulverizing, by which our assortment is improved and we prefer selling low. For the cash we make a liberal discount according to the amount ordered.

To Means and Wilder: We have an excellent assortment of Medicines on hand and will sell low for cash, lowering from our catalogue price according to the amount ordered. . . . Your friend Peter Boyd.

Some of the accounts required careful negotiation before a deal could be struck.

Union Village July 21, 1851. W. W. Brown: Estimed Friend; Your order of the 15th. Inst. is to hand and we have all the articles ordered ready, except the s. marjoram which will be ready to send in about two weeks, but some of them we cannot sell at your prices as we have to pay for some of them considerable higher in New York City for instance. Barberry bark you price at 20 cents, we pay about 10 cents higher in this instance besides the freight from New York. Poppy flowers we cannot sell at less than our catalogue price which is 75 cents. But our uniform way of doing business is where the customer purchases from $150 to $200 per year we allow a discount of 20 percent off less than that amount, 10% off and above that amount 25% off. We will delay sending your order for the present and wait your reply. Hoping to hear from you soon, I remain your friend, Peter Boyd. By W. H.

Another letter indicated that the tansy crop had failed due to a "miserable drought." Only eighteen to twenty bottles of tansy oil were available, at $1 apiece in cash.

Assistance from Other Societies

Because interest in Shaker herbs was so high, Deacon Boyd sometimes turned to herbalists at other Shaker societies for help in filling orders. In a letter dated September 12, 1850, Peter Boyd asks Edward Fowler at New Lebanon to supply at the lowest price the following: aconite root, black elder, borage, balmony leaves, cancer root, centaury *(Centaurea cyanus)*, lavender seed growth of 1851, cowparsnip root, frostwort, hardhack leaves, laurel leaves, lady's-slipper root, and fever twig (bittersweet) root.

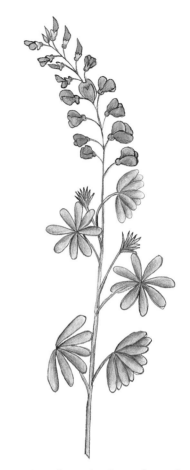

△ Lupine, drawn by Canterbury sister Cora Helena Sarle.

CASH, NOT COMMISSION

We are not in the habit of distributing our medicines on commission. We sell low for cash as you will perceive by our catalogue which we have sent you. Your order accompanied by a remittance will be personally attended to.

ACCOUNT BOOK
OF PETER BOYD, 1851–52

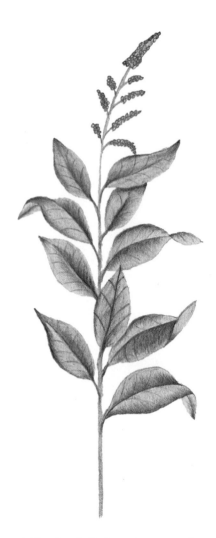

△ Hardhack *(Spiraea tomentosa)*, drawn by Canterbury sister Cora Helena Sarle.

To Chauncey Miller of Watervliet (New York) he wrote:

Dear Brother; Will you please be so kind as to affix your lowest prices to the following articles and oblidge your friend, Peter Boyd.

Prices in bulk and in paper pressed: 40 lbs. aconite leaves, 40 angelica root, 30 lbs. evans root, 40 lbs. Black elder, 10 lbs. borage, 50 lbs. Balmony leaves, 10 lbs. cancer root, 40 lbs. centaury (sabatia angularis) 40 lbs. centaury (s. paniculata), 20 lbs. coriander seed herb, growth of 1851, 20 lbs. cow-parsnip root, 10 lbs. frostwort, 5 lbs. hardhack, 20 lbs. laurel leaves, 30 lbs. lady slipper roots, 40 lbs. male fern roots, 400 lbs. pipsisaway, 20 lbs. wild indigo, 20 lbs. extract of aconite.

He wrote a letter dated December 12, 1851, to Canterbury:

Beloved Brother David Parker: We shall be glad to have your order for a large amount of oils of peppermint and wormseed. Perhaps it might answer you to make an arrangement with Jonathan Wood, New Lebanon. We are indebted there and should like our oil to pay the same. Anything that you can do that would be mutually beneficial we should be glad and thankful for. Your friend. P. B.

Dealing with Debtors

It is easy to understand the indignation of Deacon Peter when bills were not paid. To Dr. H. Snizer:

You should have a better thinking about doing business with our concern. You have our medicine, we do not have your money. The information you give in your letter is untrue and we expected a speedy correspondence with remittance to correct the situation.

He also had trouble in this respect with one H. P. Turner in Kentucky and there ensued several very brisk letters regarding some large orders without remittance.

Sir: How do you suppose we should think of them [the material] being seized on the way by your creditors when you had not paid the insurance. Henry, we shall hold you in honor bound to pay the debt to us by any bank in Cincinnati.

Again H. P. Turner gave him trouble. "Respected Friend: I would be glad to accommodate you with the drugs if I could do so and see myself safe for the payment. You owe $75. plus $23. since 12 months past." And finally Boyd sought outside help in collecting:

March 25, 1852, Postmaster, Hopkinsville, Kentucky. Respected Friend: My object of addressing you at this time is to get you to do me the favor of giving me the name of some suitable person to collect a claim I have on a man in your place by the name of P. Turner. I think he is in the drug business, perhaps he practices medicine. My claim is a note of hand given last March for $75. and $23. Any information on this subject will be thankfully received. Peter Boyd.

A Shaker Doctor and a World's Doctor

The Shakers issued a publication in 1888 titled *The Influence of the Shaker Doctor*, a ten-page illustrated advertising circular for medicines made at the Shaker village. It showed a Shaker residence; the medical laboratory, exterior and interior; and the office building. It also had pictures of Peter Boyd; a Shaker doctor, Dr. J. R. Singerland; and a doctor from the world, Dr. Louis Turner. And it said of the latter:

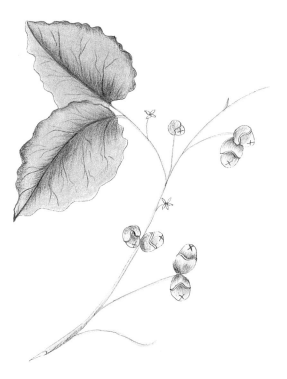

△ Witch hazel, drawn by Canterbury sister Cora Helena Sarle.

Dr. Louis Turner a regular graduate of medicine, of high repute, number of years ago, engaged in the manufacture and sale of medicines, made from the formulas he used in his extensive practice, and found to be specifics for those troubles, he recommended them for.

The merit of those remedies, having received for them a most extensive sale, it became necessary for the doctor to increase his facilities, owing to the difficulty he experienced, in supplying the demand, and at the same time attend to his other duties. The chief source of embarrassment which presented itself at this time was the trouble of obtaining a sufficient quantity of crude material, such as Roots, Barks, Buds, Berries, Blossoms and Seeds, which had been gathered at the proper time, to secure their best medical effect.

It was under these perplexing circumstances that the Doctor concluded to arrange with the Shakers, his old friends, as being the best prepared to help him out of the difficulty. . . .

From this knowledge of the Shakers, the Doctor concluded to select the Community at Union Village, Warren County, Ohio, as being the best suited for his purpose. This society is the parent community of the west, being the most important west of the Allegheny Mountains and dates from 1805, they own 4,500 acres of land in one tract, which for fertility, and other qualities, is perhaps unexceled by any body of land of equal size on the continent. The special reason Dr. Turner expected to find here exactly what he needed, was that he knew here was founded in 1833, a special Botanical Garden for raising medicinal plants, under the care of the scientific members of the Shakers, prominent among which may be mentioned Dr. Abiathar Babbitt, and Dr. Andrew Houston, who at the same time acted as physicians to the community and neighborhood.

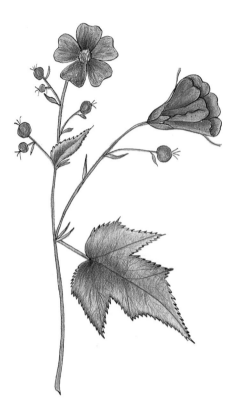

△ Mulberry, drawn by Canterbury sister Cora Helena Sarle.

CONSUMPTION CURE

Dr. Turner also advertised a consumption cure or Shaker Cough Remedy. He said that there were more than 200,000 deaths from consumption each year in the United States, and in more than two-thirds of the cases there was no trace of hereditary consumption. Most cases, he claimed, started with a slight cold that could have been cured easily by a single bottle of his consumption cure.

Dr. Turner visited the community at Union Village and toured the botanical garden, the laboratory, and the farm. Turner and Singerland worked together to produce a line of medicines that were made by the Shakers and endorsed by the doctor. Even more persuasive than the doctor's endorsement, apparently, was the Shaker name:

Right here Dr. Turner wants it understood by all, that these remedies are made by the Shakers, and they will vouch for their purity and curative action.

If anyone doubts this statement write Dr. J. R. Singerland, Union Village, Warren Co., Ohio, who will cheerfully give an endorsement wished.

Shaker Cures

The remaining pages of the booklet are devoted to Dr. Turner's Wonder Herbs, "the great Shaker Blood Cure, for all altered, changed and poisoned conditions of the blood," and Turner's Wonder of Shaker Pain Cure. These two medicines were prescribed for rheumatism; neuralgia; sick, nervous, or bilious headache; burns and scalds; diarrhea, cramps, colic, cholera morbus, and cholera; corns; earache; sprains, bruises, and cuts; sore throat and diphtheria; catarrh; inflammation of the kidneys; piles; pains in the side, breast, back, or any part of the system; asthma and phthisic; dyspepsia; contracted cords or muscles; deafness; chilblains or frosted feet; toothache; fever and ague; nervous prostration and general debility; and skin diseases. A final paragraph was directed

To the Ladies — who suffer Periodical Pains in the Back, burning sensation at the top of the head, dragging down pains below the waist, palpitation of the heart, smothering sensations and general lassitude of the system, take from ten to thirty drops in a little sweetened water from one to three times a day, at the same time using the Wonder as directed for Rheumatism, also use Singerland's Shaker Granules.

These granules were made like all the rest of Shaker medicines, the advertisement said, and for the ladies "to whom life has become a wearisome burden and whose power and nerve force seems gone," this botanic medicine was guaranteed to be "nature's proper restorer."

Despite the success of its herb business, this lovely village, this "pattern of neatness," this affluent community, suffered from unfortunate business management. Certain members plunged the society into bankruptcy, making it necessary to sell the land and eventually to liquidate the community.

NORTH UNION, OHIO

The Ministry at New Lebanon (Mount Lebanon) presided over all of the Shaker communities but was particularly concerned with the eastern brethren. It was assisted (but not exceeded in its authority) by the ministry at Union Village, Ohio, whose responsibility was the western societies, those in Ohio and Kentucky. And in 1826 the Ministry founded a community at North Union, Ohio.

From account books, journals, and letters of visiting Shaker brethren we have a picture of the life at North Union and the products raised by the families. The seed and herb gardens were large; they and the orchards took up one-third of the land of the East Family. The garden house at the East Family was spacious and was used as a dry house as well.

The garden nursery and the orchards at the Center Family farm were large, and there was also a fine toolhouse, notable for its size. A map of the lands of the Center Family in 1880 shows large gardens and orchards and a sage hedge covering an area as big as the pear orchard on the map. In all Shaker settlements sage was a major crop. It is the one herb mentioned in Elder James S. Prescott's journal when he writes that the seed garden was fenced off in 1835.

At North Union, the Shakers, like other pioneers, raised herbs and medicinal plants for their own use. Caroline Piercy in *The Valley of God's Pleasure* tells us about the cultivation of herbs at North Union:

> In the fine gardens were rows of tansy, horehound, feverfew, thyme, marjoram, marigold, foxglove, dandelion, boneset, numerous mints, roses and lavender. . . . The sisters went gathering in the wild berry-tea, penny royal and catnip for teas; poke berries for ink and sundry roots and herbs for poultices and steeps. The neatly kept rows of red roses with no thought of their beauty and fragrance, were raised to be converted into delicate rosewater with which the sisters bathed the feverish brow or flavored the crisp apple pies or the enormous silver cakes — especially produced for Christmas and Mother Ann's birthday. Nor was the making of wild-cherry bitters, various tonics or medicinal wines ever neglected

In a recent history of Shaker Heights (now a suburb of Cleveland), the North Union community is discussed and the industries of the Shakers are described. Their major area of productivity and chief source of income were, respectively, the manufacture of woolen goods and the dairy business, which supplied quantities of milk, butter, cheese, and eggs to the Cleveland market. "The seed business was carried on very extensively," the author stated, "as well as the sale of medicinal herbs which they gathered and prepared for the market."

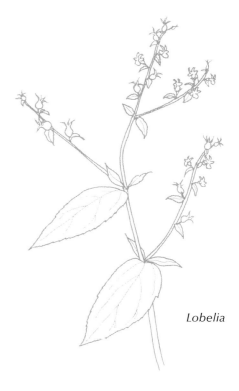

Lobelia

Maintaining Good Health

The Shakers at North Union held advanced notions about the virtues of good hygiene and fresh air. In his *History of North Union*, James S. Prescott writes:

> *Doctoring. Their former mode of practice for curing physical disease was Thomsonian more than any other, but of late years (1880) since they have paid more attention to ventilating their sleeping apartments and dwelling rooms and have become better informed with regard to the laws of life and health, sickness is almost unknown among them, consequently they have but little use for lobelia, drugs or doctors of any kind, not withstanding.*
>
> *Deaths. No pestilential diseases have ever been known among them — in time of cholera, no case has ever been known, this may be attributed in great measure to their regular habits and clanliness [cleanliness].*

PLEASANT HILL, KENTUCKY

Elisha Thomas's 140-acre farm, located on the Shawnee Run, high above the Kentucky River, was the nucleus of the Shaker society founded and organized at Pleasant Hill in 1814. Situated between Harrodsburg and Lexington in the midst of the famous bluegrass region of the state, the beautiful rolling meadows of this farm on a level limestone plateau eventually totaled over 4,300 acres.

A writer has given an account of Pleasant Hill in *The Cultivator* for September 1856. This farm journal noted that the Shaker farm at Pleasant Hill included about 5,000 acres of land and that the buildings "are excellent and commodious and several of them remarkably well proportioned, if not absolutely tasteful, their principles being opposed to extraneous show and ornament." The article praised the Shakers for being careful and systematic farmers, "among the first in giving attention to improved stock," and commented upon their self-sufficiency:

> *With the exception of cotton and sugar only, we believe they are the producers of nearly all their own foods and clothing and necessities, bringing into requisition quite a wide range of raw material and giving occasion for many labor saving contrivances, which last, like the best economists everywhere they think it the wisest policy to invent or make use of whenever possible.*
>
> *The main sales of the community are of garden seeds in which they do a large business in the south, and west, and of preserved fruits. Of the last they dispose of jars and cans to the amount of twelve to fourteen hundred dollars worth last year. They are preserved of course with the utmost neatness, and put up so that they will keep for any length of time.*

THOMSONIANISM

Several Shaker societies in their early days followed the Thomsonian practice of herbal medicine. They believed herbs could cure all ailments, as herbs were the first medicine used by man.

Samuel Thomson was born in Alstead, New Hampshire, in 1769. One of six children, he was often taken into the woods to help a botanic practitioner gather herbs and plants. When very young he experimented with the herb lobelia, which he discovered to be an emetic. He cut his leg badly when he was nineteen years old and, acting against advice to have it amputated, he applied a poultice of comfrey root and saved his leg. Having proved the emetic qualities of lobelia he advocated the necessity of eliminating waste materials from the body to restore it to the natural conditon of health. He also stressed steaming the body outwardly and using herb stimulants to produce inward heat. These were the rudiments of Thomsonian medical practices.

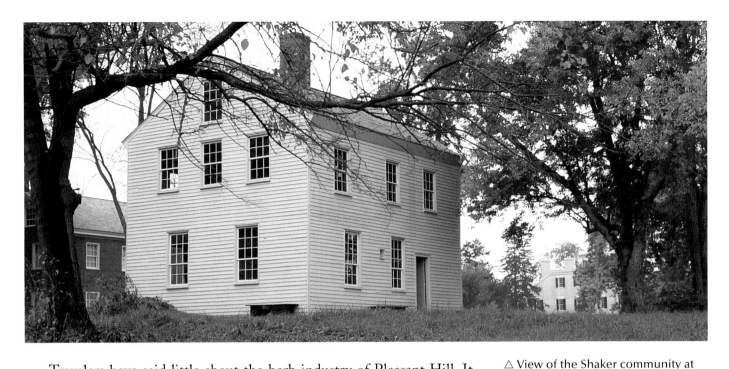

△ View of the Shaker community at Pleasant Hill.

Travelers have said little about the herb industry of Pleasant Hill. It was not conducted on the scale of the eastern societies or of Union Village, Ohio. Still, journals and diaries written from 1843 to 1888 record considerable activity in the raising and selling of herbs. The Kentucky River was a great channel of transportation that the Shakers used to ship products from their farms and shops southward.

Dr. Benjamin Dunlavy's diary for January 1843 notes: "Today we ploughed up a piece of meadow on the west side of the south shed for the purpose of removing the medical garden to that place. Same day ploughed up a piece of meadow, on the west side of the south street, twice as large, as we need more space. Medical garden by John Shain, length 28 feet by 11 feet."

A Family Journal

A family journal kept by Order of the Deaconesses of the East House between 1843 and 1871 is concerned with many events and activities:

June 1st [1843] We make a general turn out to gather herbs for sale.
June 2nd. We gather herbs again. June 3rd. We gather first meal of strawberrys.
June 29th. The sisters went to the Mill to gather elder flowers for sale.
July 13th. The sisters began to gather cherrys to dry.
Aug. 19th. The sisters went to the Shawney Springs after boneset.
Sept. 1st. Sisters gathered medical herbs.

A SHAKER PEDDLER

John Shain not only managed the medical garden but also took to the road to peddle garden seeds, herbs, and brooms. It was on these excursions that he kept an eye open for children orphaned by the cholera epidemics of 1833 and 1849, bringing them home to be cared for by the Shakers, perhaps to remain at Pleasant Hill for many years.

May 3rd [1844] Some of the sisters from each family went with John Shain and James Cooney to Harrison after hoarhound for sale. May 7th. Went after hoarhound. May 29th. The first herb was cut in John's garden.

Aug. 21st. The sisters began to dry apples. Same day went for loblia.

Produce in 1845 for sale . . . 1175 pounds of herbs.

May 5, 1846 The sisters began to gather herbs. May 12th. Five hands began to gather herbs. May 23rd. All hands turned out to gather herbs.

June 6th. All hands engaged in gathering cherries and herbs. June 17th. Gathered herbs again.

July 15th. These times are chiefly occupied in gathering herbs. July 25th. Still going on with fruits and herbs.

Aug. 20th. Another trip was taken after herbs.

Produce for sale, 1846, 550 pounds of herbs.

May 6, 1847 Gathered some herbs.

June 2nd. Gathered herbs.

Aug. 26th. Gathered lobelia in the rye field.

Sept. 30th. Gathered hops and apples.

Oct 1st. The sisters went after hoarhound. Oct. 16th. Dug and roasted meadow roots, also went after herbs.

Produce for sale, 1847, 761¾ pounds of herbs.

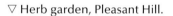

▽ Herb garden, Pleasant Hill.

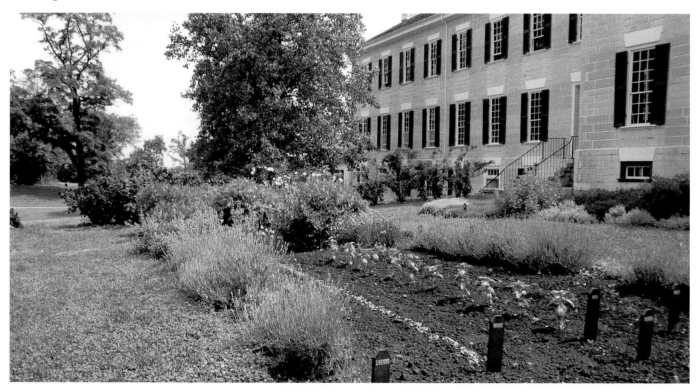

June 24, 1848 Went after elder flowers.

July 23rd. Went after wild plants.

Sept. 7th. Went to the cliff pasture after life everlasting, found lobelia there very unexpectedly. Gathered it. Sept. 8th. Gathered life everlasting and lobelia.

Oct. 24th. Began to put up herbs again.

Produce for sale, 1848. 529 pounds of herbs.

June 1, 1849 Gathered hoarhound and finished gathering herbs in the garden. June 5–22. Gathered hoarhound, catnep and elderblow. June 26th. William and the sisters went after mint and elderblows with the waggons.

Several entries follow as to picking elder blows and blackberries to make into cordials.

Sept. 28th. The brethren commenced pressing herbs.

Produce for sale, 1849, 504 pounds of herbs.

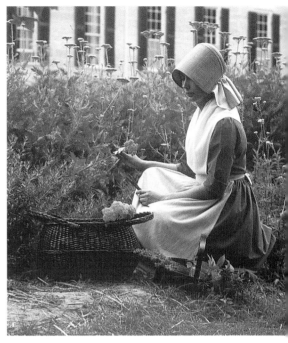

△ Garden and gardener, Pleasant Hill.

May 1, 1850 The Center and West sisters trimmed off the thyme and tanzy in John's garden. May 3rd. Gathered hoarhound in the hen lot. May 4th. Cleaned the garden house and press house.

A financial journal kept by one unidentified family lists the pounds of herbs they produced: In 1850, 417; 1851, 600; 1852, 271; 1853, 107; 1854, 160; and 1855, 282.

A journal kept by Kitty Jane Ryan commencing January 1, 1839, records an herb industry in the Center Family.

July 25, 1849 Gathered sage and other herbs in the garden. The largest cutting ever known. Gathered blackberries at the Cove spring.

Sept. 29th. Gathered hops, grapes and walnut roots for dye. Went after herb roots with Joel and three sisters and all the boys, but got none.

May 1, 1850 Trimmed off the thyme and tanzy in John's garden. May 1–4th. Cut herbs in the garden, burned caterpillars, gathered hoarhound, tanzy, bugleweed in the hen lot, cleaned herb house and press house.

June 16–19th. Gathered and shipped off catnep, gathered sage, thyme and other garden herbs.

July 31st. Gathered blackberries and mint.

Aug. 6th. The whole society of sisters went out after supper and cut sage. William went to Harrodsburg after roots. Aug. 24th. The young sisters set up the night previous and cut peaches and apples to fill dry house and press herbs.

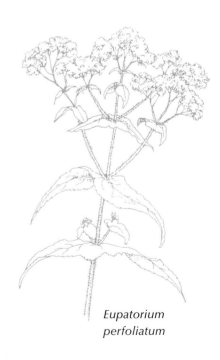

Eupatorium perfoliatum

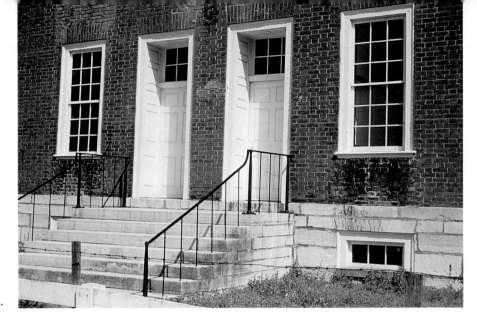

▷ East Family dwelling, Pleasant Hill.

PURE AND RELIABLE

Pure and Reliable Medicines: Manufactured and for Sale by the Shakers, Pleasant Hill. We append to our Catalogue of Preparations our Remedies, with the methods of the U.S.P. (Pharmacopaea) 1877 so that all parties concerned may compare the results of each and in this way may draw their own conclusions as to which method is the best to Secure Pure and Reliable Medicines of full strength in acts of principle and menstrums. N.B. Spurious and fraudulent imitations may be sold for much less than the Real and Pure, but are vastly more costly in the end.

1877 ADVERTISEMENT

Singing Their Products' Praises

One of the marketable medicines that traveled down the Kentucky River was the Shaker Aromatic Elixir of Malt. A broadside advertising it claimed: "Manufactured exclusively by the Shakers at Pleasant Hill, Mercer Co., Ky., under the supervision of R. B. Rupe, M.D. Pharmacist. Orders to be addressed to E. S. Sutton, General Agent, Louisville." But the manufacture of the elixir, from 1880 to 1883, was a short-lived enterprise, for the lack of profits caused the Shakers to abandon the undertaking. The label on the bottle showed a Shaker brother and stated:

> *This elegant elixir may be used in all cases where the extract is indicated and it will prove far superior, for it is Carmative, Nutrient and Tonic. It may be administered in Consumption, Debility, the Loss of Flesh and Strength, Variable Appetite, Dispepsia, Headache, Flatulence, Diarrhoea, etc., etc.*
>
> *This preparation of malt is grateful to the most delicate Stomach, and can be prescribed in many cases, where the common extract of Malt can not be taken.*
>
> *It is also a good vehicle for the administration of Quinine, iron Cod Liver Oil, etc. etc. . . . R/x Aromatic Elixir seven parts; Pure Extract of Malt (our own make) eight parts. Dose for adults one tablespoon three times a day after meals. Children less in proportion to age. Retail per bottle, $1. Six bottles for $5.*

Orders again were directed to Dunlavy and Scott.

One might feel that some of the testimonies concerning material produced by the Shakers are boastful, but the claims were justified. So much attention and care were devoted to making a perfect article that the brethren felt entitled to sell it with praise.

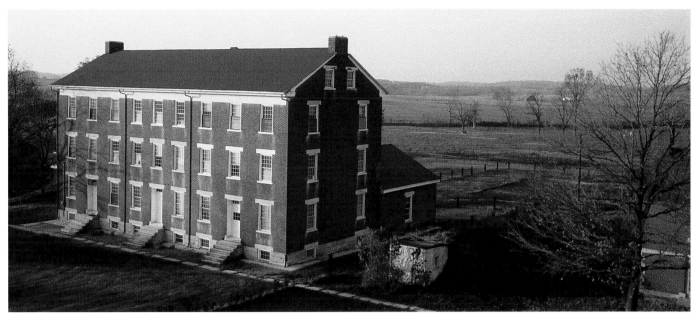

△ View of the Wash House, Center Family, South Union.

SOUTH UNION, KENTUCKY

While all of the communities in Ohio, and to a much lesser degree the eastern families, suffered from the Civil War and its aftereffects, nothing could compare to the harassment, destruction, and desolation experienced at South Union and Pleasant Hill. Nevertheless, the beautiful rich farmlands at South Union were once again producing bumper cash crops in 1873. Other sources of income were the preserved fruit business, leasing of farmland, and raising of garden seeds — an extensive operation.

During the three decades prior to the Civil War the society had been almost entirely self-sufficient and the members provided for nearly all of the food and clothing they needed. They had planted large orchards of peach, cherry, and apple trees and acres of gardens to produce vegetable seeds for the market. They grew medicinal herbs for their own use and sold the surplus along with the garden seeds.

River Trade

The Shakers had a busy river trade, peddling garden seeds, herbs, brooms, straw hats, socks, and jeans down the Red, Ohio, and Mississippi Rivers to New Orleans. Material was traded for needed commodities, and other necessities were purchased. A journal of such a trip was kept from October 6, 1831, to February 2, 1832, by Thomas Jefferson Shannon.

Brother Jefferson, or "T. J.," as he is referred to in his diaries, lists the sale of "Garden Seeds by the Box, $1,773.41," ten times the amount of any other single item sold. In the final accounting the sale of herbs is not

SHAKER REMEDIES

The South Union Shakers used herbal remedies in their nursing. There are records that herbs were gathered in the wild state but that the Shakers grew and sold sage themselves. Hervey Eades writes on June 12, 1833: *"Herb Press. Samuel McClelland finished and put up a new herb press for pressing herbs for sale."*

The Shakers' cholera remedy carried on its label: "This remedy was discovered by Dr. J. P. Holmes, deceased, last member [of the society] from whom we obtained the formula." A statement of the efficacy of this medicine in the London epidemics is signed by Dr. Holmes.

itemized, but there are fifteen references to selling herbs in the lengthy journal. Sage was sold most frequently: "A pound of sage. . . . Sage $10. . . . Sold some herb worth $9. . . . Sold 52 ozs. essential oils at 25 cents per oz., $13. . . . Sold some sage. . . . Sage to John W. Swains' Drug Store and exchanged it for some medicines."

Family Records

The records kept by Hervey L. Eades from October 1836 to April 1868 reveal the day-to-day activities of a busy family. He noted that the garden seed business continued to grow, with increasing acreage put under cultivation for this industry. "Sept. 9th. Finished boxing garden seed . . . whole amount 170,000 papers." He continues:

1847 *June 30th. White walnut bark. Brother George Rankin and Deacon Rubin Wise get it at Frazers. . . . Whole amount of wheat this year 829½ bushels.*

July 23rd. Lobelia gathering. Elder Brother S. Shannon, Olive and Lucy Shannon and Denise Barker go to Stokes' oil field for this purpose. July 27th. Eli and Sister gather lobelia again at Stokes.

1848 *October 3rd. Gardners finished putting up seed. 103,143 papers. October 6th. Gather chestnut. . . .*

1850 *October 7th. Finished papering 110,000 papers of seed. . . .*

1854 *July 12th. Blackberries. Teams and hands, Sisters especially, into the country to gather blackberries to make wine and cordial. . . .*

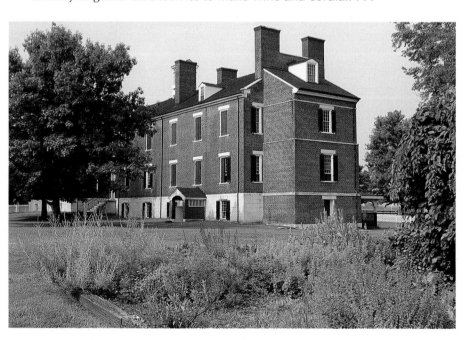

▷ Main herb garden at South Union, with 1824 Centre House in background.

For the next four years Eades's diary still covers the events in the families, but he is mostly concerned with the Civil War. Hervey Eades, now an elder, continues his record, in 1864, by stating "the money wealth of the Society, $45,000 in bonds and cash." There were also "210 souls, 1st, 2nd, and Junior Orders."

1864 February 25th. Seed trip south down the Mississippi River, the first since the War got under way. Elder H. L. Eades and Brother Jackson McGown start by Railroad to Louisville thence down Ohio and Mississippi Rivers with 150 Boxes, 30,000 papers and garden seeds. Late for a southern trip.
March 22nd. Return of Elder Hervey. Successful as could be expected. $1450. Expenses were enormous, $400.

The Civil War

The outbreak of the Civil War placed the Believers of Kentucky in a difficult position. They had never owned slaves and did not approve of the institution that permitted it, and on that account were regarded with distrust and suspicion by the pro-slavery element of the neighborhood. Meanwhile, their principles of pacifism, which forbade them to take up arms in the defense of the Union, brought them into conflict with the authorities in Washington. Much tact was required on the part of the leaders to steer safely through those troubled times. Their settlements were often occupied by Northern and Southern forces, and the bands of irresponsible guerrillas were a constant source of anxiety, but their greatest loss came from the almost total cessation of business. The seed and herb peddlers traveled in constant fear of confrontations with guerrillas. Nevertheless Eades could write in 1864:

The garden seed [business] has become good. Sales better than for many years. A large business is done in the seed line . . . and also in the Chh [Church Family] in pressed and prepared herbs and roots, besides many tons in bulk . . . considerably many tons of powdered herbs and root . . . and many tons of Extracts, both solids and fluids. The War makes great demand for all these articles. They sell in large quantities. We cannot prepare enough to meet the demand.
1865 January 30th. Ex. Elder Soloman Rankin and James Richardson started south west and west with a small load of seeds. This trip is extra hazardous having to pass through guerilla country. I do not look for them to return with their horses as one looks well and is about sure to be taken, if the guerillas come across them, we hope they may return with their lives.
February 2nd. Brother Joseph Averett started south with small load of seeds. Springlike weather.

TREATING SPIDER BITE

A Shaker record from 1804 to 1836, later transcribed by Hervey Eades in 1870, and also one of Eades's own journals contain many interesting details of the lives of the Believers and the medical procedure and herbs they used. For example:

Nov. 6th. Spider Bite! Andrew Barnett while rising was bitten by a spider and soon life despaired of. A great many things done, given Black snake root. Plantain, sweet oil clysters, warm baths, drafts of raw onions, spirit of Harts Horn. Did not get about until the next 3rd day and not entirely well for over two weeks. Note: [from H. L. Eades] The Spirits of Hart Horn perhaps was the only thing that did any good. In a precisely similar case, I gave the patient nearly a half gill of Hartshorn and Brandy mixed and though previously screaming with pain, was relieved in 5 hours and well as common next day.

February 12th. Ex-Elder Soloman Rankin and James Richardson returned this evening. Succeeded tolerably well in sales. Brought home with them $390. Were not molested by guerillas. . . .

Postwar Rebuilding — and Decline

When peace was restored after the Civil War, Elder Hervey Eades, a Shaker for all fifty-five years of his life, applied himself with great energy to building up and maintaining the size of his community, by intense recruiting and by receiving orphans. Keeping the members in good health was a constant burden and worry. Eades also had to repair the financial damage his community had suffered. He was successful at that, but as the years went on he was pained to see the steady decline in the number of members.

Julia Neal commented about the society after the war:

Practicing their economic precepts in the reconstruction years as they had in the beginning period of the society, the trustees took advantage of every possible source of income, offering for sale such nonrelated items as 181 pounds of Jamestown weed or "Strammon"; 1,121 pounds of honey "the most ever got in one season"; and tanyard leather, the 1867 sale of which brought $1,296.57.

The reference to "Jamestown weed," or *Datura stramonium,* is the only one this author has encountered in records of the western societies. It was an energetic narcotic poison and, although handled by some of the eastern Shakers in their medical departments, was eventually dropped as being too dangerous.

The vigorous and well-administered society at South Union diminished gradually in number and in prosperity. Over a long period of years, at most fifty, the members (under good leadership for the most part) worked with characteristic energy to maintain their industries and trade.

After the Thirteenth Amendment was ratified in December 1865, the Shakers were pleased to be able to hire men who had been slaves, and it was lawful to pay them directly. This came at a time when, because of their reduced membership, extra hands were needed to increase the output of the community. Even so, when Elder Henry died in 1892, there were less than fifty souls under his ministry and thirty years later, only ten.

The society closed and the property was sold in 1922. This brave band of Believers had withstood the invasions of both the Union and the Confederate Armies, raging epidemics, and national financial panics, but changes in the outer world — in material, industrial, and social conditions — were not favorable toward enticing even the most sympathetic into their society. Against this trend, the Shakers were helpless.

DANGEROUS TIMES

February 7th. Elder William Ware started from the Junior Order with a horse load of seeds, 1400 papers. He goes via Gallatin out to middle and east Tennessee. We cannot but have unpleasant forbodings for him. . . .

JOURNAL OF
HERVEY L. EADES, 1865

The Herbal Compendium

EVERY HERB EMPLOYED FOR A MEDICINAL PURPOSE, whether in its natural state or after processing, belongs to the herbal materia medica. This section of the book lists those herbs that the Shakers collected, grew, or purchased for use in their own societies or for resale. More than 350 plants, shrubs, and trees with their roots, barks, flowers, and berries have been compiled, many of which were included in the pharmacopoeia of most of the Shaker societies at some period in their history.

The botanical names and the properties ascribed to the plants were taken from Shaker catalogs, which covered a sixty-four-year period from 1830 to 1894. The major source for this herbal compendium was the *Druggist's Hand-Book of Pure Botanic Preparations, &c. sold by Society of Shakers, Mount Lebanon, Columbia County, New York,* published in 1873. That catalog listed 304 herbs with their Latin names, the medical properties ascribed by the Shakers, and a synopsis of the various diseases in which they were used. There were two indexes, one of the botanical names and the other of 860 common names that included 557 synonyms. It eliminated many of the early herbal remedies and continued to offer for sale only those herbs that were most constantly in demand and relied upon by the medical profession.

Not every Shaker medicinal herb catalog carried every plant, of course, but all of the material has been listed that the Shakers prepared and sold in five eastern states and three midwestern states.

The reader may also note minor omissions of information and discrepancies within the entries for individual herbs, and these are simply repetitions of the gaps or discrepancies in the original catalogs.

The herbs were sold in various quantities and forms; that is, as leaves, roots, bark, flowers, buds, berries, and whole herbs, and in ground, fluid, pulverized, or solid form.

A NOTE TO THE READER

The reader should regard this list of medicinal plants and their uses as an addendum to the history of the Shaker herb industry. **The botanical information given here is not intended to foster use of herbs by the amateur in cases of illness nor to replace the services of a physician.** While every herb given here was classified at some time or other as medicinal in some degree, however slight, we are quoting the evaluation given them by the Shaker herbalists of the eighteenth and nineteenth centuries and not by present-day botanists.

ELDER HENRY'S OBSERVATIONS

In the compendium beginning on page 126, the paragraphs in italics, enclosed in quotation marks, are the notations that appear on Canterbury sister Cora Helena Sarle's drawings. These are believed to be the observations of Canterbury Elder Henry Clay Blinn. Abbreviations appear as in the original.

To make this herbal a more practical guide for today's student of botany, we have, in many cases, updated the nomenclature and corrected the Shakers' early spelling, bearing in mind that fixed or rigid botanical nomenclature in Latin or the vernacular is unattainable. The sources consulted to help resolve these inconsistencies were: *A Field Guide to Wildflowers* by Roger Tory Peterson and Margaret McKenney, *A Field Guide to the Ferns and Their Related Families* by Boughton Cobb, *A Field Guide to Trees and Shrubs* by George A. Petrides, *The Herbalist* by Joseph E. Meyer, *A Modern Herbal* by M. Grieve and Mrs. C. F. Leyel, *Hortus Third*, compiled by Liberty Hyde Bailey and Ethel Zoe Bailey, and *Manual of Botany*, 8th edition, by Asa Gray.

Under each herbal entry are listed the major healing principles according to the old Shaker catalogs, listed in the order of priority given in those catalogs. The principles are defined in the glossary of medical and other terms that may be unfamiliar to readers, appearing at the back of this compendium.

To help identify the plants listed in this section we have arranged them alphabetically under their most familiar names. We have adopted this method from two English herbal authorities, Mrs. Maud Grieve, compiler of *A Modern Herbal,* and Mrs. C. F. Leyel, who edited Mrs. Grieve's monumental work. The listing in the compendium differs from some other methods. We expect that interest in Shaker herbs will be largely a historical one for the amateur botanist. We hope the professional botanist will understand that the arrangement has been made to conform to that used by the Shakers in their catalogs. The reader looking for a name such as sweet balsam, for example, and not finding it under S should check under B. In other cases, double names will be treated as a unit and will be alphabetized under the first letter of the first name. For example, lady's slipper will be found under L.

Common names listed in Shaker catalogs differed from place to place among the three major areas — Northeast, Midwest, and South — and these listings have been retained. Different parts of plants were used and different uses made of the herbs in the various communities, and the Shaker catalogs also reflected this.

Key

Properties of Herbs:*

Abortive. Capable of producing abortion.
Acrid. Biting; caustic.
Adenagic. Acting on the glandular system.
Alterative. Capable of producing a salutary change in disease through catalytic action when used with another substance.
Anaphrodisiac. Capable of blunting the sexual appetite.
Anodyne. Relieving pain or causing it to cease.
Anthelmintic. Destroying or expelling worms.
Antibilious. Correcting the bile and bilious secretions.
Antilithic. Preventing the formation of calculous matter.
Antiperiodic. Preventing periodic attacks of a disease, as in intermittent fevers.
Antiphlogistic. Counteracting inflammation.
Antiscorbutic. Opposed to scurvy.
Antiseptic. Opposed to putrefaction; checking the growth or action of microorganisms.
Antispasmodic. Correcting and relieving spasms.
Antisyphilitic. Acting against venereal disease.
Aperient. Gently moving the bowels.
Aromatic. Fragrant, spicy.
Astringent. Shrinking and driving the blood from the tissues.
Balsamic. Mild, healing, and soothing.
Carminitive. Allaying pain by expelling gas from the alimentary canal.
Cathartic. Purgative; cleansing.
Cephalic. Relating to the head.
Cholagogue. Causing the flow of bile.
Corroborant. Strengthening and giving tone.
Demulcent. Capable of soothing an inflamed mucus membrane or protecting it from irritation.
Deobstruent. Removing obstructions.
Depurative. Purifying or cleansing.
Detergent. Cleansing parts of wounds.
Diaphoretic. Promoting moderate perspiration.
Discutient. Repelling or resolving tumors.

Diuretic. Increasing the secretion of urine.
Drastic. Operating powerfully on the bowels.
Emetic. Capable of producing vomiting.
Emmenagogue. Promoting menstruation.
Emollient. Relaxing and softening inflamed parts.
Erratic. Having unpredictable results.
Excitant. Stimulant.
Expectorant. Facilitating or provoking discharge of mucus.
Febrifuge. Abating or driving away fevers.
Herpatic. Attacking cutaneous diseases.
Hydragogue. Capable of expelling serum.
Hypnotic. Promoting sleep, somniferous.
Laxative. Gently cathartic.
Mucilaginous. Resembling gum in its character.
Narcotic. Having the property of stupefying.
Nauseant. Exciting nausea.
Nephritic. Relating to the kidney.
Nervine. Acting in the nervous system.
Nutritive. Relating to nutrition.
Parturient. Inducing or promoting labor.
Pectoral. Relating to the breast.
Phrenic. Relating to the diaphragm.
Purgative. Operating on the bowels more powerfully than a laxative.
Refrigerant. Depressing the morbid temperature of the body.
Rubefacient. Causing redness of the skin.
Secernant. Affecting the secretions.
Sedative. Directly depressing the vital forces.
Sialogogue. Provoking the secretion of saliva.
Stimulant. Causing a temporary increase in vital activity.
Stomachic. Giving tone to the stomach.
Styptic. Arresting hemorrhage; stopping bleeding.
Sudorific. Provoking sweat.
Tonic. Invigorating; bracing; refreshing.
Vermifuge. Capable of expelling worms.
Vesicant. Inducing blistering.
Vulnerary. Favoring the consolidation of wounds.

In the individual herbal entries, properties are listed in order of precedence, as they were in the original catalogs.

Abscess

Polemonium reptans
   Greek Valerian. Blue Bells. Jacob's Ladder.

ROOT: Alterative. Diaphoretic. Astringent.

Serviceable in pleurisy, fevers, and inflammatory diseases.

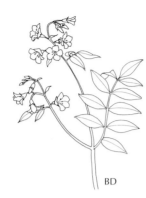

BD

Aconite

Aconitum napellus
   Monkshood. Wolfsbane.

LEAVES: Narcotic. Sedative. Antiphlogistic. Diaphoretic.
ROOT: Narcotic. Sedative. Antiphlogistic. Diaphoretic.

Used in scarlatina, inflammatory fever, acute rheumatism, neuralgia, etc. Must be used cautiously. Although monkshood in the hands of the intelligent physician is of great service, it should not be used in domestic practice. As a sedative and anodyne it is capable of many beneficial uses in the hands of a skilled person.

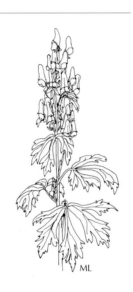

ML

Agrimony

Agrimonia eupatoria
   Cockleburr. Stickwort.

HERB: Tonic. Alterative. Astringent. Diaphoretic.

Highly recommended in bowel complaints, gravel, asthma, coughs, and gonorrhea. Used as a tea sometimes infused with licorice root. Also used as a gargle for throat and mouth irritations.

"Found by the roadsides and borders of fields, Can. and U.S. common, July."

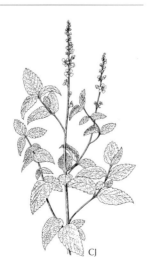

CJ

Alder, Black

Ilex verticillata (Prinos verticillatus)
   Striped Alder. Winterberry. Fake Alder.

BARK: Tonic. Alterative. Vermifuge. Astringent.
BERRIES: Cathartic. Vermifuge.

Used with good effect in jaundice, diarrhea, gangrene, dyspepsia; the berries are used for worms in children. Used by dyers, tanners, and leather dressers; the bark is powdered and used as a basis for blacks.

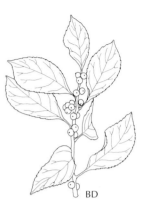

BD

Alder, Red or Tag

Alnus rugosa (A. oregona)
   Tag Alder. Smooth Alder. Brook Alder.

BARK: Alterative. Emmenagogue. Astringent. Tonic. Deobstruent.
TAGS: Alterative. Emmenagogue. Astringent.

Valuable in scrofula, syphilis, and diseases of the skin. Bark, leaves, and berries used. Used also in bitters and as an astringent.

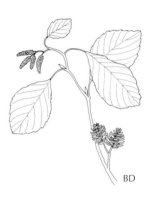

BD

Bark of black and red alder used by dyers, tanners, and leather dressers, also by fishermen for their nets. The young shoots dye yellow and when cut in March will dye a cinnamon color. The catkins dye green.

Alum Root

Heuchera pubescens
   Cranesbill. Splitrock.

ROOT: Astringent. Antiseptic. Detergent.

Wild alum root is powerfully astringent without bitterness or an unpleasant taste and is useful in diarrhea. Boiled in water and mixed with sugar and milk, it is easily administered to children. Also used as a gargle for throat irritation.

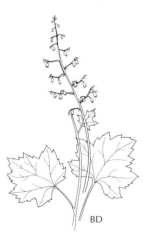

BD

Angelica

Angelica atropurpurea

Purple Angelica. Masterwort. High Angelica. Archangel.

LEAVES: Carminitive. Stomachic. Tonic. Balsamic.
ROOT: Balsamic. Aromatic. Stimulant. Carminitive. Diuretic. Stomachic. Emmenagogue.
SEED: Carminitive. Acrid. Aromatic. Stimulant.

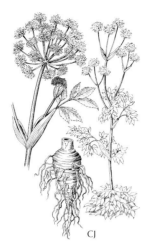

Used in flatulent colic, heartburn, and debility. The seeds are used in syrup for pain in the stomach and side. Serviceable in promoting elimination through the urine and skin.

Apple

Malus sylvestris (Pyrus malus)

BARK: Tonic. Febrifuge. Astringent.

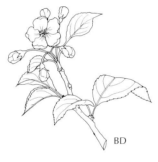

For intermittent, remittent, and bilious fevers; also for gravel.

Arnica

Arnica montana

Leopardsbane. Mountain Tobacco.

FLOWERS: Stimulant. Diaphoretic. Vulnerary.
ROOT: Stimulant. Diaphoretic. Vulnerary.

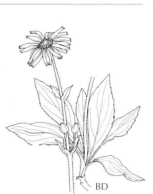

Used in gout, dropsy, and rheumatism; the tincture of arnica is used for bruises, wounds, irritation of nasal passages, chapped lips, sprains, and the bites of insects. This flower should be used externally only, as it may produce a serious reaction if taken internally.

Note: A salve, used for the same purposes, is made by heating one ounce of the flowers with one ounce of lard for a few hours. For another external use, take two heaping teaspoons of the flowers to a cup of boiling water. Apply cold to sores or wounds.

Ash, Mountain

Sorbus americana (Pyrus americana)

Roundwood.

BARK: Astringent. Tonic. Detergent.
BERRIES: Vermifuge. Antiscorbutic. Astringent.

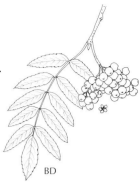

The bark is used in bilious diseases to cleanse the blood; the berries for scurvy and as a vermifuge.

Ash, Prickly

Zanthoxylum americanum

Toothache Bush. Yellow Wood. Suter Berry.

BARK: Stimulant. Tonic. Alterative. Sialogogue. Diaphoretic.
BERRIES: Stimulant. Carminitive. Antispasmodic.

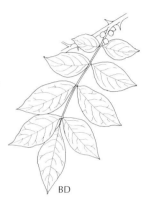

A valuable tonic in low typhoid fevers; used in colic, rheumatism, scrofula, etc. The berries are a most valuable agent in Asiatic cholera. They contain a volatile oil and are aromatic. The bark is used for flatulence and diarrhea.

Ash, White

Fraxinus americana

BARK: Tonic. Cathartic. Astringent.

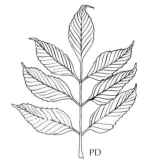

Beneficial in constipation, dropsy, ague cake, etc. The seeds are said to prevent obesity.

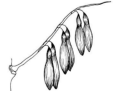

Asparagus Root
Asparagus officinalis

ROOT: Aperient.

Valuable in dropsy and enlargement of the heart.

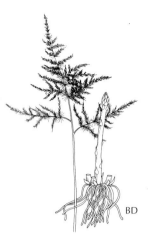

Aspen, Quaking
Populus tremuloides
Trembling Aspen.

BARK: Febrifuge. Antiscorbutic. Vermifuge.

The active principles of the bark are salicin and populin. Used as a vermifuge by veterinaries.

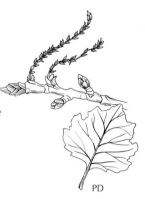

Avens, Water
Geum rivale
Chocolate Root. Throat Root. Cure-All. Evans Root.

ROOT: Tonic. Astringent. Stomachic.

Valuable in hemorrhages, chronic diarrhea and dysentery, leukorrhea, and active ulcers.

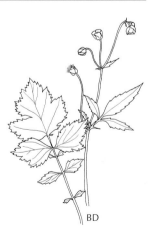

Backache Brake
Athyrium filix-femina
Female Fern. Lady Fern.

ROOT: Anthelmintic. Vermifuge. Pectoral. Demulcent.

Used to expel worms.

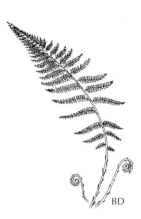

Balm, Lemon
Melissa officinalis
Bee Balm. Blue Balm. Cure-All. Dropsy Plant.

HERB: (leaves and stalk) Stomachic. Diaphoretic. Antispasmodic. Sudorific.

Useful in low fevers and to assist menstruation. A warm infusion taken freely produces sweating; is made more palatable by adding lemon juice.

Lemon balm tea, a pleasant drink; sometimes a little rosemary or spearmint may be added, and a few cloves. Alone, it is agreeable as a summer beverage iced and slightly sweetened.

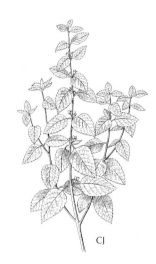

Balm, Moldavian
Dracocephalum moldavica
Sweet Balm. Tea Balm. Dragonhead.

LEAVES: Aromatic. Stomachic. Diaphoretic.

Useful in low fevers and to assist menstruation.

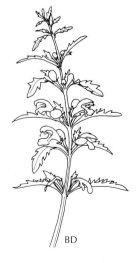

Balm of Gilead
Populus balsamifera

BUDS: Pectoral. Stimulant. Tonic. Diuretic. Antiscorbutic. Balsamic. Stomachic.
BARK: Tonic. Cathartic.

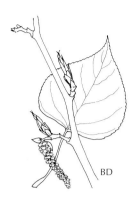

Tincture of the buds is used in affections of the chest, stomach, and kidneys, along with rheumatism and scurvy. Applied to frost and fresh wounds. The bark is useful in gout and rheumatism.

Balmony
Chelone glabra
Snakehead. Turtlebloom. Turtlehead. Salt Rheum Weed. Fishmouth. Shell Flower. Bitter Herb.

LEAVES: Tonic. Cathartic. Anthelmintic. Antibilious. Vermifuge.

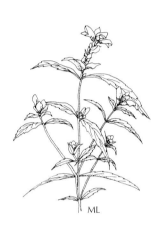

Especially valuable in jaundice and hepatic diseases, to remove worms and excite the digestive organs to action, particularly the liver. An ointment made from the fresh leaves is valuable for the itching and irritation of piles.

Balsam, Sweet
Gnaphalium obtusifolium var. *polycephalum (G. polycephalum)*
Life Everlasting. White Balsam. Indian Posy. Old Field Balsam.

HERB: Astringent. Stomachic. Diaphoretic. Sudorific. Sedative.

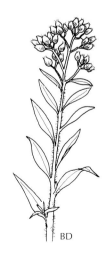

Irritations of the mouth and throat are said to be relieved by chewing the leaves and blossoms; the leaves applied to bruises and other local irritations are very efficacious.

Barberry
Berberis vulgaris
Sowberry

BARK: Tonic. Laxative. Refrigerant. Astringent.
BERRIES: Tonic. Laxative. Refrigerant. Astringent.

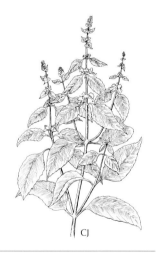

Employed in all cases where tonics are indicated; has proved efficacious in jaundice. The berries are used as a wash in canker. The berries form an agreeable acidulous drink. The bark of the root is the most active, a teaspoon of the powdered bark acting as a purgative. A decoction of the bark or berries will be found of service as a mouthwash or gargle.

Basil, Sweet
Ocimum basilicum

LEAVES: Aromatic. Stimulant.

To allay excessive vomiting. This plant is aromatic with the added advantage of value in cooking and use as a tea.

Basswood
Tilia americana
Linden. Lime-Tree. Spoonwood. Tilia Flowers.

BARK: Emollient. Discutient. Stomachic.
FLOWERS: Emollient. Discutient. Stomachic.
LEAVES: Aromatic. Stimulant. Astringent.

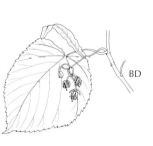

Used as a poultice in painful swellings. A tea of linden flowers and leaves promotes sweating. An admirable remedy for quieting coughs and relieving hoarseness resulting from colds.

"A common forest tree in the northern and middle states. June."

Bayberry

Myrica pensylvanica (M. cerifera)
Wax Myrtle. Wax Berry.
Candle Berry. Myrtle.

BARK: Stimulant. Astringent.
Emetic. Erratic.
BERRIES: Stimulant. Astringent.
LEAVES: Aromatic. Stimulant.
Astringent.

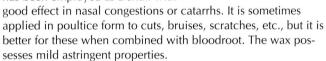

Valuable in jaundice, diarrhea,
dysentery, canker in the mouth,
throat, and bowels, and as a wash
for spongy gums. The leaves are
used to treat scurvy. Powdered, it
has been employed as a snuff with
good effect in nasal congestions or catarrhs. It is sometimes
applied in poultice form to cuts, bruises, scratches, etc., but it is
better for these when combined with bloodroot. The wax possesses mild astringent properties.

"Found in dry woods, or in open fields, Can. to Fla. May."

Beech, American

Fagus grandifolia (F. ferruginea)

BARK: Astringent. Tonic.
Antisyphilitic.
LEAVES: Astringent. Tonic.
Antisyphilitic. Alterative.

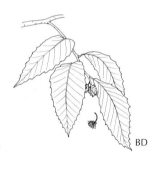

Useful in diabetes, cutaneous diseases, ulcers, and dyspepsia.

*"A common forest tree in U.S. and
Can. 50 to 80 ft. high. May."*

Beechdrops

Epifagus virginiana

WHOLE PLANT: Discutient.
Astringent.

An eminent astringent. Applied
locally to minor cuts, wounds,
and bruises.

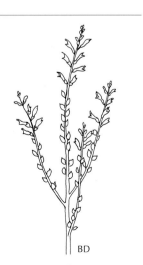

Belladonna

Atropa belladonna
Deadly Nightshade. Dwale.

LEAVES: Narcotic. Anodyne.
Diaphoretic. Diuretic.

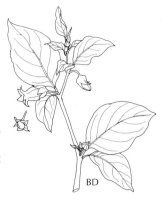

Used in convulsions, neuralgia,
rheumatism, mania, gout, and
painful conditions of the nervous
system. Requires caution in its use.
In the hands of skilled physicians
this botanical has great virtues, but
it is too powerful and dangerous
for general or home use. The
leaves should be gathered while
the plant is in flower.

Bellwort

Uvularia perfoliata
Mohawkweed.

LEAVES: Tonic. Demulcent.
Nervine. Herpatic.

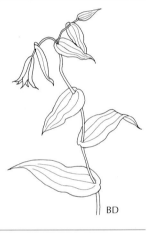

For sore throat, inflammation, and
as poultice in erysipelas and
wounds.

*"A handsome plant in the woods.
Can. and U.S. May."*

Benne

Sesamum indicum
Sesame. Gingili. Tell.

LEAVES: Demulcent. Laxative.
Emollient.
SEED: Demulcent. Laxative.
Emollient.

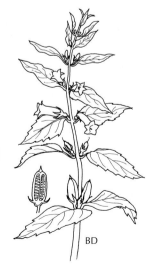

The seeds are used in cookery,
cosmetics, etc. The leaves are used
as a demulcent and emollient,
sheathing or lubricating.

Bethroot

Trillium erectum var. *album*
(T. pendulum)

Birth Root. Indian Balm.
Ground Lily. Cough Root.
Pariswort. Truelove. Wake
Robin. Purple Trillium.

ROOT: Astringent. Tonic.
Antiseptic. Pectoral.
Alterative.

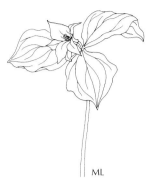

Valuable in coughs, asthma, hectic fever, bloody urine.

Betony, Wood

Pedicularis canadensis (Betononica officinalis)

HERB: Nervine. Tonic.
Discutient. Aperient.

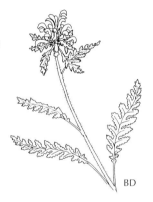

For headache, hysterics, and nervousness, and used as a cordial.

Birch, Black

Betula lenta

Cherry Birch. Sweet Birch.
Mahogany Birch. Spice Birch.

BARK: Aromatic. Tonic.
Astringent. Stimulant.
Diaphoretic. Anodyne.
Diuretic.

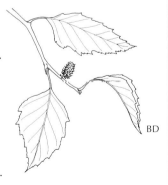

Used in diarrhea, dysentery,
cholera infantum, and to tone the
bowels after exhausting discharge.

Bird Pepper

Capsicum frutescens

Tabasco Pepper. Chillies.

FRUIT: Stimulant. Cathartic.
Rubefacient.

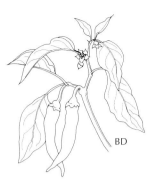

A powerful stimulant used in
colds, rheumatism, spasmodic
affections, and cholera.

Bitter Herb

Centaurium erythraea (Erythraea centaurium)

Centaury. European
Centaury.

TOP AND ROOT: Aromatic.
Tonic. Febrifuge.

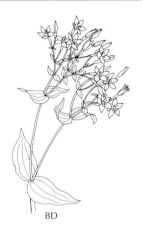

Aromatic and bitter, used to dispel fever by allaying fever heat.

Bitterroot

Apocynum androsaemifolium

Honey Bloom. Milk Ipecac.
Dogsbone. Wandering
Milkweed. Flytrap. Dogbane.

ROOT: Alterative. Sudorific.
Emetic. Diuretic. Vermifuge.
Diaphoretic. Tonic. Cathartic.

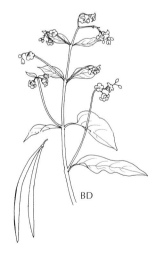

Valuable in chronic liver complaints, syphilis, scrofula, intermittent and low stages of typhoid
fever. In conjunction with yellow
parilla, it is excellent for dyspepsia.

Bittersweet

Solanum dulcamara

Garden Nightshade. Woody Nightshade. Violet Bloom. Fever Twig. Scarlet Berry.

HERB: Narcotic. Alterative. Diuretic. Sudorific. Discutient. Herpatic. Deobstruent.
TWIGS AND BARK OF ROOT: Herpatic. Deobstruent. Alterative.

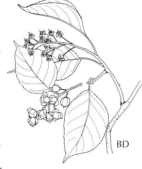

Employed in cutaneous diseases, scrofula, syphilitic diseases, jaundice, obstructed menstruation, rheumatic afflictions, and for the relief of skin irritation. It is a purifying tea and a pectoral tea.

"A well known climber with blue flower and red berries. N. Eng. to Ark. The berries are said to be poisonous. July."

Bittersweet, False

Celastrus scandens

Staff Tree or Staffvine. Waxwork. Climbing Orange Root.

BARK OF ROOT: Antibilious. Discutient. Alterative. Diaphoretic. Diuretic.
BERRIES: Emollient. Discutient. Alterative. Diaphoretic. Diuretic.

Used in scrofula, syphilis, leukorrhea, and obstructed menstruation.

Blackberry

Rubus spp.

Dewberry. Bramble. Gout Berry. Cloud Berry.

HERB: Astringent. Tonic.
ROOT: Astringent. Tonic.

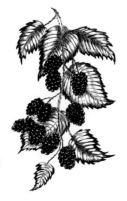

Excellent in cholera infantum, diarrhea, dysentery, and relaxed condition of intestines of children; as an injection in gleet, gonorrhea, and prolapsus uteri and ani. Also used by some for offensive saliva. The fruit was made into wine and brandy and used to treat diarrhea.

"In damp woods and by the roadside. Can. to Carolinas. Trailing several feet. May and June."

Blazing Star

Aletris farinosa

Devil's Bit. Unicorn. Stargrass. Colic Root. Ague Root. Star Root.

ROOT: Narcotic. Tonic. Emetic. Cathartic. Stomachic. Diuretic. Stimulant.

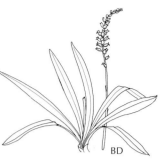

Used in chronic rheumatism, dropsy, and colic. The decoction was useful as a gargle in throat irritations.

Bloodroot

Sanguinaria canadensis

Indian Paint. Red Puccoon. Tetterwort.

ROOT: Emetic. Stimulant. Alterative. Tonic. Expectorant. Deobstruent. Acrid. Diaphoretic.

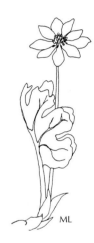

Valuable in typhoid pneumonia, catarrh, scarlatina, jaundice, dyspepsia, ringworm, and in affections of the respiratory organs. In small doses, it stimulates the digestive organs, acting as a stimulant and tonic. It appears to be used chiefly as an expectorant.

"In woods. Can. and U.S. When bruised the plant exudes an orange red fluid. The juice is emetic and purgative. Apr. May."

Blue Flag

Iris versicolor

Poison Flag. Flag Lily. Water Flag. Fleur De Lis. Liver Lily. Snake Lily.

ROOT: Diuretic. Cathartic. Alterative. Sialogogue. Vermifuge. Emetic.

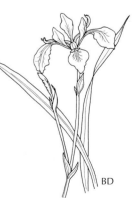

A potent remedy in dropsy, scrofula, affections of the liver, spleen, and kidneys, and secondary syphilis.

Boneset

Eupatorium perfoliatum

Thoroughwort. Feverwort. Throughstem. Vegetable Antimony. Crosswort. Sweating Plant. Indian Sage. Ague Weed. Eupatorium.

HERB: Sudorific. Emetic. Tonic. Aperient. Diaphoretic. Febrifuge.

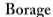

Excellent in colds, fevers, dyspepsia, jaundice, general debility of the system, fever, and ague. The cold infusion or extract is tonic and aperient. The warm infusion is diaphoretic and emetic. A strong tea of boneset sweetened with honey will break up an ordinary head cold. Also, can be made into an ointment or syrup.

"A common plant on low grounds, meadows, U.S. and Can. Abundant. The plant is bitter and used in medicine. Aug."

Borage

Borago officinalis

Burrage. Bugloss.

HERB: Stomachic. Diaphoretic. Aperient. Refrigerant.

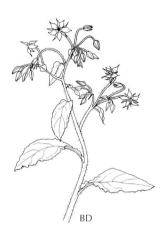

Used in catarrh, rheumatism, and diseases of the skin. It is made into a cordial and is pectoral and aperient. Also used as a culinary herb.

Boxberry

Gaultheria procumbens

Wintergreen. Checkerberry.

LEAVES: Aromatic. Diuretic. Stomachic.

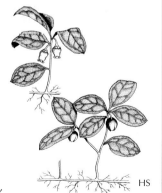

This is a diuretic. Small doses stimulate the stomach; large doses have an extreme effect and cause vomiting.

"In old woods and on mountains. N.E. to Newfoundland. May. June."

Boxwood

Cornus florida

Dogwood. Flowering Cornel. Budwood.

BARK: Tonic. Astringent. Stimulant.
FLOWERS: Emmenagogue. Sudorific.

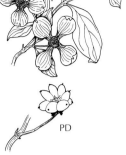

An excellent substitute for Peruvian bark. Valuable in jaundice and liver complaint. The flowers are used for accelerating the discharge of the menses. The bark should only be used in its dried state. Cornine, its active principle, seems to have been used occasionally as a substitute for quinine.

Brooklime

Veronica beccabunga

Water Pimpernel. Water Purslain. Beccabunga.

HERB: Antiscorbutic. Diuretic. Emmenagogue. Febrifuge. Discutient. Alterative.

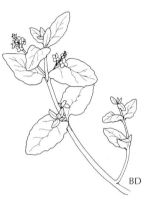

Beneficial in obstructed menstruation, scurvy, fevers, skin diseases, and coughs.

Broom

Cytisus scoparius

Link. Genista. Banal.

HERB: Emetic. Cathartic. Diuretic.

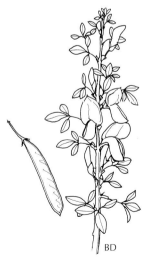

Especially beneficial in dropsy. Said never to fail in increasing the flow of urine. Broom tops are purgative and act on the kidneys. This tea is of great service. It is often used in equal parts with the root of dandelion for diuretic purposes.

Buckbean

Menyanthes trifoliata

Bogbean. Trefoil. Water Shamrock. Wind Shamrock. Bitterworm. Marsh Trefoil. Bog Myrtle.

ROOT: Tonic. Diuretic. Anthelmintic.
HERB: Tonic. Diuretic. Anthelmintic. Cathartic. Deobstruent.

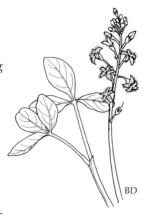

Used in the treatment of scurvy, rheumatism, jaundice, dyspepsia, hepatics, and worms. A tea of buckbean improves digestion and promotes and improves gastric juices.

Buckhorn Brake

Osmunda regalis

Male Fern. Royal Fern. King's Fern.

ROOT: Tonic. Mucilaginous. Demulcent. Styptic. Vermifuge. Astringent.

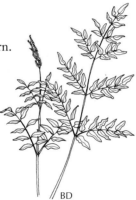

Very valuable in female weakness, cough, and dysentery; said to be a certain cure for rickets, spine complaint, and debility of the muscles.

"A large and beautiful fern in swamps and meadows. The fronds are 3 feet high. June."

Buckthorn

Rhamnus cathartica

Purging Berries. Red Root. New Jersey Tea. Arrow Wood. Alder Dogwood. Bird Cherry.

BARK: Hydragogue. Cathartic. Vermifuge.
BERRIES: Hydragogue. Cathartic. Alterative.

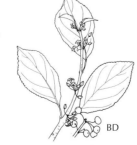

The bark should be at least one year old before using. It is purgative, its action similar to that of rhubarb. Used in rheumatism, gout, dropsy, and eruptive diseases. An ointment made of the fresh bark is excellent for skin irritation. (The syrup is made from bark and berries.)

Bugle, Bitter

Lycopus europaeus

Bugle Weed. Gipseywort. Water Hoarhound.

HERB: Styptic. Astringent. Tonic. Narcotic. Pectoral. Deobstruent.

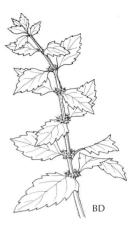

Recommended in intermittent fever and hemorrhage of lungs, bowels, or stomach.

Bugle, Sweet

Lycopus americanus

Water Bugle. Paul Betony. Water Horehound. Green Archangel.

HERB: Sudorific. Tonic. Astringent. Deobstruent. Styptic. Pectoral. Sedative. Narcotic.

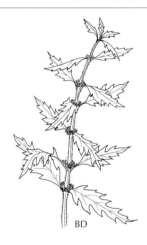

Useful in phthisis, hemorrhage of the lungs, diabetes, and chronic diarrhea. It is sedative and mildly narcotic.

Burdock

Arctium lappa

Clotbur. Bardana.

LEAVES: Sudorific. Emollient. Diaphoretic. Aperient.
ROOT: Sudorific. Herpatic. Antiscorbutic. Alterative.
SEED: Carminitive. Tonic. Diuretic.

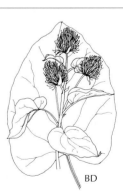

Used in gout and scorbutic, syphilitic, scrofulous, and leprous diseases; the leaves are used as a cooling poultice. The root should be dug in the fall or early spring. Only year-old roots should be used. Externally, it is valuable in salves or as a wash for burns, wounds, and skin irritations.

Burnet, Great

Sanguisorba officinalis
　　Garden or Common Burnet.

WHOLE PLANT: Astringent.
　　Tonic.

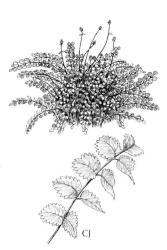

Both herb and root are administered internally in all abnormal discharges in diarrhea, dysentery, and leukorrhea. Dried and powdered, it has been used to stop purgings. A decoction of the whole herb has been found useful in arresting hemorrhage.

Buttercup

Ranunculus acris
　　Crowfoot.

HERB: Acrid. Antiseptic.

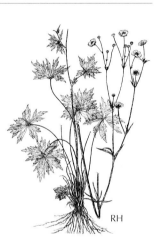

This plant is too acrid to be used internally, especially when fresh. When applied externally, it may be employed where conditions of counterirritation are indicated. Its action, however, is generally so violent that it is seldom used.

"This is the most common species in the N.E. and Can. In fields and pastures. June. Sept."

Butternut

Juglans cinerea
　　White Walnut. Oil Nut.
　　Lemon Walnut.

BARK (INNER): Cathartic.
　　Alterative. Deobstruent.
　　Tonic.
LEAVES: Cathartic. Alterative.
　　Deobstruent. Tonic.

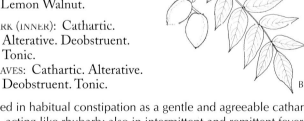

Used in habitual constipation as a gentle and agreeable cathartic, acting like rhubarb; also in intermittent and remittent fevers. The bark was used in the preparation of vegetable dyes, and candied butternut meats were an item in most of the Shaker sisters' shops.

Cancer Root

Orobanche uniflora
　　Beech Drops. Broom Rape.

ROOT: Astringent.
WHOLE PLANT: Astringent. Tonic.

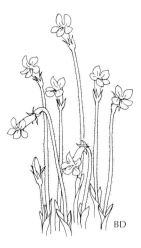

Beneficial in hemorrhage of the bowels or uterus, and in diarrhea. Valuable in erysipelas and, as a local application, to arrest the tendency of ulcers and wounds to gangrene. This is a plant that is parasitic upon the roots of beech trees. It flowers in August and September.

Canella

Canella winterana (C. alba)
　　White Wood. Wild Cinnamon.

BARK: Anodyne. Stomachic.

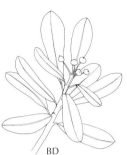

An aromatic bitter useful in enfeebled conditions of the stomach, and often given with other medicines.

Note: The Shakers bought this, as it is native only in the West Indies and Florida.

Canker Root

Prenanthes alba
　　Rattlesnake Root.

ROOT: Astringent. Tonic.

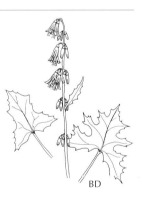

Used in diarrhea and relaxed and debilitated conditions of the bowels.

Canker Weed

Prenanthes serpentaria

HERB: Astringent. Tonic.

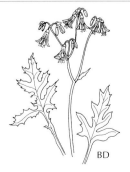

Useful as a mouthwash or gargle.

Caraway

Carum carvi

SEED: Aromatic. Carminitive. Tonic. Stomachic.

Used in flatulent colic of children, as a corrective to nauseous purgatives, and to improve flavor of disagreeable medicines. Used also as a potherb and as a spice in breads and cakes.

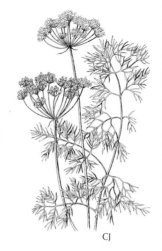

CJ

Cardamom

Elettaria cardamomum

SEED: Carminitive. Stimulant. Aromatic.

The seeds are useful in flatulency because of their warmth, but are rarely used alone. Used as a spice and also as a breath sweetener. Imported by the Shakers to resell.

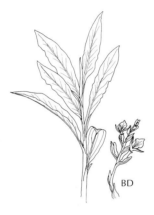

BD

Cardinal, Blue

Lobelia siphilitica
   Blue Lobelia. Blue Cardinal Flower.

HERB: Diuretic. Emetic. Cathartic. Herpatic. Deobstruent. Sudorific.

Used in gonorrhea, dropsy, diarrhea, and dysentery.

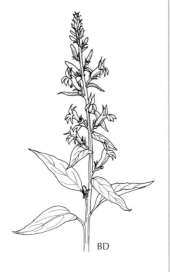

BD

Cardinal, Red

Lobelia cardinalis
   Hog Physic. Red Lobelia. Cardinal Flower. Indian Pink. Red Cardinal Flower.

HERB: Anthelmintic. Nervine. Antispasmodic. Cathartic. Diuretic. Emetic. Vermifuge.

Used in early days as a dye. Said to be useful in removing worms from the bowels.

"A fall species frequent in meadows and along streams. Can. to Car. [Carolinas] and west to Illinois. Stem from 2 to 4 feet. July and August."

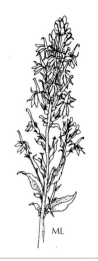

ML

Cardus, Spotted

Cnicus benedictus
   Blessed Thistle. Holy Thistle. Milk Thistle.

HERB: Tonic. Diaphoretic. Emetic. Diuretic.
ROOT: Tonic. Diaphoretic. Emetic.

Used as a tonic in loss of appetite, dyspepsia, and body coldness. Useful in producing copious perspiration when taken hot, for intermittent fevers. Taken double or triple strength, it becomes an emetic. The seeds are also considered therapeutic.

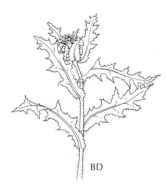

BD

Carpenter's Square

Scrophularia marilandica
   Heal-All. Square Stalk. Figwort. Scrofula.

LEAVES: Deobstruent. Tonic. Alterative.
ROOT: Deobstruent. Tonic. Alterative.

Used externally, in the form of an ointment, on bruises and scratches; internally as an alterative.

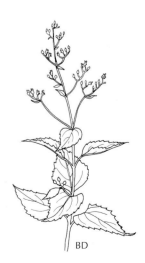

BD

Carrot, Wild

Daucus carota
Bee's Nest Seed. Queen Anne's Lace.

LEAVES: Stimulant. Diuretic. Carminitive. Emmenagogue. Deobstruent.
ROOT: Stimulant. Diuretic.
SEED: Stimulant. Diuretic. Carminitive. Emmenagogue. Deobstruent.

Used in dropsy, gravel and strangury, and as a poultice on foul and indolent ulcers.

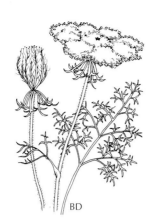

Castor Oil Plant

Ricinus communis
Castor Bean.

SEED: Cathartic.

The seeds are cathartic and yield castor oil.

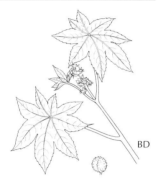

Catmint

Nepeta cataria
Catnip. Catnep.

HERB: Sudorific. Antispasmodic. Diaphoretic. Carminitive. Emmenagogue. Stomachic.

Useful in febrile, nervous, and infantile diseases; also to restore the menstrual secretions. Useful in flatulency and upset stomach. Cats eat it ravenously, being fond of it for its effect.

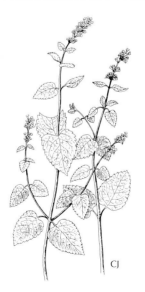

Cayenne

Capsicum annuum
Bird Pepper Chillies.

POWDER: Stimulant. Rubefacient. Erratic.

A stimulant that produces heat and redness of the skin and causes discharge at the nostrils. Used only in conjunction with other material, not alone. Grown in Africa, it was bought by the Shakers for use and resale.

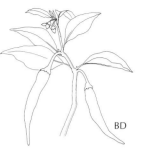

Cedar, Red

Juniperus virginiana

APPLES: Anthelmintic.
LEAVES: Stimulant. Diuretic.

Used in kidney complaints, suppression of urine, and obstructed menstruation.

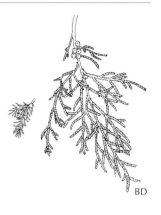

Celandine, Garden

Chelidonium majus
Tetterwort. Turmeric. Great Celandine.

HERB: Cathartic. Acrid. Alterative. Stimulant. Diuretic. Diaphoretic. Herpatic.

Used in scrofula, cutaneous diseases, piles, and affections of the spleen. The juice is used to cure warts, ringworms, and fungus growths.

"Grows by road sides and fences. Hast abundant bright yellow juice. It is used to distroy warts. May–Oct."

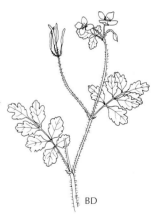

Celandine, Wild

Impatiens pallida

Jewelweed. Touch-Me-Not. Balsamweed. Slipperweed.

HERB: Antiperiodic. Diuretic. Antibilious. Stomachic.

Recommended in jaundice, dropsy, liver complaint, and salt rheum, and to cleanse foul ulcers. Used internally as decoction or tincture and externally as poultice or ointment.

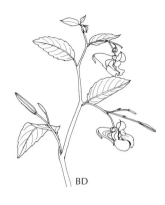

BD

Centaury, American

Sabatia angularis

Red Centaury. Rose Pink. Bitter Clover. Eyebright. Bitter Bloom. Wild Succory.

HERB: Tonic. Astringent. Stomachic.

Useful in autumnal fevers, dyspepsia, and worms, and to restore the menstrual secretion. Should be gathered during flowering season. An excellent tonic; serviceable as a bitter tonic in dyspepsia and convalescence. Should be administered in warm infusion.

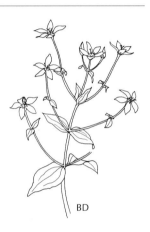

BD

Chamomile

Chamaemelum nobile (Anthemis nobilis)

Roman Chamomile. Mayweed.

FLOWERS: Tonic. Aromatic. Stimulant. Emetic. Febrifuge. Sudorific.

Used in dyspepsia, weak stomach, intermittent and typhus fevers, hysteria, and nervousness. When used as a tea, it is the flower that is used. The cold infusion is used as a hair rinse — not a dye but a brightener.

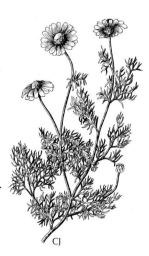

CJ

Chamomile, Low

Anthemis arvensis

Garden Chamomile. Corn Chamomile.

HERB: Tonic. Stomachic.

Employed in fevers, colds, and to produce perspiration.

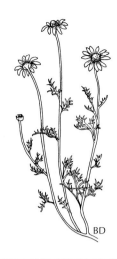

BD

Checkerberry

Gaultheria procumbens

Mountain Tea. Deer Berry. Tea Berry. Box Berry. Wintergreen.

LEAVES: Stimulant. Aromatic. Astringent. Diuretic. Stomachic. Emetic.

Valuable in dropsy and diarrhea. The oil was used to flavor other medicines. The essence was used for colic in infants.

"Common in woods and pastures. Can. to Ky. June and Sept."

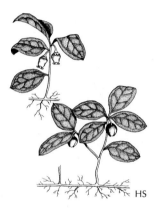

HS

Cherry, Wild

Prunus serotina

Black Cherry. Choke-Cherry. Virginia Prune.

CHERRIES: Febrifuge. Astringent. Tonic. Antiseptic. Pectoral. Stomachic. Sedative.
BARK: Astringent. Tonic. Antiseptic.

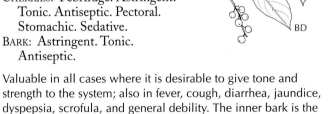

BD

Valuable in all cases where it is desirable to give tone and strength to the system; also in fever, cough, diarrhea, jaundice, dyspepsia, scrofula, and general debility. The inner bark is the part used medicinally. The outside layer of the bark should be removed; the green layer is then stripped off and carefully dried. Young thin bark is the best.

Chestnut

Castanea dentata (Cerastium vulgatum)

LEAVES: Astringent. Tonic. Febrifuge.

Used a remedy in fevers and for its tonic and astringent properties. The Shakers also used chestnut leaves in the preparation of vegetable dyes and sold them for this purpose.

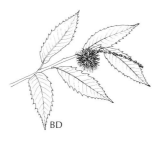

Chickweed

Stellaria media
  Mouse Ear.

HERB: Refrigerant. Emollient. Demulcent.

Used as a poultice for old and indolent ulcers and with benefit also in ophthalmia, erysipelas, and cutaneous diseases. It is a cooling demulcent. The fresh leaves are bruised and applied as a poultice. An ointment may be made by bruising young leaves in fresh lard, and used for skin irritations.

"Grows in fields and wash grounds. Can. and U.S. Flowering all summer."

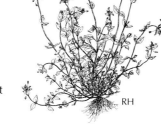

Chicory

Cichorium intybus
  Succory. Wild Succory. Endive. Centaury.

ROOT: Tonic. Diuretic. Laxative. Stomachic.
HERB: Tonic. Diuretic. Laxative.

Used in jaundice and liver complaints. A tea made of the dried root is good for sour stomach. It may be taken whenever the stomach has been upset by any kind of food.

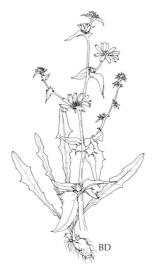

Cholic Root

Dioscorea villosa
  Colic Root. Rheumatism Root. Wild Yam.

ROOT: Antispasmodic. Diuretic. Expectorant.

Used in biliary colic. In large doses, it seems to be diuretic and to act as an expectorant.

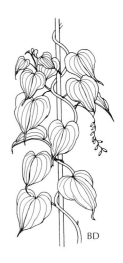

Cicely, Sweet

Osmorhiza longistylis
  Anise Root. Sweet Anise. Sweet Javril.

ROOT: Aromatic. Stomachic. Carminitive. Expectorant.

Useful in coughs and flatulence, and as a gentle stimulant tonic to debilitated stomachs.

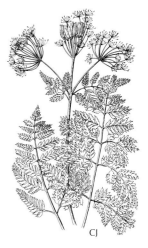

Cicuta

Conium maculatum
  Spotted Cowbane. Beaver Poison. Musquash Root. Poison Hemlock. Poison Parsley. Water Hemlock. Poison Root. Spotted Hemlock.

LEAVES: Narcotic. Anodyne. Antispasmodic. Discutient. Deobstruent.
SEED: Narcotic. Anodyne. Antispasmodic. Discutient.

Used in chronic rheumatism, neuralgia, asthma, an excited condition of the nervous system. Use cautiously; it is a virulent poison suitable for use only by a skilled physician.

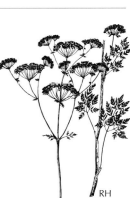

Cinchona

Cinchona pubescens (C. succirubra)
Peruvian Bark. Foso Bark. Red Bark. Crown Bark.

BARK: Tonic. Antiperiodic. Astringent. Febrifuge.

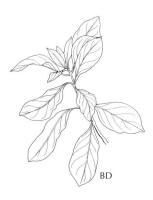

Useful as a tonic and antiperiodic; moderately astringent and eminently febrifuge. Used freely as a mouthwash and gargle and given internally as a remedy for malaria. Taken internally, it imparts a sensation of warmth to the stomach and fights fevers.

Cinnamon

Cinnamomum zeylanicum

OIL: Germicide.
POWDERED SPICE: Food preservative.

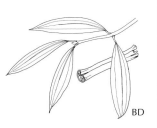

Several Shaker societies used it, but did not list it in their catalogs.

Clary

Salvia sclarea
Clammy Sage. Clarry.

HERB: Antispasmodic. Balsamic. Stomachic. Diaphoretic. Diuretic. Stimulant.

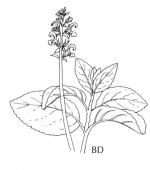

Used in night sweats, hectic fever, and flatulence. Also used in the making of wine and beer — especially the fresh flowers, which give a distinctive flavor to raisin wine and sweeten it. The leaves and flowers are more highly scented than common sage, and are used in sachets and potpourri.

Cleavers

Galium aparine
Goose Grass. Clivers. Catch Weed. Bed Straw. Rough Cleavers.

HERB: Refrigerant. Diuretic. Sudorific.

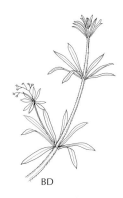

Valuable in curing suppression of urine, and to cure inflammation of kidney and bladder. As a wash it was used to remove freckles.

"Common in thickets and low ground. Can. and U.S. July."

Clover, Red

Trifolium pratense
Sweet Clover. King's Clover. Clover Blows.

BLOSSOMS: Acrid. Pectoral. Expectorant. Diuretic.

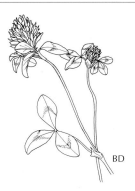

An extract of the blossoms is an excellent remedy for cancerous ulcers, corns, and burns.

Clover, White

Melilotus alba
Sweet White Clover. Sweet Melilot.

BLOSSOMS: Expectorant. Diuretic.

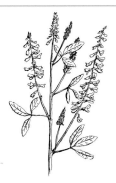

Used in chest complaints. Also used to flavor cheese and tobacco.

Clover, Yellow

Trifolium agrarium

BLOSSOMS: Expectorant. Diuretic.

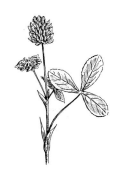

Used for the same purposes as white clover. Very sweet and pleasant in sachets and potpourri mixtures.

"In dry soils. N.H. [New Hampshire] to Va. [Virginia]. Flowers at length reflexed. June, July."

Cloves

Syzygium aromaticum (Eugenia caryophyllata)

BUD: Astringent.

Imported or bought from importers by Shakers and offered for sale. Used in cooking, for preparing foods for storage, and for astringent purposes. (See Cinnamon.)

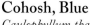
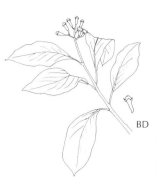

Cocash

Aster puniceus

Squaw Weed. Life Root. Cocash Weed. Red Stalked Aster. Cold Water Root. September Weed.

ROOT: Sudorific. Stomachic. Stimulant. Diaphoretic. Tonic. Astringent. Diuretic. Carminitive.

The warm infusion is used for colds, rheumatism, nervous debility, headache, and menstrual irregularities.

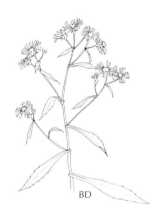

Cohosh, Black

Cimicifuga racemosa

Rattle Root. Black Snake Root. Bugbane. Rattle Weed. Squaw Root. Baneberry.

ROOT: Deobstruent. Alterative. Antiperiodic. Narcotic. Nervine. Diaphoretic. Diuretic. Sedative. Antispasmodic.

Useful for rheumatism, dropsy, epilepsy, and spasmodic affections. Valuable in female complaints and as a postpartum accelerator. Its leaves are said to drive away bugs. Boiling water absorbs the properties of the root only partially, but alcohol absorbs them completely. A purifying tea and pectoral syrup.

Cohosh, Blue

Caulophyllum thalictroides

Squaw Root. Papoose Root. Blue Berry.

ROOT: Stimulant. Antispasmodic. Diuretic. Diaphoretic. Parturient. Emmenagogue. Anthelmintic.

A favorite remedy in chronic uterine diseases. As a parturient it has proved invaluable. Also used in rheumatism, dropsy, cramps, colic, and hysterics. The seeds, which ripen in August, make a decoction that closely resembles coffee.

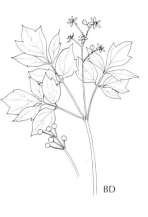

Cohosh, Red

Actaea rubra

ROOT: Diuretic. Diaphoretic. Anthelmintic. Deobstruent. Narcotic.

Used in uterine diseases, rheumatism, dropsy, and colic.

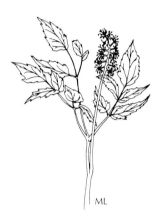

Cohosh, White

Actaea pachypoda (A. alba)

Necklace Weed. Bane Berry. Noah's Ark.

ROOT: Purgative. Emmenagogue. Deobstruent. Narcotic. Carminitive.

A decoction useful for the itch. Also used in rheumatism, flatulence, and nervous irritability.

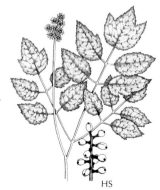

Colchicum

Colchicum autumnale
Meadow Saffron. Autumn
Crocus.

ROOT: Acrid. Narcotic. Sedative.
Cathartic. Diuretic. Emetic.
SEED: Acrid. Narcotic. Sedative.
Cathartic. Diuretic. Emetic.

Used in gout, rheumatism, palpitation of the heart, gonorrhea, and
enlarged prostate. Should be used
cautiously.

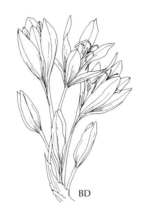

Colombo, American

Cocculus carolinis
Indian Lettuce. Pyramid
Flower. Meadow Pride. Yellow
Gentian. American Colombo.

ROOT: Tonic. Cathartic. Emetic.

An excellent tonic, which may be
used in all cases where a mild
cathartic or emetic is required.

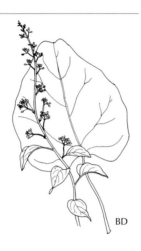

Coltsfoot

Tussilago farfara
Bullsfoot. Ginger Root.
Coughwort.

LEAVES AND FLOWERS: Emollient.
Demulcent. Tonic. Pectoral.
Expectorant.
ROOT: Emollient. Demulcent.
Tonic.

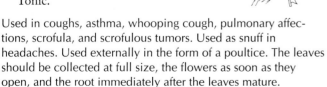

Used in coughs, asthma, whooping cough, pulmonary affections, scrofula, and scrofulous tumors. Used as snuff in
headaches. Used externally in the form of a poultice. The leaves
should be collected at full size, the flowers as soon as they
open, and the root immediately after the leaves mature.

*"In wet places, brooksides and on the shore of lakes. North and
Middle States. It grows in clayey soil. The flower appears in
early spring before a leaf is to be seen. Early Spring."*

Comfrey

Symphytum officinale
Gum Plant. Healing Herb.
Slippery Root.

ROOT: Demulcent. Astringent.
Balsamic. Pectoral.

Useful in diarrhea, dysentery,
coughs, leukorrhea, and female
debility; as an application to bruises, fresh wounds, sores, and burns,
and in nasal congestion or catarrh.

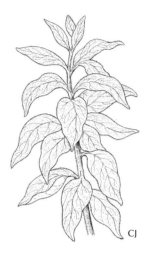

Consumption Brake

Botrychium lunaria
Moonwort.

ROOT: Astringent. Stimulant.
Tonic.

Used in diarrhea and dysentery, and
to prevent mucus discharges.

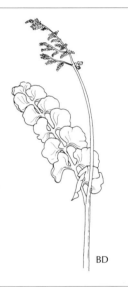

Coolwort

Mitella diphylla (M. cordifolia)
Mitrewort. Bishops-Cap.

HERB: Diaphoretic. Tonic.
Diuretic.

Valuable in strangury, diabetes,
and all kidney complaints.

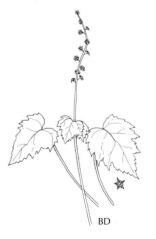

Coriander

Coriandrum sativum

SEED: Stomachic. Stimulant. Carminitive.

Used to flavor and correct the action of other medicines. In syrup, used for pain in the stomach and side. The Shakers imported it or bought it for resale.

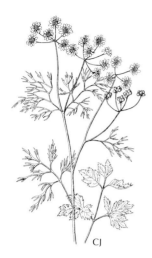

Cotton Root

Gossypium herbaceum

BARK OF ROOT: Emmenagogue. Parturient. Abortive.

Said to promote uterine contractions as efficiently as the herb ergot, and with perfect safety. The seed is used in fever and ague. It should not be employed by the unskilled. Although a native of Asia, it was cultivated in the southern portion of America more successfully than anywhere else.

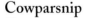

Cowparsnip

Heracleum sphondylium subsp. *montanum (H. lanatum)*

LEAVES: Nervine. Carminitive. Diuretic. Aromatic. Stomachic.
ROOT: Carminitive. Diuretic. Nervine. Narcotic. Stomachic.
SEED: Carminitive. Aromatic. Nervine. Stomachic. Diuretic.

Useful as a diuretic and to expel wind.

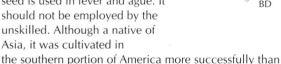

Cowparsnip, Royal

Imperatoria ostruthium
Masterwort. Golden Alexanders.

LEAVES: Antispasmodic. Tonic.
ROOT: Antispasmodic. Tonic.
SEED: Carminitive. Aromatic.

Used in asthma, colic, palsy, and apoplexy. The Shakers produced the extract in vast quantities.

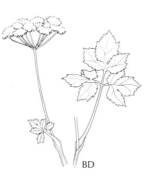

Cramp Bark

Viburnum trilobus
High Cranberry. Squawbush.

BARK: Antispasmodic.

Very effective in relaxing cramps and spasms in asthma, hysteria, pains incident to females during pregnancy, convulsions, etc. A poultice of the fruit is said to be efficacious when applied to the throat for minor irritations.

"A handsome shrub, in woods and borders of fields. Northern States and British Am. June."

Cranesbill

Geranium maculatum
Spotted Geranium. Crowfoot [not to be confounded with crowfoot of the *Ranunculus* family]. Alumroot. Dovefoot. American Tormentilla. Storksbill.

ROOT: Astringent. Styptic. Tonic.

A powerful astringent used in dysentery, diarrhea, cholera infantum, hemorrhage, canker, and also as a gargle.

"In dry rocky places. Can. to Va. Stem reddish. It has a disagreeable smell. May to Sept."

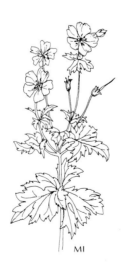

Crawley

Corallorhiza odontorhiza

Dragon's Claw. Coral Root. Fever Root. Chickentoe.

ROOT: Sedative. Febrifuge. Diaphoretic. Balsamic. Stomachic.

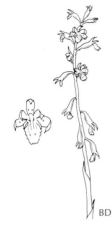

Invaluable in low typhoid fever and intermittent fever, pleurisy, and night sweats. One of the most prompt and satisfactory diaphoretics in the materia medica, but its scarcity and high price have tended to keep it from coming into general use. It can be combined with blue cohosh, and also with black root or mayapple to act upon the bowels. Mixed with colicroot, it is helpful in flatulent and bilious colic.

Cuckold

Bidens frondosa

Swamp Beggar's Tick. Beggar Lice. Harvest Lice. Spanish Needles. Cow Lice. Leafy Burr Mangold.

HERB: Astringent. Diuretic. Carminitive. Emmenagogue. Expectorant.

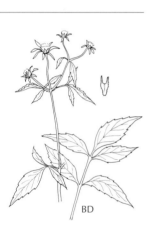

Used in palpitation of the heart, cough, and uterine derangement. Roots or seeds are also used as an expectorant in throat irritation.

Culver's Root

Veronicastrum virginicum (Leptandra virginica)

Blackroot. Tall Speedwell. Culver's Physic. Tall Veronica. Leptandra.

ROOT: Cathartic. Deobstruent. Tonic. Diuretic.

The fresh root is too irritating to be employed, but the dried root is laxative, cholagogic, and tonic. Its medicinal virtues are stronger when the roots are dug from plants growing in limestone areas. It should be gathered in the fall of its second year.

Daffodil

Narcissus pseudonarcissus

Daffy-Downdillies.

ROOT: Emetic. Cathartic.

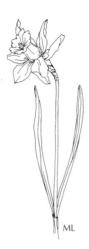

Powdered, the roots act as an emetic and afterward as a purge, and are excellent for use in all obstructions.

Daisy, White

Chrysanthemum leucanthemum (Leucanthemum vulgare)

White Weed. Ox-Eye Daisy.

FLOWERS: Tonic. Diuretic. Antispasmodic. Emetic. Vulnerary.

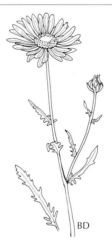

Used in whooping cough, asthma, nervousness, and leukorrhea, and as a local application to wounds and cutaneous diseases.

Dandelion

Taraxacum officinale

Blow Ball. Cankerwort.

HERB: Antibilious. Stomachic. Alterative. Tonic. Diuretic. Cathartic. Deobstruent.

ROOT: Astringent. Stomachic. Alterative. Tonic. Diuretic. Cathartic. Deobstruent.

Recommended in diseases of the liver, and in constipation, dropsy, diseases of the skin, and uterine obstructions. Should be collected when the plant is in flower. The young plant possesses some slight narcotic properties. The dried root, when fresh, is a stomachic and tonic with slightly diuretic and aperient actions.

Dill

Anethum graveolens
  Dillseed. Dilly.

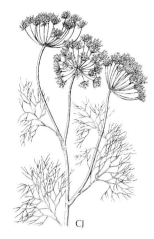

SEED: Carminitive. Aromatic. Stomachic. Expectorant.

Used in flatulence and colic, to stop hiccups, and to expel gas. Also used in cooking.

Dittany

Cunila origanoides (C. mariana)
  Stone Mint. Mountain Dittany. American Dittany. Wild Basil.

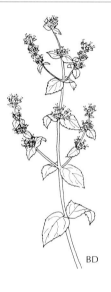

LEAVES: Diaphoretic. Stimulant. Nervine. Carminitive. Antispasmodic. Aromatic. Tonic. Sudorific.
FLOWERS: Diaphoretic. Stimulant. Nervine. Carminitive. Antispasmodic. Aromatic. Tonic. Sudorific.

Used in a warm infusion for colds, headache, fevers, colic, and nervous affections. The warm tea is diaphoretic.

Dock, Broadleaf

Rumex obtusifolius

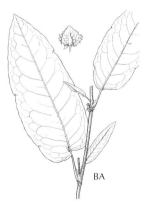

ROOT: Tonic. Cathartic. Deobstruent. Herpatic.

A purge and tonic. Useful when the blood needs purifying.

Dock, Water

Rumex aquaticus
  Great Water Dock. Sour Dock. Narrow Dock.

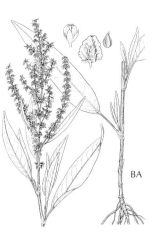

ROOT: Detergent. Alterative. Deobstruent. Herpatic. Astringent. Diaphoretic.

Useful in diseases of an eruptive nature; used in ointment form for itching.

Dock Root, Yellow

Rumex crispus
  Sour Dock. Narrow Dock. Curled Dock. Rumex.

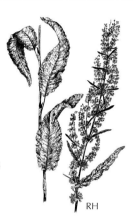

ROOT: Detergent. Alterative. Deobstruent. Herpatic. Tonic. Astringent.

Useful in scrofula, syphilis, leprosy, and diseases of an eruptive nature; as an ointment for itching and indolent glandular tumors; and in all cases where the blood needs purifying. There are two other varieties of dock, *Rumex aquaticus* (water dock) and *Rumex obtusifolius* (broadleaf dock), but yellow dock is the only one entitled to extensive consideration. It is a very rich source of digestible plant iron.

Dog Grass

Agropyron repens
  Witch Grass. Quick Grass. Couch Grass. Scratch Grass. Triticum. Durfa Grass.

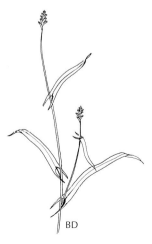

ROOT: Diuretic. Aperient. Demulcent. Tonic. Cathartic. Febrifuge.

Useful in conditions in which it is desirable to promote or increase the flow of urine. Large and frequent doses are considered a good tonic in the spring. Kills worms in children.

"A rough species. Flowers white. Can. and U.S. June."

Dogwood
Cornus sericea
> Boxwood. Green Ozier.
> Flowering Cornel. Rose Willow.

BARK: Astringent. Stimulant.
Tonic.
FLOWERS: Astringent. Stimulant.
Tonic.

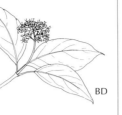

The bark should be used in its dried state. Cornine, the active principle, is used occasionally as a substitute for quinine. Dogwood exerts its virtues best in the form of an ointment.

Dragon Root
Arisaema triphyllum (Arum triphyllum)
> Jack-in-the-Pulpit. Wild
> Turnip. Indian Turnip. Wake
> Robin.

ROOT: Diaphoretic. Stimulant.
Acrid. Narcotic. Expectorant.

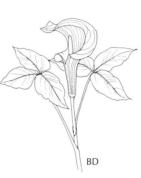

It is acrid, and used as an expectorant; it is also diaphoretic. It is used as well for lung diseases. The root should be used fresh, but must be partially dried, as it loses its strength with age.

Elder
Sambucus canadensis
> Sweet Elder. American Elder.
> Panicle Elder Sambucus.

BARK: Cathartic. Deobstruent.
Diuretic. Sudorific. Herpatic.
Nervine.
BERRIES: Cathartic. Alterative.
Aperient.
FLOWERS: Diaphoretic.
Stimulant. Diuretic.
Sudorific. Herpatic.
Alterative.

The bark is used in dropsy and erysipelas, and as an alterative in various chronic complaints; the berries are used in rheumatism and gouty affections. The flowers are used in erysipelas, fevers, and constipation.

"A common shrub 6 to 10 ft. high in hilly pastures and woods, U.S. and Can. Berries dark purple. May. July."

Elder, Dwarf
Aralia hispida
> Wild Elder. Bristlestem
> Sarsaparilla.

ROOT: Diuretic. Alterative.
Demulcent. Tonic. Diaphoretic.

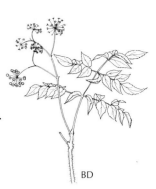

Very valuable in dropsy, gravel, suppression of urine, and other urinary disorders.

Elecampane
Inula helenium
> Scabwort.

ROOT: Diaphoretic. Diuretic.
Expectorant. Astringent.
Stomachic. Tonic. Stimulant.

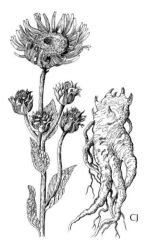

Much used in cough, colds, lung diseases, weakness of the digestive organs, and dyspepsia; also in tetter, itching, and cutaneous diseases. The root should be gathered in its second year, during the fall months.

Elm, Slippery
Ulmus rubra (U. fulva)
> Red Elm. Indian Elm. Sweet
> Elm. Moose Elm.

BARK, INNER: Emollient.
Diuretic. Demulcent.
Expectorant. Tonic.
GROUND: Emollient. Diuretic.
Demulcent. Expectorant.
Tonic.
FLOUR: Emollient. Diuretic.
Demulcent. Expectorant.
Tonic.

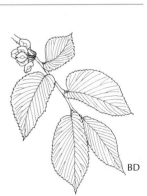

Highly beneficial in dysentery, diarrhea, and inflammation of the lungs, bowels, stomach, bladder, or kidneys; also as poultice for skin irritation. The bark is chewed for sore throats. (The tree is not to be confused with American elm.)

Ergot
Secale cereale (S. cornatum)
    Spurred Rye. Smut Rye.

SEED: (Degenerated Seeds of
    Common Rye) Acrid.

Used to promote uterine contractions.

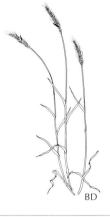

Euphorbia
Euphorbia ipecacuanhae
    Spreading Spurge. Dysentery-
    Weed. Milk Purslane.
    American Ipecac.

ROOT: Astringent. Emetic.
    Cathartic. Tonic. Diaphoretic.
    Expectorant.

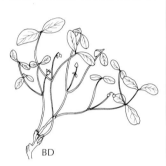

Valuable in bilious colic, dropsical affections, dyspepsia, jaundice, and sluggishness of the liver.

Fennel
Foeniculum vulgare
    Wild Fennel. Sweet Fennel.
    Large Fennel.

SEED: Aromatic. Carminitive.
    Stimulant. Diuretic. Pectoral.

Used to expel wind from the
bowels. A good aromatic; used to
flavor other medicines.

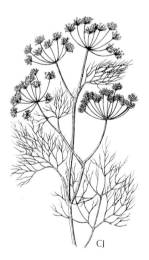

Fern, Maidenhair
Adiantum pedatum

HERB: Carminitive. Refrigerant.
    Expectorant. Tonic. Sudorific.
    Astringent. Pectoral.
    Stomachic.

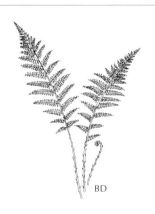

Valuable in cough, asthma,
hoarseness, influenza, pleurisy,
jaundice, febrile diseases, and
erysipelas. A decoction of the
plant is cooling and of benefit in
coughs resulting from colds, nasal congestion, catarrh, and
hoarseness. It can be used freely.

*"A beautiful fern, abounding in damp rocky woods. Stalk glossy
purple, approaching to a jet black. July."*

Fern, Male
Dryopteris filix-mas
    Male Shield Fern.

ROOT: Vermifuge. Tonic.
    Astringent.

Valuable to expel tapeworm.

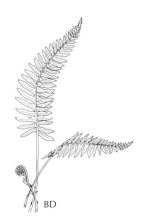

Fern, Polypody
Polypodium vulgare
    Rock Polypod. Rock Brake.
    Brake Root. Female Fern.

ROOT AND TOP: Pectoral.
    Demulcent. Purgative.
    Anthelmintic. Cathartic.

Used in pulmonary and hepatic
complaint; also used to expel
worms.

*"On shady rocks and in woods
forming tangled patches. July."*

Fern, Sweet

Comptonia peregrina
(C. asplenifolia)

Spleenwort Bush. Fern Gale.
Sweet Fern. Sweet Bush.

HERB: Tonic. Astringent.
Alterative. Stomachic.

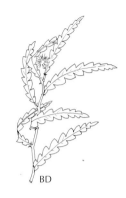

Useful in cholera infantum, dysentery, leukorrhea, and debility following fevers, bruises, and rheumatism. Also, because of its tonic and astringent properties, it is successful in diarrhea.

"A well known handsome aromatic shrub common in pastures and on hillsides. The main stem is covered with a rusty brown bark which becomes reddish in the branches, and white downy in the young shoots. Leaves numerous. Fertile flowers in a dense rounded burr or head situated below the barren ones. May."

Feverbush

Lindera benzoin

Wild Allspice. Spice Bush.
Snap Wood. Fever Wood.
Benjamin Bush.

LEAVES: Aromatic. Tonic.
Stimulant. Vermifuge.
Febrifuge. Nervine. Stomachic.

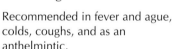

Recommended in fever and ague, colds, coughs, and as an anthelmintic.

Feverfew

Chrysanthemum parthenium
Featherfew.

HERB: Tonic. Carminitive.
Emmenagogue. Vermifuge.
Stimulant. Nervine.
Stomachic.

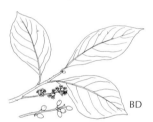

A warm infusion is used for recent colds, flatulency, worms, irregular menstruation, hysterics, and suppression of urine.

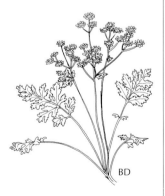

Feverroot

Triosteum perfoliatum

Wild Ipecac. Horse Gentian.
Tinker's Weed. Wild Coffee.

ROOT: Tonic. Cathartic. Emetic.
Diuretic.

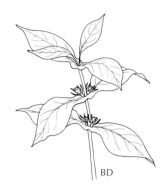

Used in fever and ague, pleurisy, dyspepsia, and rheumatism.

Fireweed

Erechtites hieracifolia
Pilewort.

HERB: Astringent. Emetic.
Cathartic. Tonic. Alterative.
Vulnerary. Deobstruent.
ROOT: Astringent. Emetic.
Cathartic. Tonic. Alterative.
Vulnerary. Deobstruent.

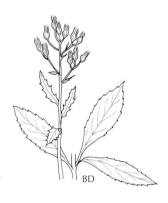

Excellent in diseases of the mucous tissues of the lungs, stomach, and bowels, summer gastric complaint of children, piles, hemorrhage, and dysentery.

Fitsroot

Monotropa uniflora

Pipe Plant. Bird's Nest. Ice
Plant. Indian Pipe. Fit Plant.
Dutchman's Pipe. Ghostflower.
Ova Ova.

ROOT: Antispasmodic. Tonic.
Sedative. Nervine.

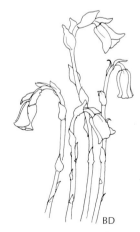

The whole plant is ivory white, resembling frozen jelly, and when handled, melts away like ice.

Five-Finger Grass

Potentilla canadensis
  Cinquefoil.

LEAVES: Tonic. Astringent.
  Emmenagogue.
ROOT: Tonic. Astringent.
  Emmenagogue.

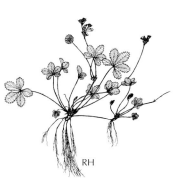

Useful in fevers, bowel complaints, night sweats, spongy gums, sore mouth, and hemorrhages, and can be brewed as a tea. Excellent as a mouthwash and gargle. The root is used for a red dye.

"Common in fields and in thickets U.S. and Canada. Apr. Aug."

Flax

Linum usitatissimum
  Linseed. Lint Bells. Toad Flax.

SEED: Demulcent. Emollient.

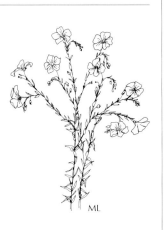

Useful internally in coughs resulting from colds. The ground seed, used in combination with elm bark, makes an excellent poultice for general use. The flowers are used for yellow dye.

"A very showy plant common by road sides, N. Eng. to Ky. and Ga. 1 to 2 ft. high, very leafy. July. Aug."

Fleabane

Erigeron canadensis (E. canadense)
  Colt's Tail. Pride Weed. Scabious. Horse Weed. Butter Weed.

HERB: Tonic. Diuretic. Styptic. Astringent. Aromatic. Narcotic.

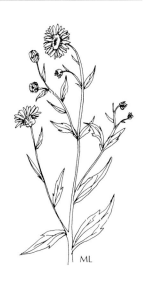

Efficient in diarrhea, gravel, diabetes, urine scald, hemorrhage of bowels or uterus, and bleeding of wounds. Should be gathered when in bloom.

"By roadsides and in fields throughout North America. Aug. Nov."

Flower De Luce

Iris sambucina
  Fleur-De-Lis. Blue Flag. Water Flag.

ROOT: Diuretic. Deobstruent. Diaphoretic. Narcotic. Alterative. Cathartic.

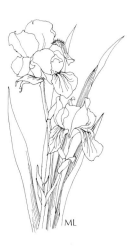

A useful cathartic and used as an alterative, often combined with mandrake, poke, or black cohosh. It will sometimes cause salivation but need cause no apprehension.

Foxglove

Digitalis purpurea

HERB: Narcotic. Diuretic. Sedative. Diaphoretic.

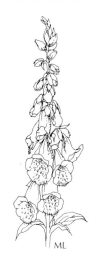

An active remedy in neuralgia, insanity, febrile diseases, acute inflammatory complaints, dropsy, palpitation of the heart, and asthma. Should be used only on the advice of a physician.

"A showy plant 2 to 4 ft. high. In woods throughout the U.S. Aug. and Sept."

Frostwort

Helianthemum canadense
  Rock Rose. Frost Plant. Scrofula Weed.

HERB: Tonic. Astringent. Antiscorbutic.

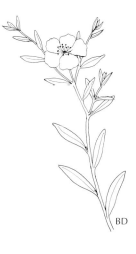

A valuable remedy in scrofula, syphilis, cancerous affections, and as a gargle in scarlatina and canker; and as a wash in ophthalmia, itching, and cutaneous diseases. Used in the form of a decoction, syrup, or fluid extract. In combination with the herb stillingia it is more valuable.

Fumitory

Fumaria officinalis
> Hedge Fumitory. Earth Smoke. Fumatory.

HERB: Tonic. Diaphoretic. Antiperiodic. Alterative. Diuretic. Laxative. Deobstruent.

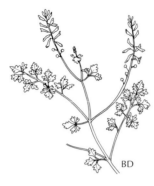

Used in jaundice, obstruction of the bowels, scurvy, and general debility of the digestive organs. A wineglass of an infusion of the leaves is usually given every four hours.

Galangal

Alpinia galangal
> East India Catarrh Root. Catarrh Root. Kassamak Root.

ROOT: Aromatic. Stimulant.

An aromatic stimulant. Has been used as a snuff in catarrh and nervous headache. Somewhat similar to ginger.

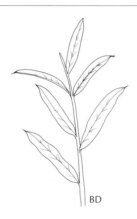

Garget

Phytolacca americana (P. decandra)
> Pigeon Berry. Poke. Poke Root. Skole. Scoke Root. Coakum.

BERRIES: Emetic. Narcotic. Cathartic. Alterative. Acrid. Deobstruent.
LEAVES: Emetic. Narcotic. Cathartic. Alterative. Acrid. Deobstruent.
ROOT: Emetic. Narcotic. Cathartic. Alterative. Acrid. Deobstruent.

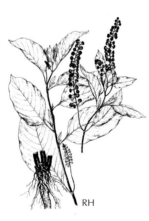

Valuable in chronic rheumatism, syphilis, scrofula, and as an ointment in itching and scab head.

Garlic

Allium sativum

BULB: Stimulant. Diuretic. Expectorant. Rubefacient. Tonic.

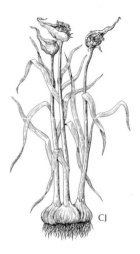

Recommended in cough, asthma, catarrh, hoarseness; promotes activity of the excretory organs. Externally it is used as a counter-irritant in pulmonary affections.

Gelsemium

Gelsemium sempervirens
> Yellow Jasmine. Wild Woodbine. False Jasmine. Yellow Jessamine.

ROOT: Sedative. Antispasmodic. Diaphoretic. Febrifuge.

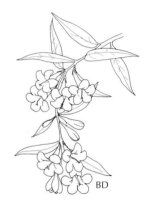

A powerful spinal depressant. A poison.

Gentian, Blue-Fringed

Gentianopsis crinita (Gentiana crinita)

ROOT: Tonic. Stomachic. Aromatic.

A powerful tonic; improves the appetite, aids digestion, and gives force to the circulation. Used in dyspepsia, jaundice, gout, scrofula, and fever and ague.

"Not uncommon in cool, low grounds. Can. to Car. August."

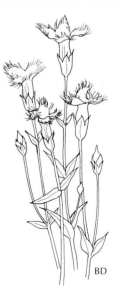

Ginger

Asarum canadense
Wild Ginger. Canada
Snakeroot.

LEAVES: Stimulant. Aromatic.
Diuretic. Emetic. Cathartic.
ROOT: Stimulant. Aromatic.
Diuretic. Purgative.

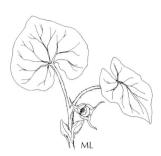

The root is useful to flavor meats
and fish. Ground, it is a reliable
digestive, which also increases
the flow of urine. The leaves and
roots act upon the bowels.

Ginger, African

Zingiber officinalis
Jamaica Ginger.

ROOT: Stomachic. Tonic.
Stimulant. Rubefacient.
Erratic. Sialogogue.

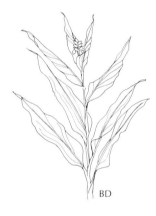

Valuable in diarrhea, dysentery,
cholera, cholera morbus, habitual
flatulency, and dyspepsia, and to
relieve pains in the bowels and
stomach. Also to prevent the griping of cathartic medicines.

Ginseng

Panax quinquefolius
Ninsin. Chinese Seng. Five
Fingers. Garantogen.

ROOT: Tonic. Stimulant. Nervine.
Sialogogue.

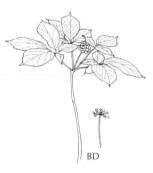

Useful in loss of appetite, nervous
debility, weak stomach, asthma,
and gravel. Also, it increases the
flow of saliva.

Goldenrod

Solidago odora
Sweet Scented Goldenrod. Blue
Mountain Tea.

HERB: Stimulant. Carminitive.
Diaphoretic. Aromatic. Diuretic.

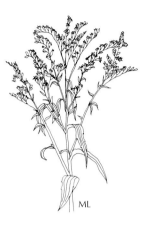

Used in flatulent colic, stomach sickness, convalescence from severe diarrhea, dysentery, cholera morbus,
dropsy, gravel, and urinary difficulties. As a tea it is diaphoretic when
taken warm. It is excellent to use to
disguise the taste of medicinal herbs.

Goldenseal

Hydrastis canadensis
Yellow Puccoon. Ohio Curcuma.
Ground Raspberry. Eye Balm.
Orange Root. Turmeric Root.

ROOT: Tonic. Stomachic. Aperient.
Antibilious. Cathartic.

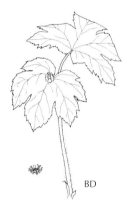

Invaluable in dyspepsia, erysipelas;
remittent, intermittent, and typhoid
fevers; torpor of the liver, ulceration
of the mouth, ophthalmia, and spermatorrhea. A good mouthwash. The
powder may be boiled in water and sniffed up into the nostrils
for nasal congestion. As a dye, goldenseal imparts a rich durable
light yellow of great brilliancy, which, when used with different
mordants, gives all the shades of yellow from pale to orange.
With indigo it imparts a fine green to wool, silk, and cotton.

Goldthread

Coptis trifolia
Mouth Root. Canker Root.
Yellow Root.

ROOT: Tonic. Astringent.
Stomachic.

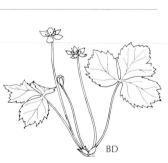

Valuable as a gargle in ulceration
of the mouth; used in dyspepsia,
and inflammation of the stomach, and with goldenseal to
destroy the appetite for intoxicating liquor. A pure, bitter tonic

*"Found from Artic Amer. to Penn. in shady woods. Stem creep-
ing, golden yellow very bitter. Peduncle bears a single, white
star like flower. May."*

Gravel Plant

Epigaea repens
> Trailing Arbutus. Winter Pink. Gravel Weed. Mountain Pink. Mayflower. Ground Laurel.

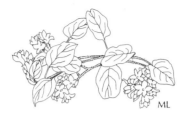

HERB: Diuretic. Astringent. Demulcent.

A remedy superior to buchu for gravel and all diseases of the urinary organs. The whole plant is used, but the leaves are especially useful.

"Found in the woods from Newfoundland to Ky. A little shrubby plant, grows flat on the ground. Flowers are very fragrant. Apr. May."

Hardhack

Spiraea tomentosa
> Meadow Sweet. White Leaf. Steeple Bush.

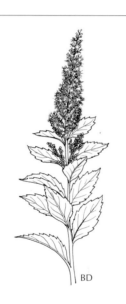

ROOT: Astringent. Tonic. Diuretic.
LEAVES: Astringent. Tonic. Diuretic.

Valuable in cholera infantum, dysentery, diarrhea, debility of the bowels, and to improve the digestion. Useful as an astringent tonic in diarrhea.

"A small shrub, common in pastures and low grounds, Can. and U.S. The fruit in winter furnishes food for the snow-birds. July. Aug."

Harvest-Lice

Bidens connata
> Cockhold Herb. Beggar's Tick. Swamp Beggar's Tick.

HERB: Astringent. Tonic.

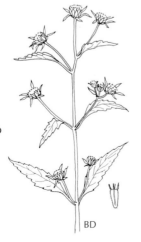

The roots and seeds are employed domestically as an emmenagogue to some extent, as well as for the purposes of an expectorant in throat irritation.

Heal-All

Prunella vulgaris
> Self-Heal. Figwort. Stone Root.

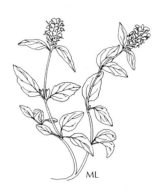

HERB: Astringent.

Valuable in hemorrhages, and for gargle in canker and sore throat.

Heart's Ease

Polygonum persicaria
> Ladies' Thump. Spotted Knot Weed.

HERB: Sudorific. Febrifuge. Diuretic.

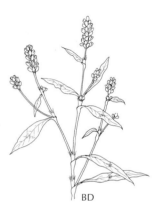

Said to be useful in asthma, colds, and fevers. Useful as a diuretic.

Hellebore, Black

Helleborus niger
> Christmas Rose.

ROOT: Drastic. Cathartic. Diuretic. Emmenagogue. Anthelmintic.

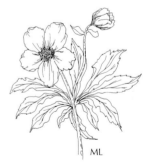

Used in palsy, insanity, apoplexy, dropsy, epilepsy, chlorosis, amenorrhea. In large doses it is a powerful poison.

Hellebore, White
Veratrum viride

Swamp Hellebore. American Hellebore. False Hellebore. Itch Weed. Indian Poke.

ROOT: Narcotic. Sedative. Diaphoretic. Emetic. Nervine. Acrid.

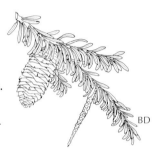

Valuable as an arterial sedative in pneumonia, typhoid fever, and itching, but only on the advice of a physician. The powder or decoction is useful to destroy insects on plants.

"A large, coarse looking plant, of our meadows and swamps. Can. to Ga. Root emetic and stimulant, but poisonous. July."

Hemlock
Abies balsamea (A. canadensis)
Balsam. Hemlock Spruce.

BARK: Astringent. Tonic.
LEAVES: Sudorific. Emmenagogue. Diaphoretic. Alterative.

The bark is used in leukorrhea, prolapsus uteri, diarrhea, and gangrene. The oil is used in liniments, the gum in plasters.

Hemlock
Pinus rigida
Pitch Pine.

BARK: Astringent. Tonic.
GUM: Astringent. Tonic.
LEAVES: Diaphoretic. Emollient. Alterative. Sudorific.

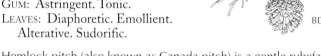

Hemlock pitch (also known as Canada pitch) is a gentle rubefacient. The oil from this tree is used in liniment.

From a manuscript, Watervliet, 1832: "Hemlock Plant grows 6' high or more, good to ease pain in open cancer which it does more powerfully than opium, used also in open tumors, ulcers, consumption, venereal ulcers, epilepsies and convulsions. Produces sweat and urine. But this plant is so very poisonous that it is imprudent to eat it. It ought not to be administered by those unskilled in medicine. Dose of the leaves in powder — or if the extract, a grain or 2. Great care ought to be taken to distinguish this plant from Water Hemlock for the latter is a deadly poison."

Henbane, Black
Hyoscyamus niger

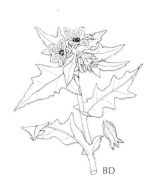

HERB: Narcotic. Nervine. Antispasmodic.

Used in gout, neuralgia, asthma, chronic rheumatism, to produce sleep, and to remove irregular nervous action.

Hollyhock
Alcea rosea (Althaea rosea)

FLOWERS: Emollient. Demulcent. Diuretic. Astringent.

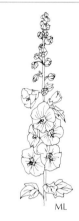

Used in coughs, female weakness, inflammation of the bladder, retention of urine, and affection of the kidneys.

Hop
Humulus lupulus

FLOWERS: Anthelmintic. Hypnotic. Febrifuge. Antilithic. Anodyne. Aromatic.

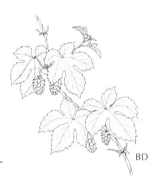

Valuable as a sedative to produce sleep and in nervousness or delirium tremens; used externally as fomentation in cramps, pains, swellings, indolent ulcers, salt rheum, and tumors.

Horehound
Marrubium vulgare

HERB: Stimulant. Tonic. Expectorant. Diuretic. Stomachic. Pectoral. Deobstruent.

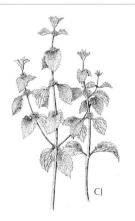

Useful in coughs, colds, chronic catarrh, asthma, and pulmonary affections; the cold infusion is used for dyspepsia and as a vermifuge.

Horsemint

Monarda punctata

HERB: Stimulant. Carminitive. Sudorific. Diuretic. Aromatic. Tonic.

Used in flatulence, nausea, vomiting, suppression of urine, and as an emmenagogue.

"An herbaceous, grayish plant 1 to 2 ft. high. Growing in muddy situations. Can. to Ky. Aromatic like pennyroyal, but less so. June. July."

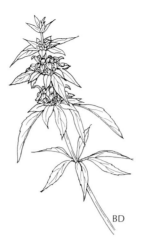

BD

Horseradish

Armoracia rusticana
(A. lapathifolia)

LEAVES: Stimulant. Diuretic. Antiscorbutic. Rubefacient. Emmenagogue. Acrid.
ROOT: Stimulant. Diuretic. Antiscorbutic. Rubefacient. Emmenagogue. Acrid.

Used with advantage for paralysis, rheumatism, dropsy, scurvy. Grated with sugar and used for hoarseness. The grated fresh root is used in cooking.

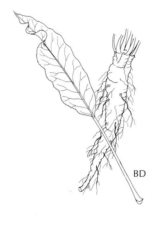

BD

Hydrangea

Hydrangea arborescens
Seven Barks. Wild Hydrangea.

ROOT: Diuretic.

Valuable to remove gravel and brick-dust deposits from the bladder, and to relieve excruciating pains caused thereby. A mild and soothing diuretic. It is reputed to be an old Cherokee remedy.

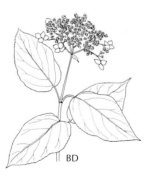

BD

Hyssop

Hyssopus officinalis

HERB: Stimulant. Aromatic. Carminitive. Tonic. Diaphoretic. Stomachic. Expectorant. Cephalic.

Valuable in quinsy, asthma, and chest diseases; the leaves applied to bruises remove pain and discoloration.

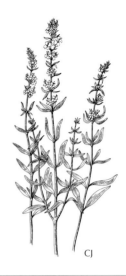

CJ

Iceland Moss

Cetraria islandica
Eryngo-Leaved Liverwort.

WHOLE PLANT: Pectoral. Demulcent. Tonic.

It is demulcent, tonic, and nutritious. Boiled with milk, it forms an excellent nutritive and tonic.

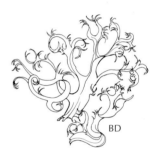

BD

Indian Cup

Silphium perfoliatum
Indian Cupweed. Ragged Cup. Prairie Dock. Compass Plant. Rosin Weed.

WHOLE PLANT: Diaphoretic. Stimulant. Alterative.

Used in coughs and painful affections of the chest.

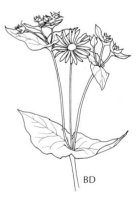

BD

Indian Hemp, Black

Apocynum cannabinum

Canadian Hemp. Indian Physic. Indian Hemp.

ROOT: Nauseant. Cathartic. Diaphoretic. Diuretic. Vermifuge. Tonic. Emetic.

Used in dropsy, remittent and intermittent fevers, pneumonia, and obstruction of the kidneys, liver, and spleen.

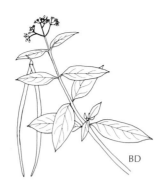

Indian Hemp, White

Asclepias incarnata

Swamp Milk Weed. Rose-Colored Silk Weed. Water Nerve Root.

ROOT: Aperient. Diuretic. Emetic. Anthelmintic. Vermifuge. Cathartic. Alterative.

Recommended in rheumatic, asthmatic, catarrhal, and syphilitic affections, and as a vermifuge.

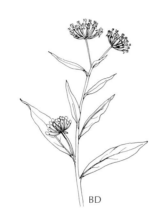

Indian-Physic

Gillenia trifoliata

Bowman's Root. Dropwort.

ROOT: Emetic. Cathartic. Sudorific. Tonic.

Valuable in amenorrhea, rheumatism, dropsy, costiveness, dyspepsia, worms, and fevers.

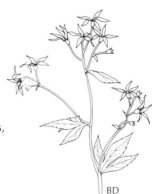

Indian Turnip

Arisaema triphyllum (Arum triphyllum)

Wake Robin. Milk Turnip. Dragon Root. Dragon Turnip. Jack-in-the-Pulpit. Pepper Turnip. Bog Onion. Marsh Turnip. Wild Turnip.

ROOT: Acrid. Expectorant. Diaphoretic. Stimulant. Narcotic. Aromatic.

Recommended internally in croup and low typhoid, and externally in scrofulous tumors and scald head (a Shaker term meaning scabs on the scalp).

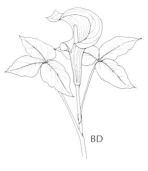

Indigo, Wild

Baptisia tinctoria

Horsefly Weed. Rattle Bush. Indigo Weed. Indigo Broom. Yellow Broom.

HERB: Purgative. Emetic. Stimulant. Antiseptic. Tonic. Diaphoretic.

ROOT: Purgative. Emetic. Stimulant. Antiseptic. Tonic. Diaphoretic.

Valuable as a wash in all species of ulcers, such as malignant sore mouth and throat, mercurial sore mouth, scrofulous or syphilitic ophthalmia, fetid leukorrhea, and discharges.

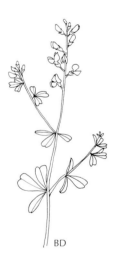

Ipecac, Carolina

Euphorbia ipecacuanhae

Indian Physic. Bitter Root. Ipecac Milk. Fever Root. Emetic Root. Blooming Spurge.

ROOT: Emetic. Cathartic. Tonic. Expectorant.

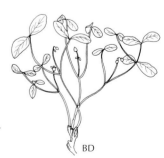

Iris

Iris x *germanica* var. *florentina*
(I. florentina)
   Orris Root.

ROOT: Aromatic. Cathartic.

Used mostly as a sachet for its
violetlike odor. The fresh root is
a powerful cathartic; its juice is
used in dropsy.

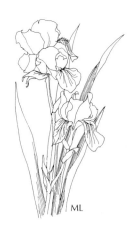

ML

Ironweed

Vernonia fasciculata

ROOT: Tonic.

A bitter tonic used to improve the
blood.

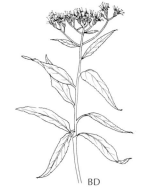

BD

Ivy, Ground

Glechoma hederacea (Nepeta glechoma)
   Gill Run. Alehof. Cat's-Paw. Gill-Go-Over-the-Ground.
   Field Balm. Turnhoof. Ground Joy.

LEAVES: Demulcent. Stomachic. Tonic. Emmenagogue.

A stimulant, tonic, and pectoral. An infusion of the leaves is very
beneficial in lead colic, and painters very often make use of it.
The fresh juice sniffed up the nose often relieves nasal congestion and headache. Used in diseases of the lungs and kidneys,
asthma, and jaundice.

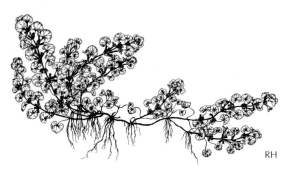

RH

Jacob's Ladder

Polemonium caeruleum

HERB: Antilithic. Diuretic.
   Emmenagogue. Nervine.
   Sialogogue.

Valuable in kidney diseases, stones
in the bladder, and falling of the
womb.

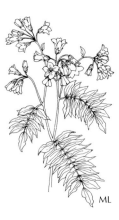

ML

Jalap

Ipomoea jalapa
   Bindweed.

ROOT: Cathartic.

This is an irritant and cathartic,
operating energetically.

*"Thickets. Can. and U.S. Climbing
over bushes. July and Sept."*

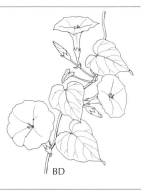

BD

Job's Tears

Coix lacryma-jobi
   Gromwell. False Gromwell.

SEED: Diuretic.

Said to dissolve calculi; used also in
dropsy and incontinence of urine.

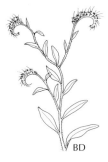

BD

Johnswort

Hypericum perforatum
   St. Johnswort.

HERB: Astringent. Sedative. Diuretic.
   Balsamic.

Used to cure suppression of urine,
chronic urinary affections, diarrhea,
dysentery, worms, and jaundice. As an
ointment, used for wounds, ulcers,
caked breast, and tumors.

*"In dry pastures. Can. and U.S. June,
July."*

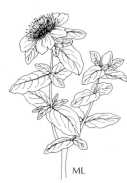

ML

Juniper

Juniperus communis
Juniper Bush.

BERRIES: Stimulant. Carminitive. Diuretic.

Efficacious in gonorrhea, gleet, leukorrhea, affections of the skin, scorbutic diseases, dropsy, and many kidney complaints.

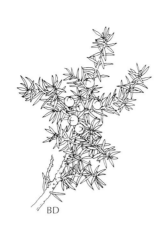

BD

King's Clover

Melilotus officinalis
Melilot. Sweet Clover.

HERB: Emollient. Diuretic. Discutient.

The leaves and flowers boiled in lard are useful in all kinds of ulcers, inflammations, and burns.

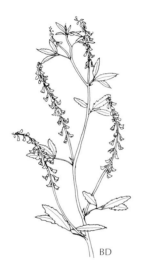

BD

Knot Grass

Triticum repens
Dog Grass. Couch Grass. Quickens. Witch Grass.

ROOT: Diuretic. Antiperiodic. Nervine. Carminitive.

Valuable in kidney diseases, irritation of the bladder, and spasmodic affections. The juice is used to heal wounds, cuts, and bruises.

"Found in wet grounds. Can. to Ga. It has very large halbert shaped leaves. June. July."

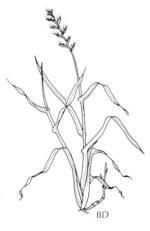

BD

Labrador Tea

Ledum groenlandicum
(L. latifolium)

HERB: Diuretic. Balsamic. Pectoral. Tonic.

Useful in coughs, dyspepsia, dysentery, and skin diseases. It is sometimes used as a table tea.

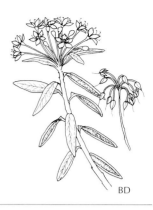

BD

Lady's Slipper

Cypripedium acaule
Pink Lady's Slipper. Pink Moccasin Flower. Nerve Root.

ROOT: Tonic. Diaphoretic. Antispasmodic. Nervine. Anodyne.

Beneficial in cases of nervous headache when administered with other remedies such as catnip or sweet balm in equal parts, taken as a tea about every half hour when needed. Preparations made from these roots are tonic, diaphoretic, and antispasmodic. They have been referred to as gentle nervous stimulants.

"In dark woods. Car. to Arc. Amer. May. June."

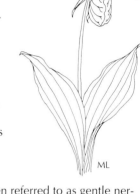

ML

Lady's Slipper, Yellow

Cypripedium calceolus var. *pubescens*
Nerve Root. American Valerian. Umbel. Yellow Moccasin Flower. Noah's Ark.

ROOT: Nervine. Anodyne. Tonic. Diaphoretic. Antispasmodic. Stimulant. Sedative.

Useful in ordinary nervous headache. A gentle nervous stimulant or antispasmodic. The roots should be gathered in August or September and carefully cleansed.

"Woods and meadows. Can. to Wis. and south to Georgia. May. June."

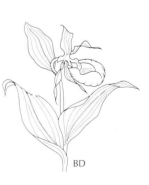

BD

Larkspur

Consolida regalis (Delphinium consolida)
    Stave's Acre.

HERB: Emetic. Cathartic. Diuretic. Narcotic. Acrid.
SEED: Diuretic. Narcotic. Acrid.

Used externally as an ointment in cutaneous diseases and to destroy insects on the body, such as lice.

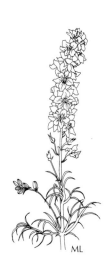

Laurel, Sheep

Kalmia angustifolia
    Laurel. Lambkill.

LEAVES: Antisyphilitic. Sedative. Astringent. Herpatic. Antiseptic.

Used in syphilitic diseases, scalp scabs, cutaneous affections, hemorrhages, diarrhea, flux, and neuralgia. When stewed with lard, it is serviceable as an ointment for various skin irritations.

"Sheep poison — Calico bush. Found in woods and by the road side from Can. to Car. Said to be poisonous to cattle. June."

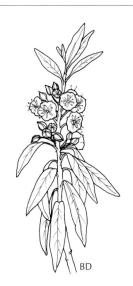

Lavender, English

Lavandula angustifolia (L. vera)

FLOWERS: Carminitive. Tonic. Stimulant. Aromatic. Pectoral. Nervine.

Valuable in flatulency, fainting, and to arrest vomiting; usually combined with other medicines.

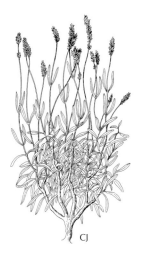

Leatherwood

Dirca palustris
    Moosewood. American Mezereon.

BARK: Emetic. Acrid. Rubefacient. Sudorific. Expectorant.

A poultice of the bark will produce vesication. It is used in combination with alteratives.

"Grows near mountain streams or rivulets. U.S. and Can. Every part of the shrub is very tough. Apr. May."

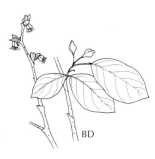

Lettuce, Garden

Lactuca sativa

HERB: Diuretic. Narcotic. Hypnotic. Anodyne.

Used as a narcotic where opium is objectionable.

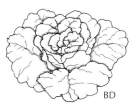

Lettuce, Wild

Lactuca serriola (L. virosa)
    Poison Lettuce. Acrid Lettuce.

HERB: Diuretic. Antiscorbutic. Narcotic.

Similar to garden lettuce in effect.

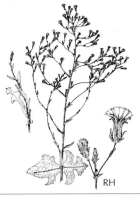

Life Everlasting

Gnaphalium obtusifolium var. *polycephalum*, *Anaphalis margaritacea*
    White Balsam. Indian Posy. Field Balsam. Sweet Balsam.

HERB: Astringent. Diaphoretic. Stomachic. Sudorific.

Used for bowel complaints, coughs, colds, bleeding of the lungs, and to produce perspiration. (Note in Watervliet manuscript, 1832: "Made into a tea good for ulcers in mouth.")

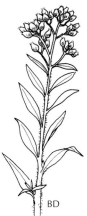

Life Root

Senecio aureus

Ragwort. Golden Senecio. Uncum. Squaw Weed. Female Regulator. Cocash Weed. False Valerian.

HERB AND ROOT: Aromatic. Stomachic. Diuretic. Diaphoretic. Tonic. Febrifuge.

Valuable in profuse menstruation, gravel, and strangury.

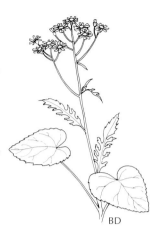

Lily, White Water

Nymphaea odorata

Toad Lily. Pond Lily. Sweet-Scented Water Lily.

THE FRESH ROOT: Astringent. Demulcent. Alterative. Pectoral. Tonic. Emollient.

Useful in dysentery, diarrhea, leukorrhea, and scrofula. Combined with cherry bark, it is used for bronchial affections. Used externally as a poultice for boils, tumors, and scrofulous ulcers.

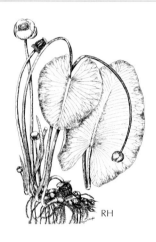

Lily, Yellow Pond

Nuphar advena

Spatterdock. Frog Lily. Beaver Root.

THE FRESH ROOT: Astringent. Demulcent. Alterative. Pectoral. Emollient. Tonic.

The properties are very similar to those of the white water lily. It is mucilaginous, demulcent, tonic, and astringent. Boiled in milk, it is also useful for external purposes.

"Found in meadows and wet places. Can. and U.S. July."

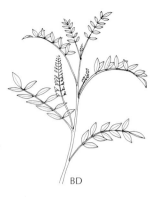

Liquorice

Glycyrrhiza glabra

Licorice.

ROOT: Nutritive. Demulcent. Expectorant. Laxative.
EXTRACT: Nutritive. Demulcent. Expectorant. Laxative.

Useful in coughs, catarrh, irritation of the urinary organs, pain of the intestines in diarrhea, and bronchial affections.

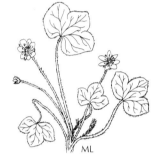

Liverwort

Hepatica americana

Noble Liverwort. Kidney Liver Leaf. Liver Leaf.

HERB: Mucilaginous. Astringent. Pectoral. Deobstruent. Narcotic. Demulcent.

Used in fevers, hepatic complaints, bleeding of the lungs, and coughs.

"This little plant is one of the earliest harbingers of the spring, often putting forth its neat and elegant flowers in the neighborhood of some lingering snow bank. Found in the woods from Can. to Ga. and west to Wis."

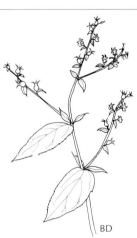

Lobelia

Lobelia inflata

Wild or Indian Tobacco. Emetic Root. Puke Weed. Eye-Bright. Asthma Weed.

HERB: Antispasmodic. Emetic. Expectorant. Diaphoretic. Narcotic. Diuretic.
SEED: Antispasmodic. Emetic. Expectorant. Diaphoretic.

Invaluable in spasmodic asthma, croup, pneumonia, catarrh, epilepsy, hysteria, cramps, and convulsions. Externally it is used as a poultice in sprains, bruises, ringworm, erysipelas, insect stings, and poison ivy.

"In fields and woods. Can. and U.S. The species of Lobelia are more or less poisonous. The milky juice is narcotic, producing effects similar to those of tobacco. July. Sept."

Lovage

Levisticum officinale
    Smellage. Lavose.

LEAVES: Aromatic. Carminitive. Diaphoretic. Stomachic. Narcotic. Emmenagogue.
ROOT: Carminitive. Diaphoretic. Stomachic.
SEED: Aromatic. Carminitive. Diaphoretic. Stomachic.

Combined with other drugs, it is used as a corrective and for its flavor. Sometimes used in female complaints and nervousness.

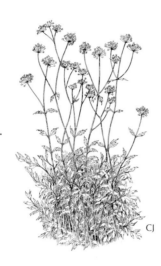

Lungwort

Pulmonaria officinalis (Mertensia virginica, P. virginica)
    Virginia Cowslip. Maple Lungwort.

WHOLE PLANT: Pectoral. Stomachic. Demulcent. Tonic.

Used in diseases of the lungs, coughs, influenza, and catarrh.

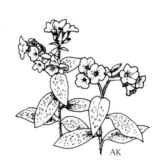

Mallow, Low

Malva rotundifolia
    Cheeses. Cheese Plant. Maller.

LEAVES: Diuretic. Demulcent. Pectoral.
ROOT: Diuretic. Demulcent. Pectoral.

Used for cough, irritation of the bowels, kidneys, and urinary organs, and as a poultice for boils.

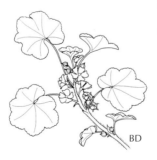

Mallow, Marsh

Althaea officinalis

FLOWERS: Astringent. Demulcent. Diuretic.
LEAVES: Demulcent. Diuretic.
ROOT: Demulcent. Diuretic. Emollient.

Valuable in hoarseness, catarrh, pneumonia, gonorrhea, irritation of the veins, dysentery, strangury, gravel, and all kidney complaints; used as a poultice in all painful swellings.

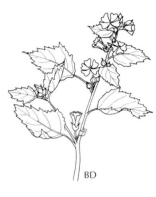

Man Root

Ipomoea pandurata (Convolvulus panduratus)
    Wild Jalap. Man-in-the-Ground. Man-in-the-Earth. Wild Potato. Bind Weed. Wild Scammony.

ROOT: Cathartic. Diuretic. Pectoral.

Has been recommended in dropsy, strangury, calculous affections, and diseases of the lungs, liver, and kidneys.

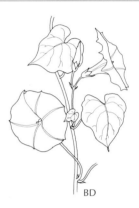

Mandrake

Podophyllum peltatum
    May Apple. Wild Lemon. Raccoon Berry. Wild Mandrake.

ROOT: Deobstruent. Cathartic. Alterative. Anthelmintic. Hydragogue. Sialogogue. Antibilious. Diuretic. Narcotic.

Valuable in jaundice, bilious and intermittent fevers, scrofula, syphilis, liver complaints, rheumatism, and where a powerful cathartic is required.

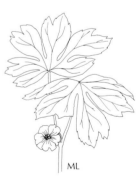

Maple, Red

Acer rubrum

Soft Maple. Whistle Wood.

BARK: Tonic. Astringent. Anthelmintic. Vermifuge.

Used for worms, as a gentle tonic, and as a wash for sore eyes.

"Common in the woods of New England. Flowers are crimson. Apr."

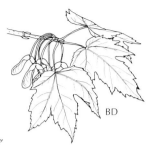

Maple, Striped

Acer pensylvanicum

Canada Maple. Moosewood.

BARK: Vermifuge. Tonic. Stimulant.

Used for worms and as an eyewash.

"A small tree 10 or 15 ft. high. In woods. May."

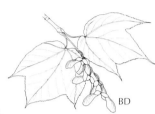

Marigold

Calendula officinalis

Pot Marigold. Marygold.

FLOWERS: Stimulant. Diaphoretic. Stomachic. Aromatic.

Valuable in controlling eruptions; the tincture is used for cuts, bruises, sprains, wounds, etc. It is unequaled in preventing gangrene.

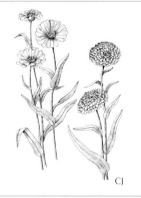

Marjoram, Sweet

Origanum majorana

HERB: Stimulant. Tonic. Emmenagogue. Stomachic. Aromatic. Diuretic. Sudorific.

Promotes perspiration, promotes menstruation when recently stopped, and relieves eruptive disease.

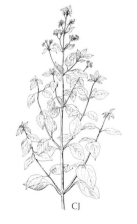

Marsh Rosemary

Limonium carolinianum (Statice caroliniana)

Sea Lavender. Ink Root. Meadow Root. American Thrift. Sea Thrift.

ROOT: Astringent. Tonic. Antiseptic.

A domestic remedy for dysentery, diarrhea, canker, leukorrhea, and gleet.

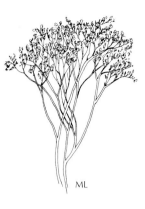

Masterwort

Imperatoria ostruthium

Cowparsnip. Royal Cow Parsnip.

ROOT: Stimulant. Antispasmodic. Carminitive. Diuretic. Tonic. Aromatic. Nervine.
SEED: Stimulant. Antispasmodic. Carminitive. Diuretic. Tonic.
LEAVES: Stimulant. Antispasmodic. Carminitive. Diuretic. Tonic. Aromatic. Nervine.

Used in flatulency, dyspepsia, epilepsy, asthma, amenorrhea, colic, dysmenorrhea, palsy, and apoplexy.

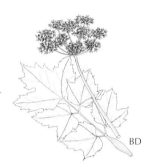

Matico

Piper angustifolium

Soldier's Herb.

LEAVES: Aromatic. Stimulant. Astringent.

An aromatic stimulant with astringent properties for internal use in arresting hemorrhages and treating diarrhea. Externally it is used in local applications to ulcers. Bought by the Shakers for resale.

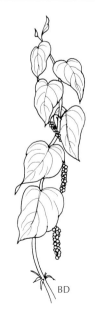

Mayweed

Anthemis cotula

Wild Chamomile. Dog Fennel.

HERB: Tonic. Emetic. Antispasmodic. Emmenagogue. Diaphoretic. Stomachic.

Used in colds to induce perspiration; also used for sick headache, amenorrhea, and convalescence from fevers.

"Found in waste places in hard soils, especially by road sides in large patches. The plant is ill scented. June and Sept."

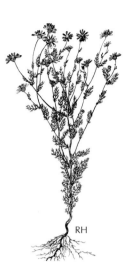

Meadow Saffron

Colchicum autumnale

Colchicum.

CORMS: Nervine. Emetic. Cathartic.
SEED: Nervine. Emetic. Cathartic.

It is a sedative, a cathartic, a diuretic, and an emetic, but great care should be used in its employment, as serious results, such as violent purging, may follow an overdose.

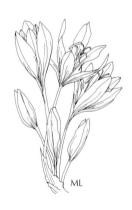

Melilot

Melilotus officinalis

Sweet Clover. Yellow Clover. Sweet Melilot.

FLOWERS: Demulcent. Tonic. Expectorant. Diuretic.

An expectorant and a diuretic. Used to flavor tobacco, cheese, and other products. Used also in sachets and potpourri mixtures.

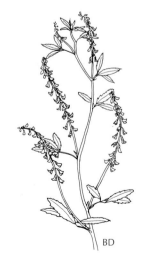

Mezereum

Daphne mezereum

Spurge Olive. American Mezereon. Leather Wood.

BARK OF ROOT AND STEM: Stimulant. Alterative. Diuretic. Narcotic. Diaphoretic.

In small doses used in syphilis, scrofula, chronic rheumatism, and diseases of the skin.

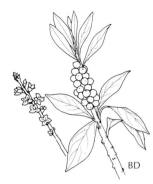

Milkweed

Asclepias syriaca

Silk Weed.

ROOT: Anodyne. Emmenagogue. Diuretic. Alterative. Aromatic. Sudorific. Tonic. Laxative. Expectorant.

Valuable in amenorrhea, dropsy, retention of urine, dyspepsia, asthma, and scrofulous diseases. Capable of producing vomiting; promotes moderate perspiration. It is tonic and acts upon the bowels.

"A common, very milky herb, 3 to 4 ft. high on hedges and road sides. Pods full of seeds with their long-silk. July."

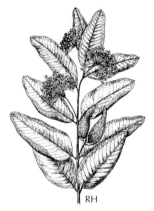

Milkwort

Polygala lurea (P. vulgaris)

European Seneca.

ROOT: Diaphoretic. Expectorant. Pectoral.

This is a bitter and used in coughs and chest ailments.

"In woods and swamps from Can. to Ca. Stem from 3 to 4 inches high. Bears from 2 to 4 flowers. May."

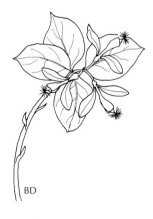

Monarda

Monarda punctata

Horsemint.

HERB: Diuretic. Stomachic. Tonic. Aromatic.

Aromatic and pungent, it contains volatile oil. Useful as a carminitive and diuretic in flatulent colic, upset stomach, and nausea.

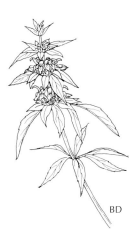

Moss, Haircap

Polytrichum juniperinum

Robin's Eye. Ground Moss. Bear's Bud.

WHOLE PLANT: Diuretic. Cathartic.

Relieves urinary distress and used to advantage with the hydragogue cathartics.

"Shady places common. Plant 6 inches high."

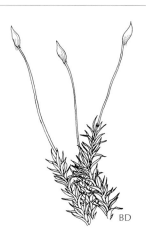

Motherwort

Leonurus cardiaca

Roman Motherwort. Lion's Tail. Throwwort.

HERB: Emmenagogue. Nervine. Antispasmodic. Laxative. Stomachic. Diaphoretic.

Valuable in female complaints, nervousness, colds, delirium, wakefulness, disturbed sleep, liver affections.

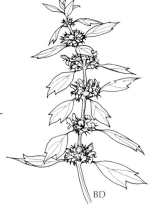

Mountain Dittany

Cunila origanoides

Wild Basil. Stone Mint. American Dittany.

LEAVES: Stimulant. Tonic. Nervine. Sudorific. Diaphoretic.
FLOWERS: Stimulant. Tonic. Nervine. Sudorific. Diaphoretic.

The warm tea is diaphoretic.

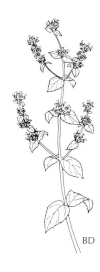

Mountain Mint

Pycnanthemum montanum

Basil. Wild Marjoram.

HERB: Stimulant, Tonic. Emmenagogue. Stomachic. Aromatic. Sudorific.

Used for obstructed menstruation, to produce perspiration, and in colds, fevers, and eruptions.

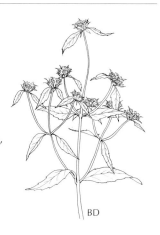

Mouse Ear*

Gnaphalium uliginosum

Dysentery Weed. Cud Weed. Everlasting.

HERB: Sudorific. Stomachic. Mucilaginous. Diuretic.

Used in coughs, diarrhea, and obstructions.

"Fields and pastures. U.S. and Can. May."

This Mouse Ear is not to be confused with the hawkweed that is called mouse ear.

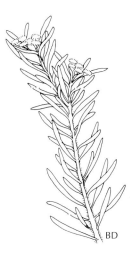

Mugwort

Artemisia vulgaris

HERB: Diaphoretic.
Emmenagogue. Nervine.
Antibilious. Deobstruent.
Tonic.
ROOT: Diaphoretic.
Emmenagogue. Nervine.
Antibilious. Deobstruent.
Tonic.

Useful in epilepsy, hysteria, and
amenorrhea; promotes perspiration;
and increases the flow of urine and
menses.

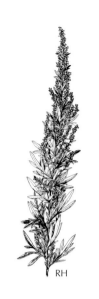

Mulberry

Morus rubra
Red Mulberry.

BARK: Vermifuge. Cathartic.

The infusion of pulverized bark is
useful as a cathartic and to dispel
worms.

*"A fine flowering shrub, in upland
woods, U.S. and Brit. Amer. common. Fruit bright red, sweet. Fruit
ripe in Aug. Flowers in June and
July."*

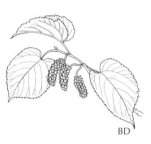

Mullein

Verbascum thapsus

FLOWERS: Astringent. Demulcent.
Emollient.
HERB: Demulcent. Diuretic.
Anodyne. Antispasmodic.
Emollient. Astringent.
ROOT: Demulcent. Diuretic.
Anodyne. Antispasmodic.
Emollient. Astringent.
SEED: Narcotic.

Used in cough, catarrh, diarrhea,
dysentery, piles, etc. Also as a poultice in white swellings, mumps, and
sore throats.

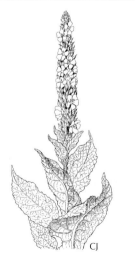

Mustard, Black

Brassica nigra

SEED: Diuretic. Vesicant.
Stimulant. Rubefacient.
Emetic.

It is used in large doses as an emetic. In cases of poison, it should be
administered immediately in luke-
warm water. Ground, it is used as a
condiment.

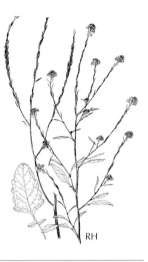

Mustard, White

Brassica hirta (B. alba)

SEED: Stimulant. Rubefacient.
Vesicant. Antiscorbutic.

The whole seed was used as a tonic
in dyspepsia. In large doses it acts as
an emetic; externally, as a poultice
to rouse the system to activity,
relieve pain, and mitigate inflammation. Ground, it is used as a
condiment.

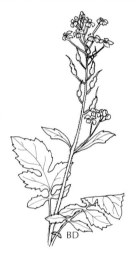

Nanny Bush

Viburnum lentago
Sheep Berry. Sweet Viburnum.
Nanny Berry.

BARK: Tonic.

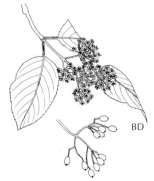

Nettle

Urtica dioica

Stinging Nettle.

FLOWERS: Tonic.
HERB: Astringent. Tonic.
Diuretic.
ROOT: Astringent. Tonic.
Diuretic.

Valuable in diarrhea, dysentery, hemorrhoids, hemorrhages, gravel, and scorbutic affections. The seeds reduce corpulence.

"A common weed in waste and cultivated grounds in Southern States. Stem covered with deflexed bristles. Internodes thickened upwards. June, July."

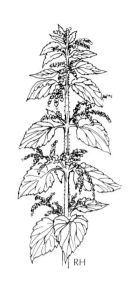

Nightshade, Black

Solanum nigrum

Black Cherry. Garden Nightshade.

LEAVES: Narcotic. Anodyne.
Antispasmodic.

This is an energetic narcotic. It is anodyne, antispasmodic, calmative, and relaxant. It is too powerful for general or domestic use and should be confined to the hands of skilled herbal physicians only.

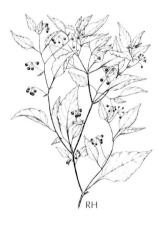

Oak, Black

Quercus velutina (Q. tinctoria)

BARK: Astringent. Tonic.

Used in sore throats, offensive ulcers, obstinate chronic diarrhea, hemorrhage, gargles, injections, leukorrhea, prolapsus ani, and piles.

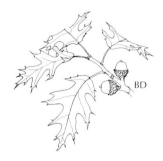

Oak, Red

Quercus rubra

BARK: Astringent. Tonic.
Stimulant.

Used in sore throats, offensive ulcers, obstinate chronic diarrhea, hemorrhage, gargles, injections, leukorrhea, prolapsus ani, and piles.

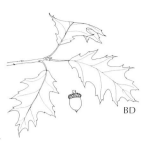

Oak, White

Quercus alba

BARK: Tonic. Astringent.
Antiseptic.

Used in sore throats, offensive ulcers, obstinate chronic diarrhea, hemorrhage, gargles, injections, leukorrhea, prolapsus ani, and piles.

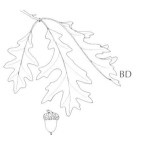

Oak of Jerusalem

Chenopodium botrys

Worm Seed. Jesuit Tea. Jerusalem Tea. Jerusalem Oak.

HERB: Anthelmintic.
Antispasmodic. Vermifuge.
Stomachic. Emmenagogue.
SEED: Anthelmintic.
Antispasmodic. Vermifuge.
Stomachic. Emmenagogue.

Used to expel worms in children; also reputedly beneficial in amenorrhea.

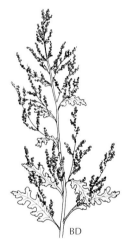

Orange

Citrus sinensis

FLOWERS: Aromatic.
Antispasmodic.
PEEL: Aromatic. Tonic.
Stomachic.

Used to cover the taste of disagreeable medicines and lessen their tendency to nauseate. The fruit is given after fevers where acids are craved, as in scurvy.

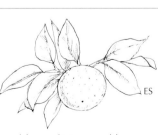

Osier, Green
Cornus alternifolia (C. circinata)

Broad-Leaved Dogwood. Dogachamus. Alder-Leaved Dogwood. Round-Leaved Cornel.

BARK: Astringent. Tonic. Stomachic. Herpatic. Diuretic. Deobstruent.

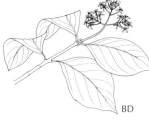

Useful in diarrhea and dysentery; as gargle in sore throats; and in typhoid fever and ague.

Oswego Tea
Monarda didyma

Mountain Balm. High Balm. Bee Balm. Bergamot Monarda.

HERB: Febrifuge. Stimulant. Carminitive. Sudorific. Diuretic. Stomachic. Aromatic. Tonic.

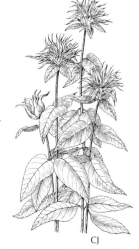

The infusion is used in flatulence, nausea, vomiting, and suppression of urine and menstruation.

Papooseroot
Caulophyllum thalictroides

Blue Cohosh. Blueberry Root. Squaw Root.

ROOT: Deobstruent. Narcotic. Emmenagogue.

A favorite remedy in chronic uterine diseases, and as a parturient it has proved invaluable. Also used in rheumatism, dropsy, colic, and hysterics.

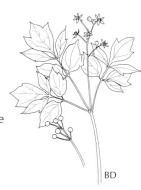

Parilla, Yellow
Menispermum canadense

Canadian Moonseed. Vine Maple.

ROOT: Tonic. Laxative. Alterative.

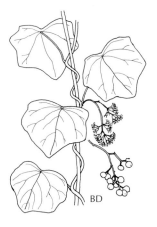

A superior laxative bitter, used in scrofula, syphilis, rheumatism, gout, and cutaneous diseases.

Parsley
Petroselinum crispum (P. sativum)

Rock Parsley.

LEAVES: Demulcent. Diuretic. Diaphoretic.
ROOT: Demulcent. Diuretic. Diaphoretic.
SEED: Demulcent. Carminitive. Diaphoretic.

The root is useful in dropsy, retention of urine, strangury, and gonorrhea. Leaves were bruised to use as fomentation for bites and stings of insects. Seeds were used to destroy vermin in the hair.

Peach
Prunus persica (Amygdalis persica)

BARK: Tonic. Stomachic. Cathartic.
KERNELS: Tonic. Stomachic.
LEAVES: Tonic. Vermifuge. Laxative.

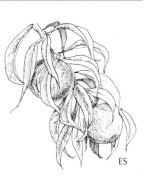

Bark and kernels recommended in intermittent fever, leukorrhea, dyspepsia, and jaundice. The leaves were used in irritability of the bladder and urethra, and inflammation of the stomach and abdomen.

Pennyroyal

Hedeoma pulegioides

Tick Weed. Squaw Mint.

HERB: Stimulant. Diaphoretic. Emmenagogue. Carminitive. Stomachic. Aromatic.

Promotes perspiration, restores suppressed lochia, promotes the menstrual discharge.

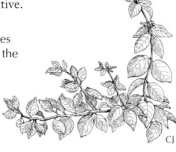

"Fragrant, a small sweet scented herb, and held in high repute. Abundant in dry pasture. Can. and U.S. Flowering all summer.

Peony

Paeonia lactiflora

FLOWERS: Antispasmodic. Tonic. Nervine. Vermifuge.
ROOT: Antispasmodic. Tonic. Nervine. Vermifuge.

Valuable in St. Vitus's dance, epilepsy, spasms, nervous diseases, and whooping cough. The seeds are reputedly effective in preventing nightmares of dropsical persons.

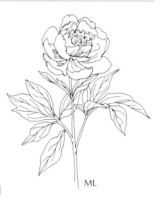

Peppermint

Mentha x piperita

HERB: Stimulant. Antispasmodic. Carminitive. Stomachic. Sudorific. Aromatic.

Used in flatulent colic, hysterics, and spasm cramps in the stomach; to allay nausea and vomiting; also to flavor other medicines.

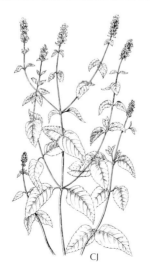

Pilewort

Ranunculus ficaria
(A. hypochondriacus)

Prince's Feather. Lovely Bleeding. Red Cockscomb.

HERB: Astringent. Herpatic.

Recommended in severe menorrhagia, diarrhea, dysentery, hemorrhage of the bowels, leukorrhea, and ulcers.

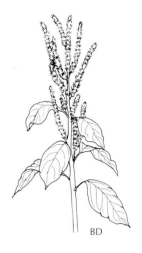

Pine, White

Pinus strobus

Spanish Pine.

BARK: Stimulant. Diuretic. Pectoral. Laxative. Diaphoretic. Demulcent. Balsamic.
PITCH: Stimulant. Diuretic. Pectoral. Laxative. Diaphoretic. Demulcent. Balsamic.

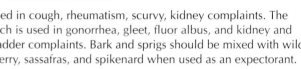

Used in cough, rheumatism, scurvy, kidney complaints. The pitch is used in gonorrhea, gleet, fluor albus, and kidney and bladder complaints. Bark and sprigs should be mixed with wild cherry, sassafras, and spikenard when used as an expectorant.

Pink Root

Spigelia marilandica

ROOT: Sudorific. Anthelmintic.

An active and certain vermifuge combined with senna and manna.

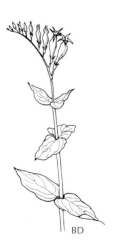

Pipsissewa

Chimaphila umbellata

Prince's Pine. Noble Pine. Ground Holly. Pyrola. Rheumatic Weed. False Wintergreen.

HERB: Diuretic. Tonic. Alterative. Astringent. Stimulant.

Useful in scrofula, chronic rheumatism, kidney diseases, strangury, gonorrhea, catarrh of the bladder, and cutaneous diseases.

"A common little evergreen in Can. and U.S. Found in the woods. Used in medicine. July."

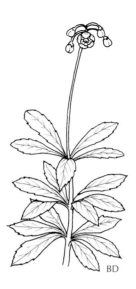

Pitcher Plant

Sarracenia purpurea

Huntsman's Cup. Eve's Cup. Fly Trap.

WHOLE PLANT: Cathartic. Deobstruent. Tonic. Stomachic.

Useful for its tonic and beneficial action on the stomach.

"In bogs & wet meadows throughout Can. and U.S. June."

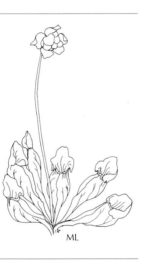

Plantain

Plantago major

Common Plantain. Greater Plantain. Bitter Plantain.

LEAVES: Alterative. Diuretic. Antiseptic. Refrigerant. Deobstruent. Astringent.
ROOT: Alterative. Diuretic. Antiseptic.

Beneficial in syphilitic, mercurial, and scrofulous diseases, leukorrhea, and diarrhea. The leaves are used in ointments.

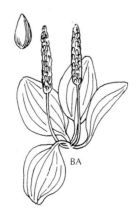

Plantain, Downy Rattlesnake

Goodyera pubescens

Adder's Violet. Rattlesnake Leaf. Spotted Plaintain. Rattlesnake Root.

HERB: Detergent.
ROOT: Detergent.

Reputed to have cured scrofula; also used in leukorrhea, in prolapsus uteri, and as a wash in scrofulous ophthalmia.

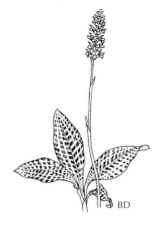

Pleurisy Root

Asclepias tuberosa

Butterfly Weed. Wind Root. Tuber Root.

ROOT: Diaphoretic. Diuretic. Carminitive. Tonic. Emetic. Cathartic. Sudorific. Anodyne. Expectorant.

Used in pleurisy, febrile diseases, flatulency, indigestion, acute rheumatism, dysentery, coughs, inflammation of the lungs, etc. Most often used in decoction or infusion for the purpose of promoting perspiration and expectoration.

"Dry fields. Can. and U.S. A medicinal plant. Aug."

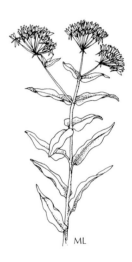

Poison Ivy

Rhus toxicodendron

Poison Vine.

LEAVES: Irritant Poison.

Has been used in chronic paralysis, chronic rheumatism, cutaneous diseases, paralysis of the bladder.

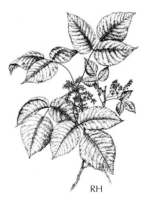

Poke

Phytolacca americana (P. decandra)

Garget. Pigeon Berry. Scoke. Coakum. Inkberry. Scokeroot.

BERRIES: Deobstruent. Alterative. Acrid.
LEAVES: Deobstruent. Alterative.
ROOT: Deobstruent. Cathartic.

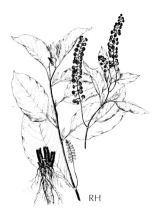

Poke is cathartic, alterative, and slightly narcotic. It is a slow-acting emetic, but is not favored for this purpose. It has superior power as an alterative, if properly gathered and prepared.

Pomegranate

Punica granatum

RIND OF FRUIT: Astringent. Tonic.

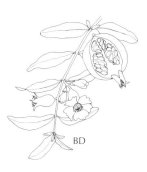

Reputed valuable in removing tapeworm, and in intermittent fever, night sweats, passive hemorrhages, diarrhea, and canker in the mouth.

Poplar

Populus tremuloides

White Poplar. Aspen. American Poplar. Trembling Poplar.

BARK: Tonic. Febrifuge. Astringent. Aromatic. Alterative. Stomachic. Antiscorbutic.
BUDS: Tonic. Febrifuge. Astringent. Aromatic. Alterative.

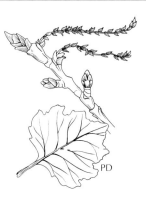

The active principles of the bark are salicin and populin. Used in intermittent fever, emaciation and debility, impaired digestion, chronic diarrhea, worms, gleet, etc. Used as a vermifuge by veterinaries.

Poppy

Papaver somniferum

Opium Poppy. White Poppy.

CAPSULES: Emollient. Anodyne. Stimulant. Narcotic.
FLOWERS: Narcotic. Anodyne. Stimulant.
LEAVES: Narcotic. Anodyne. Stimulant.

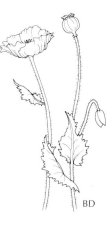

Valuable to promote rest, and as a poultice for painful swellings; the syrup was given to restless children to induce sleep.

Privet

Ligustrum vulgare

Privy. Prim.

LEAVES: Astringent. Antiscorbutic.

The leaves are astringent and may be used in a decoction as a mouthwash and gargle.

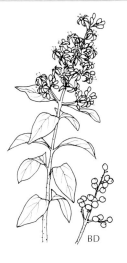

Ptelea

Ptelea trifoliata

Wingseed. Wafer Ash. Shrubby Trefoil.

BARK OF ROOT: Tonic. Anthelmintic.

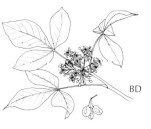

Recommended in intermittent and remittent fevers, asthma, pulmonary affections, indigestion, and dyspepsia.

Pumpkin

Cucurbita pepo

SEED: Mucilaginous. Diuretic.

Used in scalding of urine and affections of the urinary passages; is said to remove tapeworm effectually.

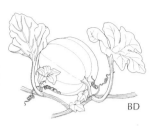

Queen of the Meadow

Eupatorium purpureum
> Joepye. Trumpet Weed. Gravel Root. Purple Boneset.

HERB: Anodyne. Diuretic. Stimulant. Tonic. Antilithic. Diaphoretic.
ROOT: Diuretic. Stimulant. Tonic.

A valuable remedy in dropsy, strangury, gravel, and all urinary disorders.

"Dry fields and woods, common. Stem 3 to 6 ft. high. Aug. Sept."

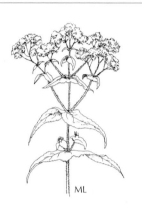

Queen's Root

Stillingia sylvatica
> Queen's Delight. Yaw Root. Silver Leaf. Cock-Up-Hat. Stillingia.

ROOT: Alterative. Emetic. Cathartic.

Invaluable in scrofula, syphilis, liver and cutaneous diseases, bronchitis, laryngitis, and lung complaints.

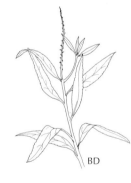

Raspberry

Rubus idaeus var. *strigosus*
> Red Raspberry.

LEAVES: Astringent. Tonic.

An excellent remedy in diarrhea, dysentery, cholera infantum, hemorrhage from the stomach, bowels, or uterus, and as an injection in gleet, leukorrhea, and canker.

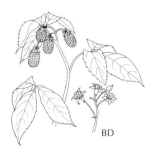

Red Root

Ceanothus americanus
> New Jersey Tea. Jersey Tea. Wild Snowball.

BARK: Astringent. Expectorant. Sedative.

Used in gonorrhea, dysentery, asthma, chronic bronchitis, whooping cough, and as a gargle for canker, sore mouth, etc.

"A small shrub, found in woods and groves, U.S. and Can. June."

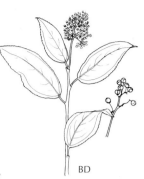

Rhubarb

Rheum rhabarbarum

ROOT: Cathartic.

Cathartic principle limited to lower bowel.

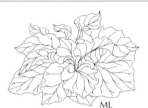

Richweed

Collinsonia canadensis
> Stone Root. Hardrock. Horseweed. Wild Citronella. Oxbalm.

HERB: Diuretic. Stomachic. Stimulant. Tonic.
ROOT: Diuretic. Stomachic. Stimulant. Tonic.

A fair stimulant, and a gentle tonic and diuretic. It is used externally, especially the leaves in fomentation and poultices for bruises, wounds, blows, sprains, and cuts.

Rockbrake

Pellaea atropurpurea, Pteris atropurpurea
> Winter Fern. Cliff Brake. Indian Dream.

HERB: Astringent. Anthelmintic.
ROOT: Astringent. Anthelmintic.

Efficacious in diarrhea, dysentery, night sweats, to remove worms, and as a vaginal injection in leukorrhea, suppression of the lochia, etc.

"Abundant in woods, pastures and waste grounds."

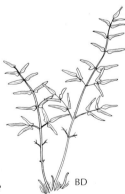

Rose, Cabbage
Rosa centifolia
> Hundred-Leaved Rose.

PETALS OF THE FLOWER:
Astringent. Tonic.

Mildly tonic and astringent.

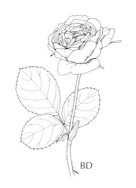

Rose, Damask
Rosa damascena
> Pale Rose.

PETALS OF THE FLOWER:
Astringent. Tonic.

Tonic and mildly astringent. Used in hemorrhages, excessive mucus discharges, and bowel complaints; the infusion with pith of sassafras for inflammation of the eyes, etc. Also used in potpourri and sachets. Considered best source of rose petals, as the blossom of the flowers is very full.

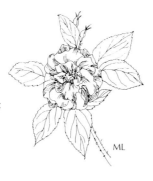

Rose, Red
Rosa gallica

FLOWERS: Aromatic. Tonic.
Astringent. Fragrant.

Tonic and mildly astringent. Used in hemorrhages, excessive mucus discharges, and bowel complaints; the infusion with pith of sassafras for inflammation of the eyes. It was also called the apothecary rose and was used extensively for making rose water.

Rose, White
Rosa x *alba*
FLOWERS: Astringent. Tonic

Tonic and mildly astringent. Used in hemorrhages, excessive mucus discharges, and bowel complaints; the infusion with pith of sassafras for inflammation of the eyes, etc.

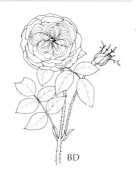

Rosemary
Rosmarinus officinalis

LEAVES AND ROOT: Astringent.
Tonic. Diaphoretic. Stimulant.
Antispasmodic. Emmenagogue.

The warm infusion for colds, colic, and nervous conditions; the oil in liniment and plasters as an external stimulant.

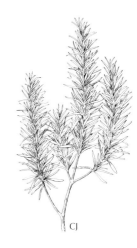

Rosin-Weed
Silphium laciniatum
> Compass Plant. Polar Plant.

ROOT: Alterative. Diaphoretic.
Diuretic. Tonic.

The resin has diuretic properties. The root has been used as an expectorant. It is also an emetic.

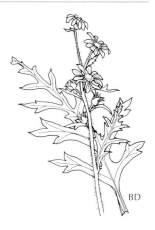

Rue
Ruta graveolens

HERB: Tonic. Anthelmintic.
Stimulant. Emmenagogue.
Antispasmodic. Diuretic.
Stomachic.

A narcotic acrid poison, used medically in flatulent colic, hysterics, epilepsy, and as a vermifuge.

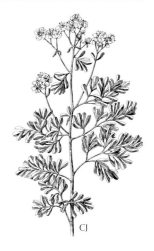

Saffron
Carthamus tinctorius (Crocus sativus)

FLOWERS: Emmenagogue. Diaphoretic. Stomachic. Aromatic. Diuretic.

Has been used beneficially in amenorrhea, dysmenorrhea, chlorosis, hysteria, suppression of the lochial discharges, febrile diseases, scarlet fever, and measles.

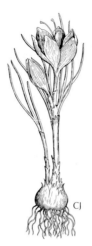

Sage
Salvia officinalis

HERB: Tonic. Astringent. Expectorant. Diaphoretic. Stomachic. Balsamic. Sudorific.

Valuable in coughs, colds, night sweats, worms, spermatorrhea, and as a gargle for ulcerated sore throats; also to produce perspiration.

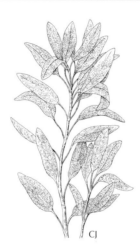

Sage Willow
Lythrum salicaria

> Rainbow Weed. Purple Willow Herb. Loosestrife.

HERB: Mucilaginous. Astringent. Demulcent. Aromatic. Stomachic. Balsamic.

Mucilaginous, astringent, demulcent.

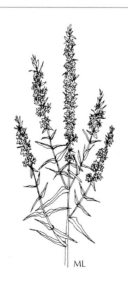

Sanicle, Black
Sanicula marilandica

> Pool Root. American Sanicle. Self-Heal.

ROOT: Diaphoretic. Antispasmodic. Expectorant. Aromatic. Deobstruent. Stomachic. Tonic. Nervine. Anodyne.

Used in ague, stomach complaints, dysentery, erysipelas, cholera, inflammation of the bladder, nervous disease, and pulmonary affections. Resembles valerian.

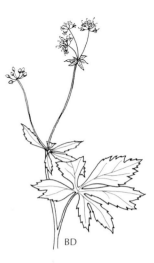

Sarsaparilla, American Wild
Aralia nudicaulis

> Wild Licorice. Small Spikenard. Dwarf Elder. Bristly Stem.

ROOT: Alterative. Diuretic. Demulcent. Deobstruent. Diaphoretic.

Used in chronic diseases of the skin, rheumatic affections, dropsy, venereal complaints, and all cases where alteratives are required.

"A well known plant found in woods. Most abundant in rich and rocky soils. Can. to Car. It has a leaf stalk, but no proper stem. June. July."

Sassafras
Sassafras albidum (S. officinale)

BARK AND BARK OF THE ROOT: Diuretic. Aromatic. Stimulant. Alterative. Diaphoretic. Stomachic. Aperient. Tonic.
PITH: Demulcent. Mucilaginous.

Valuable in scrofula and eruptive diseases, and as a flavor. The pith was used as an eyewash in ophthalmia, and as a drink in disorders of the chest, bowels, kidneys, and bladder. Useful as a spring tonic when made into a tea.

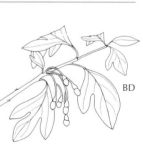

"Grows in the U.S. and Can. Every part of the tree has a pleasant fragrance and an aromatic taste. Apr. June."

Savin

Juniperus sabina

LEAVES: Emmenagogue. Diuretic. Diaphoretic. Anthelmintic. Stimulant. Acrid. Deobstruent.

Used in kidney complaints, suppression of urine, and obstructed menstruation.

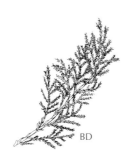

Savory, Summer

Satureja hortensis

Bean Herb. Bohnenkraut.

HERB: Stomachic. Aromatic. Stimulant. Carminitive. Emmenagogue.

A warm infusion is beneficial in wind colic. Summer savory tea is a good remedy for the nervous headache; drink it hot just before going to bed. Beneficial in colds, menstrual suppression, flatulent colic, and as a gentle stimulating tonic after fevers. The oil is used to relieve toothache.

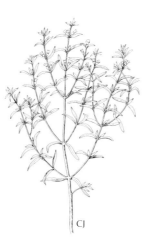

Savory, Winter

Satureja montana

LEAVES: Stomachic. Stimulant. Aromatic. Carminitive.

Possesses qualities similar to summer savory. The leaves have an aromatic odor and taste like thyme. Both winter and summer savory are cultivated for culinary purposes as well as medicinal.

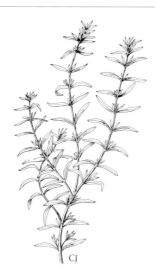

Scabbish

Oenothera biennis

Tree Primrose. Wild Evening Primrose.

HERB: Vulnerary. Mucilaginous. Demulcent. Stomachic.

Valuable in cough, tetter, and eruptive diseases.

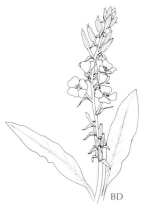

Scabious

Succisa pratensis (Scabiosa succisa)

Sweet Scabious. Devil's Bit. Primrose Scabious.

HERB: Diaphoretic. Demulcent. Febrifuge. Diuretic. Astringent. Herpatic.

An enduring remedy for promoting moderate perspiration and correcting acrid conditions in the humors. Also valuable in abating or driving away fevers.

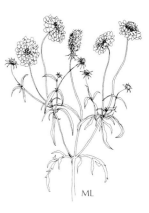

Scrofula

Scrophularia marilandica

Heal-All. Square Stalk. Carpenter's Square. Figwort.

HERB: Deobstruent. Alterative. Diuretic. Anodyne. Tonic. Demulcent. Stomachic.

Valuable in scrofula, cutaneous diseases, dropsy, and ulcers.

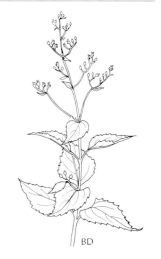

Self-Heal
Prunella vulgaris
>   Blue Curls. Wound Wort.
>   All Heal. Brown Wort. Healall.

HERB: Diuretic.

Self-heal is pungent and bitter. It increases the secretion of the urine.

"It is a member of the mint family. North America. Lat. 33° to the Arctic Sea. Flowering all summer."

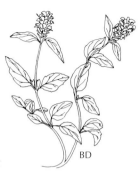

BD

Senna, American
Cassia marilandica
>   Locust Plant.

LEAVES: Cathartic. Deobstruent.
>   Diuretic.

A mild cathartic.

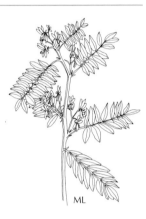

ML

Shepherd's Purse
Capsella bursa-pastoris
>   Shepherd's Heart.

HERB, WHOLE PLANT:
>   Diuretic. Antiscorbutic.

Useful for increasing the secretion of urine, and in controlling scurvy. One of best known specifics for stopping hemorrhages of all kinds.

"A common weed, found every-where in fields, pastures and road-sides. Stem 6–8–12 inches high. Stem leaves are smaller than the root leaves and are half clasping at the stems. Silicle smooth, triangular. Apr.–Sept."

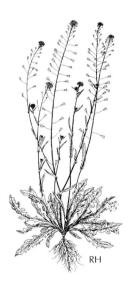

RH

Shield Fern
Dryopteris austriaca var. spinulosa
(Aspidium spinulosum)

RHIZOME: Vermifuge.
>   Anthelmintic.

Capable of destroying and expelling worms, especially tape-worms.

"Common in rocky shades. June–Aug."

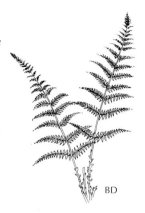

BD

Silver Weed
Potentilla anserina
>   Silver Cinquefoil. Cramp
>   Weed. Goose Tansy.
>   Moor Grass.

HERB: Astringent.

As a tea it is used for diar-rhea. The root is used as a red dye.

"A fine species on wet grounds, meadows and by roadsides. New Engl. to Arctic Amer. Leaves silvery white beneath. June. Sept."

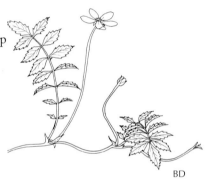

BD

Skullcap
Scutellaria lateriflora
>   Mad-Dog. Hoodwort. Blue
>   Scullcap. Virginia Scullcap.

HERB: Tonic. Nervine.
>   Antispasmodic. Sudorific.

Valuable in all nervous com-plaints, chorea, wakefulness, delirium tremens, convulsions, and excitability.

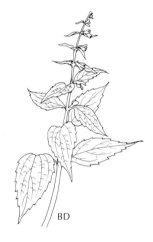

BD

Skunk Cabbage

Symplocarpus foetidus

Meadow Cabbage. Skunk Weed. Polecat Weed.

ROOT: Stimulant. Antispasmodic. Expectorant. Nervine. Acrid. Vermifuge.
SEED: Stimulant. Antispasmodic. Expectorant. Nervine. Acrid. Vermifuge.

Successfully used in whooping cough, asthma hysteria, chronic rheumatism, spasms, convulsions during pregnancy, and nervous irritability.

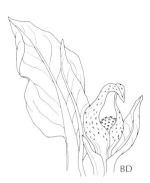

Snakehead

Chelone glabra

Balmony. Bitter Herb. Shell Flower. White Turtlehead. Turtlebloom.

LEAVES: Antibilious. Tonic. Aperient. Vermifuge.

A gentle laxative. A tonic with a beneficial effect on the liver. An ointment made from the fresh leaves is valuable for the itching and irritation of piles.

"A plant of brooks and wet places. Can. and U.S. with flowers shaped like the head of a snake, the mouth open and tongue extended. Aug. Sept."

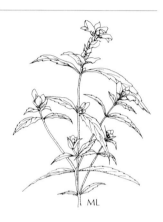

Snakeroot, Black

Cimicifuga racemosa

Black Cohosh. Rattleroot.

ROOT: Narcotic. Sedative. Antispasmodic.

It is slightly narcotic, sedative, and antispasmodic. Too-large doses cause nausea.

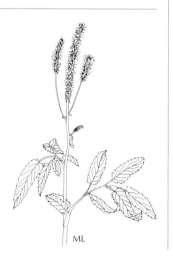

Snakeroot, Button

Liatris spicata

Gayfeather. Devil's Bit. Blazing Star. Colic Root.

ROOT: Diuretic. Tonic. Emmenagogue. Stimulant. Balsamic.

Valuable in scrofula, dysmenorrhea, amenorrhea, gleet. Also in Bright's disease, combined with bugle and unicorn.

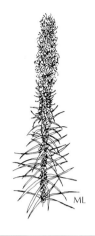

Snakeroot, Canada

Asarum canadense

Indian Ginger. Vermont Snake Root. Heart Snake Root.

ROOT: Stimulant. Aromatic. Diaphoretic. Nervine. Herpatic.

Valuable in causing perspiration; promotes expectoration, and possesses carminitive properties. Used in colic.

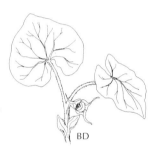

Snakeroot, Seneca

Polygala senega

Mountain Flax. Seneca Root. Senega Root.

ROOT: Sialogogue. Expectorant. Diuretic. Emetic. Cathartic. Emmenagogue. Stimulant. Diaphoretic.

Used in chronic catarrh, croup, asthma, and lung diseases, as an expectorant. In large doses it is emetic and cathartic.

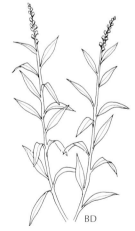

Snakeroot, Virginia

Aristolochia serpentaria

Snake Root. Snake Weed. Snagrel.

ROOT: Stimulant. Tonic. Diaphoretic. Sudorific.

Used to produce perspiration and to strengthen the stomach and appetite.

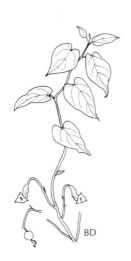

Soapwort

Saponaria officinalis

Bouncing Bet. Old Maid's Pink. London Pride.

HERB: Tonic. Diaphoretic. Alterative. Sudorific. Aromatic. Demulcent. Astringent.

Valuable in syphilis, scrofula, cutaneous diseases, jaundice, and liver complaints.

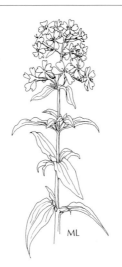

Solomon's Seal, Giant

Polygonatum multiflorum

ROOT: Tonic. Mucilaginous. Astringent. Demulcent. Balsamic. Pectoral.

Much used in female debility, leukorrhea, piles, pectoral affections, and erysipelas, and as a wash to counter the poison from ivy.

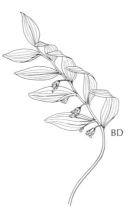

Solomon's Seal, False

Smilacina racemosa

Seal Root. Dropberry. False Spikenard.

ROOT: Tonic. Mucilaginous. Astringent. Demulcent.

Much used in female debility, leukorrhea, piles, pectoral affections, and erysipelas, and as a wash to counter the poison from ivy.

"A small plant upon the edges of woodlands. Can. and N. Eng. and West to Wis. Berries pale red, speckled with purple. May."

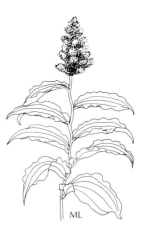

Sorrel, Lady's

Oxalis acetosella

Wood Sorrel. Common Sorrel.

LEAVES: Refrigerant. Antiseptic. Diaphoretic. Diuretic.

Uses similar to sheep sorrel. Beneficial when eaten green.

"Woods and shady places. Can. and U.S. June."

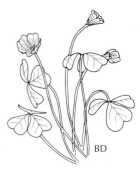

Sorrel, Sheep

Rumex acetosella

Red Top Sorrel. Field Sorrel.

LEAVES: Refrigerant. Diuretic. Antiscorbutic. Tonic.

Used in scurvy, scrofula, and skin diseases; as a poultice for tumors, wens, boils; as an extract said to cure cancers and tumors.

"A common weed in pastures and waste grounds throughout the U.S. preferring dry, hard soils. June, Aug."

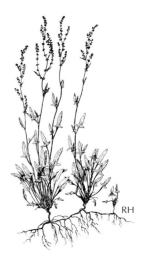

Southernwood

Artemisia abrotanum

Old Man's Tree. Boy's Love.

HERB: Stimulant. Nervine. Tonic. Anthelmintic. Detergent.

Valuable in obstructions and to remove worms.

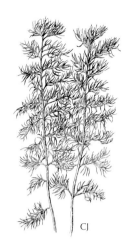

CJ

Spearmint

Mentha spicata (M. viridis)

HERB: Febrifuge. Antispasmodic. Carminitive. Stimulant. Diuretic. Aromatic.

Valuable in colic, spasms, dropsy; to prevent vomiting, gravel, suppression of urine, scalding of urine; and as a local application to piles.

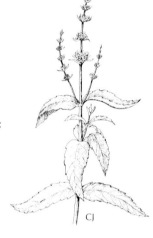

CJ

Speedwell, Common

Veronica officinalis

Paul Betony.

HERB: Expectorant. Alterative. Tonic. Diuretic. Diaphoretic.

Recommended in croup, catarrh, renal and skin diseases, jaundice, and scrofula.

"In meadows, valleys and in grass by the road side. U.S. and Can. May. Aug."

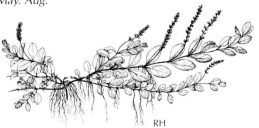

RH

Spicebush

Lindera benzoin

Fever Bush. Feverwood.

TWIGS: Aromatic. Febrifuge. Vermifuge. Stimulant.

Useful in reducing fever and expelling worms.

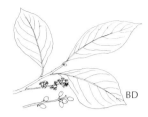

BD

Spikenard

Aralia racemosa

Life-of-Man. Petty Morrel. Spignet.

ROOT: Pectoral. Balsamic. Stomachic.

Used in coughs, colds, pulmonary affections, gout, skin diseases, and to purify the blood.

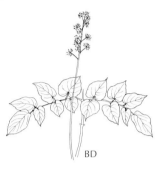

BD

Spleenwort, Silvery

Diplazium pycnocarpon (Asplenium angustifolium)

HERB: Demulcent. Pectoral. Diuretic.

Used in pectoral and lung diseases and to cure an enlarged spleen.

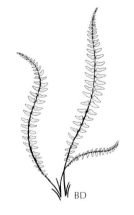

BD

Spurred Rye

Secale cereale

Smut Rye. Ergot (*Claviceps purpurea*).

THE DEGENERATED SEED: Abortive. Narcotic.

Its chief use as a medicine is to promote uterine contractions. It is too powerful and dangerous for domestic use or self-medication.

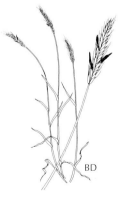

BD

Squaw Vine

Mitchella repens

> Partridge Berry. Winter Clover. Deer Berry. One Berry. Checkerberry.

HERB: Parturient. Diuretic. Astringent. Emmenagogue.

Highly beneficial in diseases of the uterus, parturition, dropsy, suppression of urine; a powerful uterine tonic. Similar in effect to pipsissewa.

"A little prostrate plant, found in woods throughout the U.S. and Can. Fruit well flavored but dry. Used by the Indians hence its name. June."

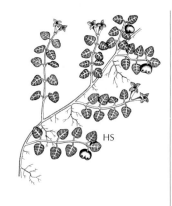

Squaw-Weed

Senecio aureus

> Life Root. Golden Ragwort. Female Regulator. Blue Cohosh. Cocash Weed. Coughweed.

ROOT: Deobstruent. Narcotic.
HERB: Tonic. Herpatic. Acrid. Deobstruent. Narcotic. Emmenagogue.

A female tonic and regulator.

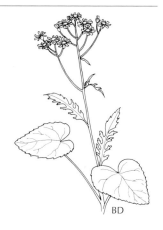

Squill

Urginea maritima (U. scilla)

> Scilla. Sea Onion.

BULB: Tonic.

Resembles digitalis in physiological action and is a poison in overdoses, causing death by heart paralysis. Used as a rat poison.

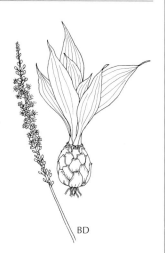

Star Root

Aletris farinosa

> Star Grass. Ague Root. Colic Root.

ROOT: Tonic.

This is of great utility in flatulent colic; a valuable bitter tonic.

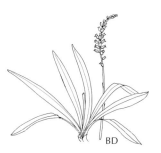

Starflower

Aster novae-angliae

> Starwort. New England Aster.

THE WHOLE HERB: Herpatic. Stomachic. Nervine. Tonic.

As a tonic it acts similarly to chamomile.

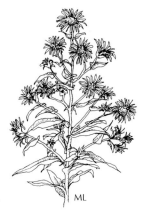

Steeplebush

Spiraea tomentosa

> Meadowsweet. Hardhack.

LEAVES: Astringent. Tonic. Antiseptic. Febrifuge.
ROOT: Astringent. Tonic. Antiseptic. Febrifuge.

Useful as an astringent, and it is tonic in diarrhea.

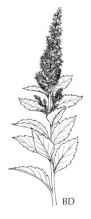

Stillingia

Stillingia sylvatica

> Queen's Root. Queen's Delight. Silver Leaf.

ROOT: Cathartic. Alterative.

Invaluable in scrofula, syphilis, liver and cutaneous diseases, bronchitis, laryngitis, and lung complaints.

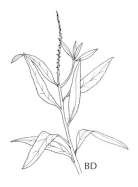

Stone Brake

Eupatorium purpureum

Queen of the Meadow. Gravel Root. Joe-Pye.

FLOWERS: Diuretic. Tonic.
ROOT: Antilithic. Diaphoretic. Astringent.

In decoctions the flowers are diuretic and tonic. The roots are astringent and useful in diarrhea.

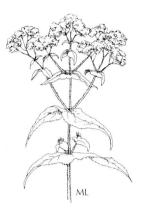

Stone Root

Collinsonia canadensis

Horse Weed. Rich Weed. Ox Balm. Wound Wort.

ROOT AND PLANT: Diuretic. Stomachic. Stimulant.

Used in chronic catarrh of the bladder, fluor albus and debility of the stomach, lithic acid, and calculous deposits.

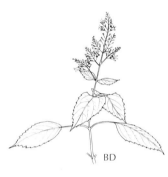

Strawberry

Fragaria virginiana

LEAVES: Astringent. Febrifuge. Refrigerant.
VINES: Astringent. Febrifuge. Refrigerant.

Useful in diarrhea, dysentery, intestinal debility, and night sweats. The fruit is used in calculous disorders and gout.

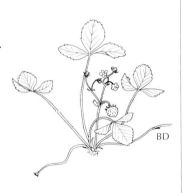

Sumach

Rhus glabra

Upland Sumach. Smooth Sumach. Pennsylvania Sumach.

BARK: Tonic. Astringent. Antiseptic.
BERRIES: Astringent. Refrigerant. Diuretic.
LEAVES: Tonic. Astringent. Antiseptic. Diuretic.

Valuable in gonorrhea, leukorrhea, diarrhea, hectic fever, and scrofula. The berries are used in diabetes, bowel complaints, febrile diseases, canker, and sore mouth.

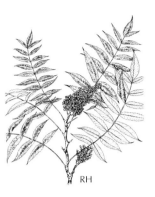

Sunflower, Garden

Helianthus annuus

SEED: Expectorant. Astringent. Diuretic.
LEAVES: Astringent.

Used in coughs and pulmonary affections, dysentery, and inflammation of the bladder and kidneys.

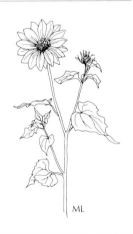

Sunflower, Wild

Helianthus divaricatus

SEED: Expectorant. Diuretic. Carminitive. Antispasmodic. Laxative.

Useful in treatment of bronchial and pulmonary affections.

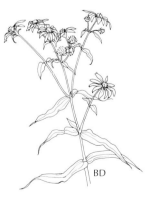

Sweet Clover

Melilotus officinalis

King's Clover. Melilot. Yellow Sweet Clover.

HERB: Emollient. Discutient.

The leaves and flowers boiled in lard are useful in all kinds of ulcers, inflammations, and burns.

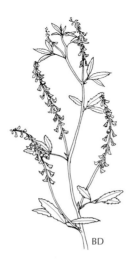

Sweet Flag

Acorus calamus

Calamus. Sweet Rush.

ROOT: Carminitive. Stomachic. Stimulant. Aromatic.

Used in flatulent colic, dyspepsia, and feeble digestion, and to aid the action of Peruvian bark in intermittents. Externally it is used to excite the discharges from blistered surfaces, indolent ulcers, and issues.

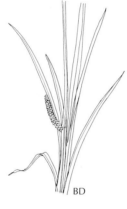

Sweet Gale

Myrica gale

Meadow Fern. Bog Myrtle. Gale Fern. Sweet Willow.

BUDS: Pectoral. Astringent. Aromatic. Herpatic.
LEAVES: Pectoral. Astringent. Aromatic. Herpatic.

This is a stimulant, alterative, depurative, and vulnerary.

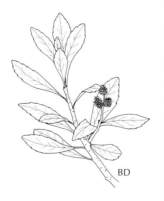

Sweet Gum

Liquidambar styraciflua

Red Gum. Star-Leaved Gum.

BARK: Pectoral.

Used as a household remedy for coughs resulting from colds. It is also useful when made into an ointment to rub on the throat.

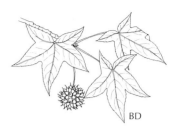

Tamarack

Larix laricina (L. americana)

Hackmatack. American Larch.

BARK: Laxative. Tonic. Diuretic. Alterative. Aperient. Expectorant. Balsamic.

Recommended in obstructions of the liver, rheumatism, jaundice, and cutaneous diseases.

"A beautiful tree in forests from Canada to Pennsylvania, April and May."

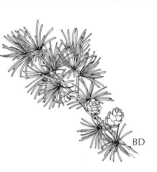

Tansy

Tanacetum vulgare

Double Tansy. Sweet Tansy.

HERB: Tonic. Emmenagogue. Diaphoretic. Vermifuge. Stomachic. Sudorific. Aromatic.

Used in fevers, agues, hysterics, dropsy, and worms, and as a fomentation in swellings, tumors, and inflammations.

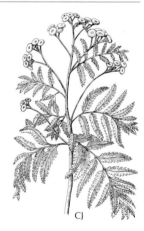

Thimble Weed

Rudbeckia laciniata

Cone-Disk. Cone-Flower.

HERB: Diuretic. Tonic. Balsamic.

Valuable in Bright's disease, wasting of the kidneys, and urinary complaints generally.

"In the edges of swamps & ditches. Can. and U.S. Aug."

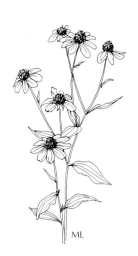

Thistle Root

Cirsium arvense

Canada Root. Canada Thistle. Cursed Thistle.

ROOT: Tonic. Astringent. Diuretic.

Boiled with milk for dysentery and diarrhea.

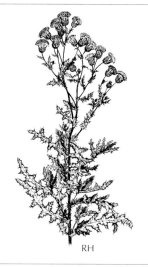

Thorn Apple

Datura stramonium

Apple. Peru. Jamestown Weed. Jimson Weed. Stink Weed. Stramonium.

LEAVES (poisonous): Antispasmodic. Narcotic. Sedative. Acrid.
SEED (poisonous): Antispasmodic. Narcotic. Acrid.

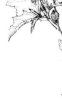

Used in epilepsy, tic douloureux, nervous affections, and ophthalmic operations. The leaves are smoked to relieve spasmodic asthma. The seeds are administered to prevent abortion. In large doses it is an energetic narcotic poison. Its victims suffer the most intense agonies and die in maniacal delirium. In medicinal doses it is reported to have been used as a substitute for opium.

Thyme

Thymus serpyllum

American Wild. Mother of Thyme. Creeping Thyme.

HERB: Stomachic. Aromatic. Tonic.

Used in dyspepsia, weak stomach, hysteria, dysmenorrhea, flatulence, colic, and headache, and to produce perspiration.

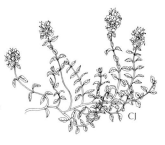

Thyme, English

Thymus vulgaris

Common Thyme. Garden Thyme.

HERB: Aromatic. Stomachic. Stimulant. Sudorific. Tonic. Carminitive. Emmenagogue. Antispasmodic.

Used in dyspepsia, weak stomach, hysteria, dysmenorrhea, flatulence, colic, and headache, and to produce perspiration.

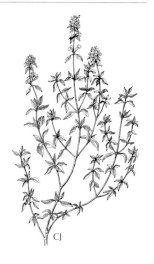

Tilia

Tilia americana

Lime Tree. Linden.

FLOWERS: Sudorific. Antispasmodic. Nervine.
LEAVES: Sudorific. Antispasmodic. Nervine.

The flowers and leaves are stomachic. A tea of linden, tilia flowers, and leaves is admirable for promoting perspiration. It quiets coughs and relieves hoarseness resulting from colds.

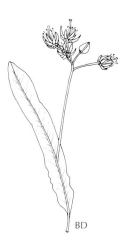

Tomato

*Lycopersicon lycopersicum
(Hycopersicon esculentum)*

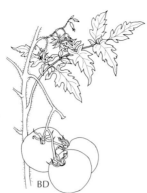

Extract of tomato was sold in several communities and was handled by the medical departments because it was used in many preparations to make them more palatable.

"Tomato Pills: Take Wild Turnip, Lady Slipper and Caraway Seed, equal parts, ½ quantity castor oil and the same of rhubarb mixed with the extract of tomato."

Trillium, Purple

Trillium erectum (T. purpureum)
  Bath Flower. Bethroot.

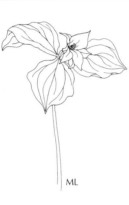

ROOT: Astringent. Tonic.

An astringent and, when boiled in milk, of eminent benefit in cases of diarrhea. The root, made into a poultice, is very useful in stings of insects. The leaves boiled in lard are a good external application for skin affections.

Turkey Corn

Dicentra canadensis
  Corydalis. Turkey Pea.
  Stagger Weed. Squirrel Corn.

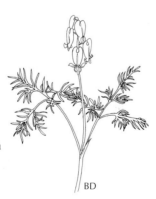

ROOT: Tonic. Diuretic.
  Alterative.

One of the best remedies in syphilitic diseases; also in scrofula and cutaneous affections.

Turmeric

Curcuma domestica (C. longa)

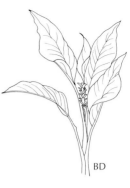

ROOT: Aromatic. Tonic. Laxative.
  Stimulant.

Used as a condiment, yellow dye, and medicine.

Twinleaf

Jeffersonia diphylla
  Ground Squirrel Pea.
  Rheumatism Root. Helmet
  Pod.

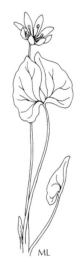

ROOT: Stimulant. Diaphoretic.
  Diuretic. Alterative.
  Antispasmodic.

Successfully used in chronic rheumatism, secondary syphilis, mercurial syphilis, dropsy, nervous affections, spasms, and cramps; also as a gargle in diseases of the throat, scarlatina, and indolent ulcers.

Unicorn Root, False

Chamaelirium luteum
  Drooping Starwort. Starwort.
  Star Root. Helonias.

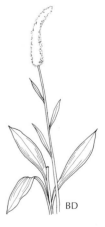

ROOT: Tonic. Diuretic. Vermifuge.
  Stomachic.

Invaluable as a uterine tonic, imparting tone and vigor to the reproductive organs; used in leukorrhea, amenorrhea, and dysmenorrhea, and to remove the tendency to miscarriage.

Uva-Ursi

Arctostaphylos uva-ursi

Bearberry. Upland Cranberry. Mountain Cranberry. Mountain Box. Arbutus Uva Ursi.

LEAVES: Tonic. Diuretic. Astringent. Antilithic.

Used in chronic affections of the kidneys and urinary passages, strangury, diabetes, fluor albus, and excessive mucus discharges with the urine, lithic acid, etc.

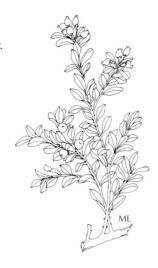

Valerian, American

Cypripedium calceolus var. *pubescens*

Nerve Root. Yellow Moccasin Flower. Yellow Lady's Slipper.

ROOT: Sudorific. Nervine. Anodyne. Stimulant.

Used in cholera, nervous debility, hysteria, and low forms of fever where a nervous stimulant is required.

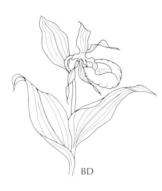

Valerian, English

Valeriana officinalis

Great Wild Valerian. Vandal Root.

ROOT: Antispasmodic. Tonic. Stimulant. Sudorific. Stomachic.

Used in cholera, nervous debility, hysteria, and low forms of fever where a nervous stimulant is required.

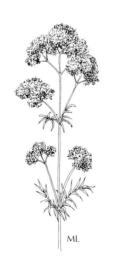

Valerian, Greek

Polemonium reptans

ROOT: Sudorific. Astringent. Febrifuge.

Used in cholera, nervous debility, hysteria, and low forms of fever where a nervous stimulant is required.

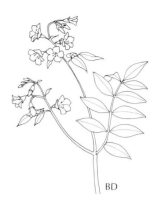

Vervain

Verbena hastata

Wild Hyssop. Simpler's Joy. Erect Vervain. Blue Vervain.

HERB: Tonic. Emetic. Expectorant. Sudorific.
ROOT: Tonic. Emetic. Expectorant. Sudorific.

Used in intermittent fevers, colds, obstructed menses, scrofula, gravel, and worms.

"Frequently by roadsides and in low grounds, mostly throughout the U.S. and Can. July. Sept."

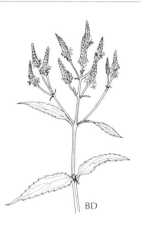

Violet

Viola pedata

Bird's-Foot Violet.

HERB: Pectoral. Expectorant. Tonic. Mucilaginous. Emollient. Demulcent. Laxative. Aperient. Antisyphilitic. Sudorific.

Used in colds, coughs, and sore throats.

"This is one of the most common kinds of violet, found in low grassy woods from Arctic Amer. to Florida. Apr. May."

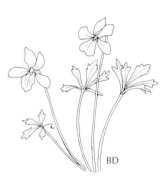

Violet, Canker
Viola rostrata

HERB: Demulcent. Tonic. Diuretic. Aperient.

Said to be useful in pectoral and cutaneous diseases; also in syphilis.

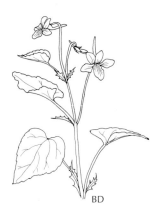

Virgin's Bower
Clematis virginiana
    Travellers' Joy. Clematis.

LEAVES: Stimulant. Nervine.

Used in severe headache, in cancerous ulcers, and as ointment in itches.

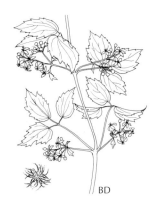

Wa-A-Hoo
Euonymus atropurpurea
    Euonymous. Indian Arrow-Wood. Burning Bush. Spindle Tree.

BARK: Tonic. Laxative. Alterative. Diuretic. Cathartic. Expectorant.

Useful in intermittent fever, dyspepsia, torpid liver, constipation, dropsy, and pulmonary affections. (This is not recommended for home use.)

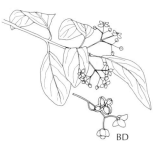

Walnut
Juglans cinerea, J. nigra
    Shagbarks. White Walnut. Butternut Bark. Oil Nut.

BARK: Styptic. Tonic. Alterative. Cathartic.
LEAVES: Styptic. Tonic. Alterative. Cathartic.

Used in scrofula, debility, and diarrhea; as a gentle cathartic; and as a wash for ulcers and sore eyes.

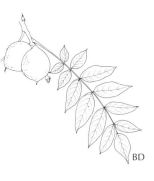

Water Hoarhound
Lycopus europaeus, L. virginicus
    Water Bugle. Gipsy Wort.

HERB: Tonic. Astringent. Sedative. Narcotic.

This is a tonic and is mildly narcotic; it has a quieting effect.

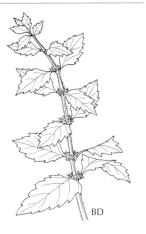

Water Pepper
Polygonum hydropiperoides
    Smart Weed. Arsmart. Heartweed.

HERB: Expectorant. Sudorific. Vesicant. Antiseptic. Diaphoretic. Stimulant. Diuretic. Emmenagogue. Acrid. Pectoral.

Used in amenorrhea, gravel, colds, coughs, milk sickness, bowel complaints, and erysipelas.

"The leaves are marked with a brownish spot. Common around buildings and fences, wet grounds. Leaves two to four inches long. Stem leafy, one to two feet high. June–Aug."

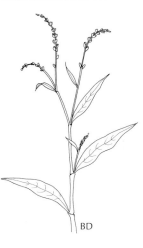

Watercup

Sarracenia purpurea

Side-Saddle Flower. Pitcher Plant. Fly-trap. Huntsman's Cup. Small-Pox Plant.

HERB: Tonic. Stimulant. Diuretic. Laxative. Nervine.

Used in chlorosis, all uterine derangements, dyspepsia, and gastric difficulties; said to be useful in smallpox.

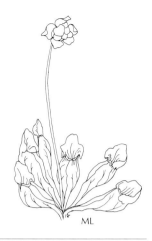

ML

Watermelon

Citrullus lanatus (Cucurbita vulgaris)

SEED: Mucilaginous. Diuretic. Demulcent. Refrigerant.

Valuable in strangury, urinary affections, and dropsy.

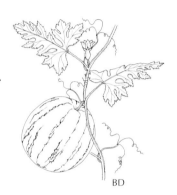

BD

White Root

Erigeron philadelphicus

White Weed. Ox Eye Daisy. White Daisy.

FLOWERS: Aromatic. Stomachic.
LEAVES: Aromatic. Stomachic.

White root is chiefly employed as an insect powder for fleas, etc. The fresh leaves or flowers will destroy or drive them away.

"Woods and pastures throughout North America. June to Aug."

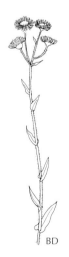

BD

Whitewood

Liriodendron tulipifera

Tulip Tree. Cucumber Tree. Tulip Poplar.

BARK: Antiperiodic. Tonic. Stimulant. Stomachic. Aromatic.

Useful in intermittent fever, low condition of the system, dyspepsia, diarrhea, and hysteria.

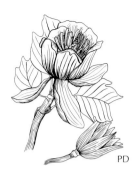

PD

Whortleberry

Vaccinium myrtillus

Bilberry. Blue Berry. Burren Myrtle.

BERRIES: Astringent.
LEAVES: Astringent.

The leaves are strongly astringent and somewhat bitter. They are of great value in diarrhea. A mixture of equal parts of bilberry leaves, thyme, and strawberry leaves makes an excellent tea.

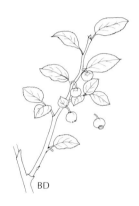

BD

Wickup

Epilobium angustifolium

Mare's Tail. Rose Bay. Willow-Herb. Fireweed.

HERB: Astringent. Antiseptic. Emetic.
ROOT: Astringent. Antiseptic. Emetic.

Used in dysentery, diarrhea, and where an astringent is required.

"In newly cleared lands, low waste grounds. Penn. to Arc. America. July. August."

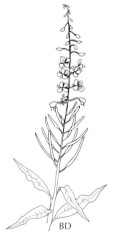

BD

Wild Turnip

Arum triphyllum

 Wake Robin. Jack-in-the-Pulpit. Dragon Root.

ROOT: Stimulant. Expectorant. Acrid. Tonic. Narcotic.

It is acrid, an expectorant and diaphoretic, and is violently irritating if improperly used by one unfamiliar with its peculiarities.

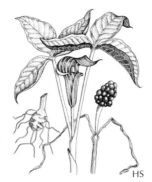

HS

Wild Yam

Dioscorea villosa

 Colic Root.

ROOT: Antispasmodic.

Successfully used in bilious colic, spasms, cramps, flatulence, after pains, and affections of the liver.

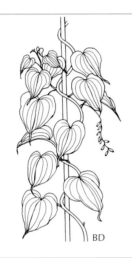

BD

Willow, Pussy

Salix discolor

BARK: Tonic. Astringent. Anthelmintic. Antiseptic.

Used in indigestion, in weak and relaxed condition of the bowels, diarrhea, worms, gangrene, and indolent ulcers. The buds are aphrodisiac.

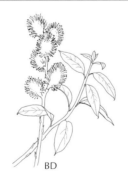

BD

Willow, Rose

Cornus sericea

 Red-Rod. Swamp Dogwood.

BARK: Astringent. Tonic.

Bitter, astringent, detergent, and antiperiodic. Used occasionally as a substitute for quinine.

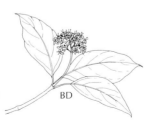

BD

Willow, White

Salix alba

BARK: Tonic. Antiperiodic. Astringent.

Used in intermittent fever, debility of the digestive organs, hemorrhages, chronic mucus discharges, diarrhea, and dysentery. Exerts its virtues in the form of an ointment.

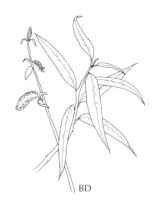

BD

Wintergreen

Gaultheria procumbens

 Tea Berry Plant. Checkerberry. Pipsissawa. Spicey Wintergreen. Box-Berry.

WHOLE PLANT: Diuretic. Stimulant. Stomachic. Emmenagogue.

Increases flow of urine. Stimulates the stomach when used in small doses. Large doses are emetic.

"In woods, Can. and Northern States. Common, June. July."

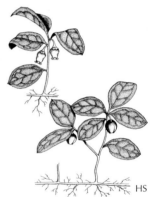

HS

Witch Hazel

Hamamelis virginiana

 Winter Bloom. Snapping Hazle. Snapping Hazle Nut. Spotted Alder.

BARK: Tonic. Astringent. Sedative. Herpatic.

LEAVES: Tonic. Astringent. Sedative.

Valuable in diarrhea, dysentery, and excessive mucus discharges; also as a wash in painful swellings, gargle for canker, and injection for fluor albus.

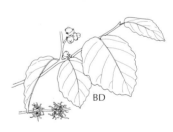

BD

Wormseed

Chenopodium ambrosioides

> Oak Jerusalem Seed. Goose-Foot.

Seed: Anthelmintic. Antispasmodic. Vermifuge. Stomachic. Antibilious.

Valuable to expel worms from children.

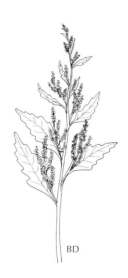

BD

Wormwood, Common

Artemisia absinthium

Herb: Anthelmintic. Tonic. Narcotic. Stimulant. Vermifuge. Antibilious. Stomachic.

Used in intermittent fever, jaundice, and worms; to promote the appetite; and externally in bruises and inflammations.

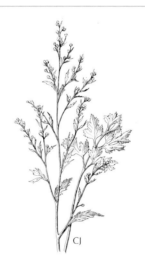

CJ

Wormwood, Roman

Corydalis sempervirens

> Ragweed. Hogweed.

Herb: Emollient. Antiseptic. Stimulant. Tonic. Vermifuge.

Used as fomentation in wounds and bruises, and as ointment in piles, in ulcers, to reduce painful swellings, etc.

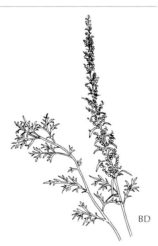

BD

Yarrow

Achillea millefolium

> Millefoil. Noble Yarrow. Lady's Mantle.

Herb: Tonic. Astringent. Alterative. Diuretic. Aromatic. Stomachic. Acrid. Stimulant. Cathartic. Detergent.

Used in hemorrhages, incontinence of urine, diabetes, piles, dysentery, and flatulence, and as injection in leukorrhea.

"In fields and pastures. N.E. to Or. and to the Arctic Sea. Flowers are white or rose colored. July. Sept."

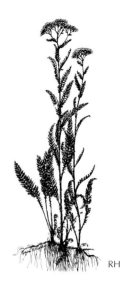

RH

Yellow Jessamine

Gelsemium sempervirens

> Wild Jessamine. Woodbine.

Root: Febrifuge.

A valuable febrifuge in all fevers, except congestive; also used in nervous irritability, headaches, and lockjaw.

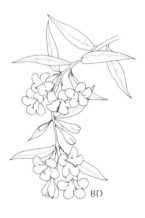

BD

Notes

In these Notes, the references for the illustrations (owner and photographer) follow the page number. The references for the text begin on the following line.

Front Matter

Page i. Lobelia cardinale, drawn by Sister Cora Helena Sarle, Canterbury, photographed by Bill Finney; used by permission of Canterbury Shaker Village, Canterbury, New Hampshire.

Page ii. (Frontispiece). "The Tree of Light or Blazing Tree," by Sister Hannah Cohoon, Hancock; Collections of Hancock Shaker Village, Pittsfield, Mass. (hereafter "Hancock Shaker Village Collections").

Page iii. (Title Page). Photograph taken at Hancock Shaker Village by Paul Rocheleau.

Page v. (Dedication). Photograph taken at Hancock Shaker Village by Paul Rocheleau.

Page vii. (Table of Contents). Lupine drawn by Sister Cora Helena Sarle, Canterbury, photographed by Bill Finney; used by permission of Canterbury Shaker Village, Canterbury, New Hampshire.

Introduction

Page 1. Apothecary cabinet photographed by Dr. M. Stephen Miller; collection of Dr. M. Stephen and Miriam Miller (hereafter "Miller Collection").

Page 2. Growth of Shaker society discussed in Charles Nordhoff, *The Communistic Societies of the United States* (New York: Harper & Brothers, 1875). Nordhoff also totals the land owned by the Shakers in 1875 to be 49,335 acres and says this is incomplete because of real estate in distant states, for which he could get no precise returns. If Shaker holdings in mills, wood lots, and "out farms" were added, the figure would certainly well exceed 60,000 acres. One farm in Kentucky owned by the Watervliet, New York, society was 30,000 acres in size and was operated by tenants.

Page 3. Journal of the Harvard Shakers photographed by Paul Rocheleau; Hancock Shaker Village Collections. *Millennial Laws,* recorded at New Lebanon, New York, August 7, 1781.

Page 4. Millennial Laws, pages 30 and 31. Nordhoff account in Nordhoff, *The Communistic Societies of the United States,* p. 160. Frederick W. Evans, an Englishman by birth, came to America in 1820. He joined the Shakers in 1830 and was in the Elders Order from 1836 to his death in 1893 at the age of eighty-five.

Watervliet (Chapter 1)

Page 5. Brick shop, Robert F. W. Meader photo, Hancock Shaker Village Collections.

Hocknell account in Anna White and Leila S. Taylor, *Shakerism: Its Message and Meaning* (Columbus, Ohio: Press of J. Heer, 1904), p. 82.

Page 6. South Family barns, Robert F. W. Meader photo, Hancock Shaker Village Collections.

Lists of herbs in Account Book kept by Brother Harvey Copley, 1830, and in Herb Journals, 1830–1848, kept by William Charles Brackett; both in collection of Western Reserve Historical Society, Cleveland.

Page 7. 1837 Watervliet catalog, Miller Collection.

1830 Catalog of Medicinal Plants and Vegetable Medicines, Watervliet, Cleveland, Western Reserve Historical Society.

Page 8. NOTE: The Shakers used the variety *Aralia nudicaulis* as sarsaparilla, rather than *Similax officinalis,* the true sarsaparilla of South America.

Page 10. Wrapper for herb cake, Miller Collection.

Peach Water and extracts in 1833 Catalog of Medicinal Plants and Vegetable Medicines, Watervliet, Cleveland, Western Reserve Historical Society.

Orders recorded in Herb Catalog issued by Watervliet Society, 1835, Cleveland, Western Reserve Historical Society.

Pages 10-11. Brackett observations in 1832 Account Book kept by Shakers at Watervliet, 1832, Cleveland, Western Reserve Historical Society.

Page 12. House of Representatives report cited in Margaret B. Keig, *Green Medicine* (Chicago: Apollo, 1971), p. 93.

Pages 12–14. 1837 Catalog of Medicinal Plants and Vegetable Medicines, Miller Collection.

Page 15. Fleabane label.
  Three herb catalogs, 1843, 1845, 1847, and 1850 Catalog of Herbs, Medicinal Plants, and Vegetable Medicines; all in Collection of Western Reserve Historical Society, Cleveland.

Page 16. Sarsaparilla label, Miller Collection.

Page 17. 1860 Catalog of Medicinal Plants, Barks, Roots, Seeds, and Flowers, Western Reserve Historical Society, Cleveland.

Page 18. Labels, Miller Collection; "Bought of Chaucy Miller" broadside, Hancock Shaker Village Collections. Photographed by Paul Rocheleau.

New Lebanon (Chapter 2)

Page 19. Kitchen garden, Hancock Shaker Village Collections. Photographed by Paul Rocheleau.

Page 20. Norwood's Veratrum Viride, Miller Collection.
  Silliman account in Benjamin Silliman, "Remarks Made on a Short Tour between Hartford and Quebec in the Autumn of 1819," *Christian Monthly Spectator* (New Haven, 1820), pp. 41–53. Dickens account in Charles Dickens, *American Notes for General Circulation Written After His First Visit in 1842* (New York: D. Appleton and Co., 1872), 2:211.

Page 21. North Family buildings, Hancock Shaker Village Collections. Photographed by Paul Rocheleau.
  Carr account in Sister Frances Carr, "The Shakers as Herb Growers," in *The Shaker Quarterly* III, 2 (Summer 1963), p. 39.

Page 22. Herb chart in account book, n.d., Emma B. King Library, Shaker Collection, Shaker Museum at Old Chatham, N.Y. Peddler's letter in Journal and letter kept at New Lebanon, 1860, Western Reserve Historical Society, Cleveland.

Page 23. Poppy label, Miller Collection. Sage label, Opium label, Hancock Shaker Village Collections. Photographed by Paul Rocheleau.

Formula for the Shaker digestive cordial, anon., Emma B. King Library, Shaker Museum at Old Chatham, N.Y.

Journals of the church deaconesses at New Lebanon, N.Y., January 1, 1843–June 23, 1864, Hancock Shaker Village Collections.

Shaker sister's account attributed to Sister Marcia Bullard, "Shaker Industries," *Good Housekeeping* (July 1906), 43:33–37.

Page 24. Photograph by Paul Rocheleau.

Page 25. Philemon Stewart records in Three Journals, Philemon Stewart, New Lebanon, 1826–1831, Library of Congress, Washington, D.C.
  Duyckinck account in Evert A. Duyckinck, *The Literary World,* vol. 9 (September 13, 1851), 11:201, 202.
  Fowler quoted in *American Journal of Pharmacy,* n.s., vol. 18, no. 24 (1852), American Pharmaceutical Association, Washington, D.C.

Page 26. Asthma Cure label, Miller Collection.
  1969 account of Tilden and Company, *Chatham Courier,* January 9, 1969, p. 12, Emma B. King Library, Shaker Museum, Old Chatham, N.Y. See also Tilden advertising circular, Tilden and Company, 1849, Shaker Collection, Western Reserve Historical Society, Cleveland.

Page 27. Syrup of Black Cohosh label, Miller Collection.
  Notebook of medical receipts and cures from the nurses' shop, New Lebanon, 1815, Hancock Shaker Village Collections.
  1836 Catalogue of Medicinal Plants and Vegetable Medicines, 1837 Catalogue of Herbs, and 1838 Catalogue of Medicinal Plants and Vegetable Medicines, Western Reserve Historical Society, Cleveland.
  Catalogues of Medicinal Plant and Vegetable Medicines, 1841, 1848, 1850, American Antiquarian Society, Worcester, Mass.
  1851 Catalogue of Medicinal Plants, Barks, Roots, Seeds, Flowers, and Select Powders, Western Reserve Historical Society, Cleveland.

Page 28. Violet drawn by Sister Cora Helena Sarle, Canterbury, photographed by Bill Finney; used by permission of Canterbury Shaker Village, Canterbury, New Hampshire. Catalogues of Medicinal Plants, Barks, Roots, Seeds, Flowers, and Select Powders, 1860, 1866, Cleveland, Western Reserve Historical Society.

Page 28 continued
"List of Fluid and Solid Extracts," n.d., Cleveland, Western Reserve Historical Society.

"List of Fluid Extracts," 1871, Hancock Shaker Village Collections.

Page 29. The Shaker Family Pills, Miller Collection. 1874 Price List, Miller Collection.

"Wholesale List for Dealers Only," 1874 American Antiquarian Society, Worcester, Mass.

"Price List of Medicinal Preparations," Emma B. King Library, Shaker Museum, Old Chatham, N.Y.

Page 30. "Shakers' Fluid Extracts," Miller Collection.

"List of Fluid Extracts," 1871, Hancock Shaker Village Collections.

Page 31. Sarsaparilla and Deadly Nightshade labels, Miller Collection.

Apothecary account in Journal kept at New Lebanon, May 23, 1789, Hancock Shaker Village Collections.

Diary of Benjamin Gates, New Lebanon, 1827, Andrews Collection, Henry Francis du Pont Museum, Winterthur, Del.

Pages 32–33. Diary of Milton Homer Robinson, New Lebanon, 1832, Library of Congress, Washington, D.C.

Page 34. "Syrup of Sarsaparilla" label, Miller Collection.

Journal of Barnabas Hinckley, New Lebanon, 1836, Andrews Collection, Henry Francis du Pont Museum, Winterthur, Del. Garrett Lawrence's death was possibly due to intestinal cancer. For a description of Lawrence's autopsy, see Giles Avery's Journal (Western Reserve Heritage Society, Cleveland, Ohio, WRHS VB:106).

DeRobigne Mortimer Bennett, mentioned on page 35, was born on December 23, 1818, died on December 6, 1882, and was received into the New Lebanon Society when he was fourteen years old. He worked in the seed gardens and learned the primitive pharmacy of roots, barks, and herbs. He became the physician of the community fourteen years later and left in 1846. He then became a purveyor of a number of spurious concoctions: Dr. Bennett's Quick Cure, Golden Liniment, Worm Lozenges, and Root and Plant Pills. He was an amalgam of quack, crank, and idealist.

Page 35. Illustration of Barnabas Hinckley in Benson John Lossing, "The Shakers," *Harper's New Monthly Magazine,* vol. 15, no. 86 (1857), 172–75.

Page 37. Autobiographical sketch of DeRobigne Mortimer Bennett in *The World's Sages, Thinkers, and Reformers,* 2nd ed. rev. (New York: Liberal and Scientific Publ. House, 1876), p. 192.

Page 36. Cornus canadensis drawn by Sister Cora Helena Sarle, Canterbury, photographed by Bill Finney; used by permission of Canterbury Shaker Village, Canterbury, New Hampshire.

Shaw account in Journal of Levi Shaw, n.d., Shaker Collection, Library of Congress, Washington, D.C.

Deaconesses' record in A Journal of Domestic Events and Transactions, January 1, 1842, to October 1864, at New Lebanon, N.Y., kept by Deaconesses, Ch[urch], 2nd order. Hancock Shaker Village Collections.

Travel record, South Union ministry, 1865–1871, vol. 1, Shaker Collection, Library of the University of Southern Kentucky, Bowling Green.

Page 37. Travel account in Eldress Betsy Smith's journal, South Union, Ky., 1854, Library of the University of Southern Kentucky, Bowling Green.

Pages 37–41. Lossing account and illustrations in Benson John Lossing, "The Shakers," *Harper's New Monthly Magazine,* vol. 15, no. 86 (1857), 172–75.

Page 41–42. Description of amounts of plant material processed in Account book of the extract herb industry, Church Family, New Lebanon, 1860–1862, Andrews Collection, Henry Francis du pont Museum, Winterthur, Del.

Page 42. Lobelia cardinale, drawn by Sister Cora Helena Sarle, Canterbury, photographed by Bill Finney; used by permission of Canterbury Shaker Village, Canterbury, New Hampshire.

Page 43. "Norwood's Tincture of Veratrum Viride" box and bottle, Miller Collection.

Sisters' work described in *The Shaker Manifesto,* February 10, 1892, Hancock Shaker Village Collections.

Shaker booklet on *Veratrum Viride,* 4th ed. (New York, 1858), Hancock Shaker Village Collections.

Formula for tincture of *Veratrum viride,* March 1934. Emma B. King Library, Shaker Museum, Old Chatham, N.Y.

Page 44. 1905 almanac advertising "Seven Barks," Miller Collection.

Benjamin Gates description of Pain King, with formula, in Benjamin Gates to "Our Seneca II," n.d., Hancock Shaker Village Collections.

Asthma promotion in Catalogue for Shaker Asthma Cure, 1886, Cleveland, Western Reserve Historical Society.

Page 45. "Syrup of Bitter Bugle," Miller Collection.

Benjamin Gates formula for Pain King in Benjamin Gates to "Our Seneca II," n.d., Hancock Shaker Village Collections.

Page 46. Letter from Peek and Velsor, botanic druggists, to Edward Fowler, Oct. 10, 1877. Williams College Archives and Special Collections, Williamstown, Mass.

Smith Brothers situation recounted in Letter from Benjamin Gates to Henry Clough, August 20, 1884, Hancock Shaker Village Collections.

Page 47. "Seigel's Curative Syrup," Hancock Shaker Village Collections, photographed by Paul Rocheleau.

Gates to Clough, September 23, 1882, Hancock Shaker Village Collections.

Gates to Clough, October 31, 1885, Hancock Shaker Village Collections.

Letter from "David at New Lebanon, to the World" (the people of the world), 1807, Williams College Archives and Special Collections, Williamstown, Mass.

Account of Indians in Journal kept at New Lebanon, anon., 1842, Cleveland, Western Reserve Historical Society.

Page 48. False hellebore *(Veratrum viride),* drawn by Sister Cora Helena Sarle, Canterbury, photographed by Bill Finney; used by permission of Canterbury Shaker Village, Canterbury, New Hampshire.

Record book kept by James Vail at New Lebanon 1841–1857, Cleveland, Western Reserve Historical Society, Shaker Collection.

Order for herbs, May 9, 1876, Emma B. King Library, Shaker Museum at Old Chatham, N.Y.

Page 49. A. J. White editorial and Hepworth Dixon testimonial in 1882 Almanac (New York: A. J. White), Hancock Shaker Village Collections.

Page 50. Vegetable seed catalogues (1881, 1884, 1885, 1887, 1888), Cleveland, Western Reserve Historical Society, Shaker Collection.

Page 51. Letter from Amelia J. Calver to Henry Clough, April 23, 1890, Hancock Shaker Village Collections.

Page 52. Butterfly weed drawn by Sister Cora Helena Sarle, Canterbury, photographed by Bill Finney; used by permission of Canterbury Shaker Village, Canterbury, New Hampshire.

Announcement of Henry Clough's return in Letter from Alonzo Hollister to "Esteemed Friend," February 19, 1909, Hancock Shaker Village Collections.

Account of vegetarianism in Martha J. Anderson, "History of Dietetic Reform as Practiced at the North Family, Mt. Lebanon and Canaan, Columbia County, New York," *Food, Home and Garden* (Philadelphia, Jan. 1894, pp. 6–7), Library of Fruitlands Museum, Harvard, Mass.

Accounts of sisters' expeditions in Deaconesses journal, 1843–1864, Hancock Shaker Village Collections.

Norwood visit recorded in Journal, Church Family (2nd Order), 1858–1867, Hancock Shaker Village Collections.

Groveland (Chapter 3)

Page 53. Photograph of Groveland meetinghouse and brick dwelling in collection of Hancock Shaker Village, Pittsfield, Mass.

History of founding of Sodus Bay community in Anna White and Leila S. Taylor, *Shakerism: Its Message and Meaning* (Columbus, Ohio: Press of Fred J. Heer, 1904), p. 155.

Recipes in "Receipts of Materia Medica written at Groveland, May 1842," Cleveland, Western Reserve Historical Society.

Hancock Bishopric (Chapter 4)

Page 55. Photograph of round stone barn, Hancock Shaker Village Collections.

Page 56. Hancock seed list and photograph of brick dwelling and sisters' gift shop, Hancock Shaker Village Collections. Photograph by Paul Rocheleau.

Account book for the seed business at Hancock, Mass. (1824–1829), 80 pp., Cleveland, Western Reserve Historical Society.

1813 Broadside, 1 p., Emma B. King Library, Shaker Museum at Old Chatham, N.Y.

Paul W. Gates, Hancock broadside, 1839, *The Farmers' Age, 1815–1860* (New York: Holt, Rinehard & Winston, 1960), facing p. 300.

Page 56 continued

    Description of Shaker herbs in Samuel W. Bush, *A History of the County of Berkshire* (Pittsfield, Mass.: 1829), pp. 55, 59, 65, 68, 69, 71, 79.

    West family journal, New Lebanon, N.Y., 1867, Emma B. King Library, Shaker Collection, Museum at Old Chatham, N.Y.

Page 57. "Floral Wreath" spirit drawing, attributed to Sister Polly Collins, Hancock Shaker Village Collections.

    Receipt book, Church Family at Hancock, 1828–1846, Cleveland, Western Reserve Historical Society.

Page 58. Photograph of Church Family, Tyringham, Hancock Shaker Village Collections.

    Tyringham herbal remedies in Darias Herrick, "Hints and Recipes" (1845), pp. 66–67, Cleveland, Western Reserve Historical Society.

Page 59. Coltsfoot drawn by Sister Cora Helena Sarle, Canterbury, photographed by Bill Finney; used by permission of Canterbury Shaker Village, Canterbury, New Hampshire.

    1826 seed catalogue, Tyringham, Emma B. King Library, Shaker Museum at Old Chatham, N.Y.

    1850 seed catalogue, Tyringham, Library of Fruitlands Museum, Harvard, Mass.

Page 60. Photograph of Church Family, Enfield, Hancock Shaker Village Collections.

Page 61. "Fresh Herbs" broadside, Hancock Shaker Village Collections. Photographed by Paul Rocheleau.

    A book of prescriptions given by Dr. Hamilton, family physician to the Shakers, Enfield, Conn., 1825. Cleveland, Western Reserve Historical Society.

    For more about Jefferson White see Deborah E. Burns, *Shaker Cities of Peace, Love, and Union* (Hanover, N.H.: University Press of New England, 1993).

Page 62. "Genuine Shaker Healoline," Miller Collection.

    Belden catalog in Rudy J. Favretti, *Early New England Gardens* (Meriden, Conn.: Meriden Gravure Co., 1962), p. 14.

Harvard and Shirley, Mass. (Chapter 5)

Page 63. Photograph of Harvard Church Family, Hancock Shaker Village Collections.

Page 64. Fruit tree records cited in Clara Endicott Sears, *Gleanings From Old Shaker Journals* (Boston: Houghton Mifflin Co., 1916), p. 235.

Physician's journal, January 1, 1834–November 8, 1842, Cleveland, Shaker Collection, Western Reserve Historical Society.

    Herbal expeditions recorded in Journal kept by the sister of the Church Family, Harvard, Mass. (1824), Library of Fruitlands Museum, Harvard, Mass.

Page 65. Photograph of Harvard Shaker community, collection of Hancock Shaker Village, Pittsfield, Massachusetts. 1854 Harvard catalog, Miller Collection.

    Hammond account in Daybook kept by Joseph Hammond, May 1, 1820–July 15, 1822, Harvard Society, Harvard, Mass., Library of Fruitlands Museum, Harvard, Mass.

    Harvard catalogs, Library of Fruitlands Museum, Harvard, Mass.

Page 66. "Herbs, Roots, Barks, Powdered Articles, &c.," Harvard broadside, Miller Collection.

    Harvard catalogs, Library of Fruitlands Museum, Harvard, Mass.

Page 67. Photograph of herb house by Paul Rocheleau; Hancock Shaker Village Collections.

    Elisha Myrick, *Day Book kept for the Convenience of the Herb Department,* Harvard Church Family, 1850, Harvard, Mass., Hancock Shaker Village Collections.

    Arthur T. West, "Reminiscences of Life in a Shaker Village," *The New England Quarterly* (June 1938), p. 347.

Pages 68–72. Elisha Myrick, *Day Book kept for the Convenience of the Herb Department,* Harvard Church Family, 1850, Harvard, Mass., Hancock Shaker Village Collections.

Page 68. Page from *Harvard Journal,* Hancock Shaker Village Collections. Photographed by Paul Rocheleau.

Page 69. Thoroughwort, drawn by Sister Cora Helena Sarle, Canterbury, photographed by Bill Finney; used by permission of Canterbury Shaker Village, Canterbury, New Hampshire.

Page 72. Eupatorium purpureum (queen of the meadow) drawn by Sister Cora Helena Sarle, Canterbury, photographed by Bill Finney; used by permission of Canterbury Shaker Village, Canterbury, New Hampshire.

Scroll from Kew Gardens acknowledging contribution of herbs from Elisha Myrick, 1857, Library of Fruitlands Museum, Harvard, Mass.

Page 73. Broadside with illustration of Simon Atherton, Miller Collection.

Account book, herb branch of medical department, January 1847–December 1853, Harvard, Mass. Andrews Collection, Library of Henry Francis du Pont Museum, Winterthur, Del.

Travel journal kept by Eldress Betsy Smith, Ministry of South Union, Ky., May 1, 1869–September 1869, Shaker Collection, Library of Congress, Washington, D.C.

Broadside printed by Elijah Myrick with Elder Simon T. Atherton's picture on cover, Library of Fruitlands Museum, Harvard, Mass.

Page 74. A sister's work recorded in *A Journal of Domestic Work of Sisters, Kept by the Deaconesses,* February 1867–April 1876, Library of Fruitlands Museum, Harvard, Mass.

Sage orders recorded in Account Book, January 1879–1888, Harvard, Mass. Church family, Library of Fruitlands Museum, Harvard, Mass.

Page 75. Growing accounts described in Account Book, January 1879–1888, Harvard, Mass. Church family, Library of Fruitlands Museum, Harvard, Mass.

Harvard history in Henry S. Norse, *History of the Town of Harvard, Massachusetts,* printed for Warren Hapgood, 1894, Library of Fruitlands Museum, Harvard, Mass., p. 257.

Page 76. Photograph of North Family broom shop, collection of Stephen J. Paterwic.

Bentley account in Diary of Rev. William Bentley, D.D., Gloucester, Mass., 1962, vol. 2, pp. 149–51, Peter Smith Collection, Yale University Library, New Haven, Conn.

Brocklebank account in Record book, Asa Brocklebank, 1805, Library of Fruitlands Museum, Harvard, Mass.

Page 77. Clara Endicott Sears quotation in *Gleanings From Old Shaker Journals* (Boston: Houghton Mifflin Co., 1916), p. XII.

1806 Record book, Library of Fruitlands Museum, Harvard, Mass.

1810 Broadside, garden seeds, signed by Oliver Burt, Shirley Society, Williams College Archives and Special Collections, Wiliamstown, Mass.

Page 78. Cayenne label, Miller Collection. Photograph of Shirley trustees' office, collection of Stephen J. Paterwic.

Herbal remedies in "Medical Formulae Prepared for the Use of the Nurse-Sisters at The Infirmary, Shirley Village, July 12, 1866," Library of Fruitlands Museum, Harvard, Mass.

The New Hampshire Societies (Chapter 6)

Page 79. Hand-colored postcard of Canterbury community, Hancock Shaker Village Collections. Photographed by Paul Rocheleau.

Page 80. Rose Water label, Miller Collection.

Description of William Tripure in *The Farmer's Monthly Visitor,* Concord, N.H., August 31, 1840. Dartmouth College Library, Hanover, N.H.

Page 81. Bottle of Corbett's Pectoral Syrup, with package, Miller Collection. Photograph of Elder Henry Blinn and beehives. Hancock Shaker Village Collections.

Page 82. Photograph of Sister Cora Helena Sarle, Canterbury from a late 19th-century photograph, Collection of the United Society of Shakers, Sabbathday Lake, Maine. Sister Helena's notebooks are in the collection of Canterbury Shaker Village, Canterbury, New Hampshire. Photograph by Bill Finney.

Hill account in *The Farmer's Monthly Visitor,* Concord, N.H., August 31, 1840. Dartmouth College Library, Hanover, N.H.

Page 83. Modern view of Canterbury Shaker community, collection of Hancock Shaker Village, Pittsfield, Massachusetts. St.-John's-wort drawn by Sister Cora Helena Sarle, Canterbury, photographed by Bill Finney; used by permission of Canterbury Shaker Village, Canterbury, New Hampshire. Hand colored postcard "The Family Garden" in collection of Hancock Shaker Village, Pittsfield, Mass.

Page 84. Sarsaparilla drawn by Sister Cora Helena Sarle, Canterbury, photographed by Bill Finney; used by permission of Canterbury Shaker Village, Canterbury, New Hampshire. Corbett's Syrup of Sarsaparilla bottle, Miller Collection.

1835 *Catalogue of Medicinal Plants and Vegetable Medicines* at Emma B. King Library, Shaker Museum at Old Chatham, N.Y.

Page 85. "Dyspepsia Cure" display card, Miller Collection. Description of origins of Corbett's syrup in *The Granite Monthly—A New Hampshire Magazine* (September–October 1885), 8:310–11.

Amount of sarsaparilla sold described in Record of 1841, Canterbury, N.H., Shaker Society, in Phyllis Shimki, *Sarsaparilla Bottle Encyclopedia* (Aurora, Ore.: 1969), p. 54.

Page 86. 1854 Catalog and "Corbett's Shaker Dyspepsia Cure" packing box, Miller Collection.

Handbill circulated by Trustee David Parker of the Canterbury Society, 1853, at Emma B. King Library, Shaker Museum at Old Chatham, N.Y.

Page 87. Bittersweet drawn by Sister Cora Helena Sarle, Canterbury, photographed by Bill Finney; used by permission of Canterbury Shaker Village, Canterbury, New Hampshire.

1854 "Catalogue of Medicinal Plants and Vegetable Medicines," Miller Collection.

Mary Whitcher's Shaker House-Keeper (Boston, 1882), Williams College Archives and Special Collections, Williamstown, Mass.

Page 88. Mother Seigel's Almanac and package, Miller Collection. Photograph of Church Family, collection of Hancock Shaker Village, Pittsfield, Mass.

Hill account in *The Farmer's Monthly Visitor,* Concord, N.H., September 20, 1839. Dartmouth College Library, Hanover, N.H.

Page 89. Brown's Extract broadsheet, label, and package, Miller Collection.

Description of Shaker products in Advertising circular for Brown's Shaker Extract English Valerian, 1879, Cleveland, Western Reserve Historical Society.

Labels on medicine bottles, Canterbury Shaker Village, Canterbury, N.H.

Page 90. Witch Hazel package (Canterbury) and Oil of Valerian bottle (Enfield), Miller Collection.

The Maine Societies (Chapter 7)

Page 91. Photograph of Church Family, Sabbathday Lake, in Collection of The United Society of Shakers, Sabbathday Lake, Maine.

History of Maine communities in Sister R. Mildred Barker, *The Sabbathday Lake Shakers: An Introduction to the Shaker Heritage* (Sabbathday Lake, Maine: The Shaker Press, 1985), and Sister R. Mildred Barker, *Holy Land: A History of the Alfred Shakers* (Sabbathday Lake, Maine: The Shaker Press, 1986).

Page 92. Alfred Daybook, Hancock Shaker Village Collections. Photographed by Paul Rocheleau.

Barker history in *The Shaker Quarterly,* vol. 3, no. 4 (Winter 1963), pp. 114, 115, 116, Collection of the United Society of Shakers, Sabbathday Lake, Maine.

Alfred broadside listing 47 vegetable and herb seeds, 1850, Cleveland, Western Reserve Historical Society.

Hill account in *The Farmer's Monthly Visitor,* Concord, N.H., July 31, 1840. Dartmouth College Library, Hanover, N.H.

Page 93. Bloodroot drawn by Sister Cora Helena Sarle, Canterbury, photographed by Bill Finney; used by permission of Canterbury Shaker Village, Canterbury, New Hampshire. Photograph of Church Family buildings with flower garden, Hancock Shaker Village Collections.

History of community in Barker, *The Sabbathday Lake Shakers.*

Travel description, Diary of Eldress Betsy Smith, July 1869, Pleasant Hill, Shaker Collection, Library of Congress, Washington, D.C.

Page 94. Photograph of 1794 meeting house, Collection of the United Society of Shakers, Sabbathday Lake, Maine.

1840 Broadside listing 83 herbs, Collection of the United Society of Shakers, Sabbathday Lake, Maine.

The Farmers' Books, 1771–1856, vol. 1 (1850), 81 pp.; vol. 2 (1853), 152 pp.; vol. 3 (1856), 44 pp., Collection of the United Society of Shakers, Sabbathday Lake, Maine.

Page 95. Photograph of Elder William Dumont, Collection of the United Society of Shakers, Sabbathday Lake, Maine.

Description of sage industry in Journal of Elder Otis Sawyer for 1873, Collection of the United Society of Shakers, Sabbathday Lake, Maine.

Origins of Shaker Tamar Laxative in *Church Record,* vol. 2 (1881), Shaker Society, p. 57, Collection of the United Society of Shakers, Sabbathday Lake, Maine.

Page 96. Photograph of 1821 Herb House, Collection of the United Society of Shakers, Sabbathday Lake, Maine.

Formula for Shaker Tamar Laxative in *The Shaker Quarterly,* vol. 2, no. 1 (Spring 1962), p. 40, Collection of the United Society of Shakers, Sabbathday Lake, Maine.

Page 97. Tamar Laxative display card, Miller Collection.

Sisters' activities described in Gretchen Belanger, "Herbalist Brings Growth to Sabbathday Lake Shaker Community." *Countryside,* January 1977, p. 26.

John S. Williams, *The Shakers* (Old Chatham, NY: Shaker Museum Foundation, 1956), n.p.

Page 98. Photographs of packaged herbs and present-day herb gardens, Collection of the United Society of Shakers, Sabbathday Lake, Maine.

Revival of Sabbathday Lake herb industry described in Sister Frances A. Carr, *Shaker Your Plate: Of Shaker Cooks and Cooking* (Sabbathday Lake, ME: United Society of Shakers, 1985), p. 41.

First sale of tarragon vinegar described by Sister R. Mildred Barker, correspondent, in "News and Notes," *Shaker Quarterly* XI, 3 (Fall 1971), p. 118.

Page 99. Photograph of herb tins, Collection of the United Society of Shakers, Sabbathday Lake, Maine.

Herb production line described by Sister R. Mildred Barker, correspondent, in "News and Notes," *Shaker Quarterly* XIII, 4 (Winter 1973), p. 146.

Hectic activity described by Sister R. Mildred Barker, correspondent, in "News and Notes," *Shaker Quarterly* XIV, 2 (Summer 1974), p. 59, p. 65.

Page 100. Photograph of Sister Frances Carr and Brother Arnold Hadd, Collection of the United Society of Shakers, Sabbathday Lake, Maine.

The Western and Southern Societies (Chapter 8)

Page 101. Photograph of Centre House, Pleasant Hill, Robert F. W. Meader photo, Hancock Shaker Village Collections.

Page 102. Herb drying room, Pleasant Hill, Collection of Shaker Museum at Pleasant Hill, Kentucky. North Family dwelling, Union Village, Robert F. W. Meader photo, Hancock Shaker Village Collections.

Journal compiled from other journals made between March 1805 and 1894 by O. H. Hampton, added to in 1856 and 1857 by anonymous editor. Shaker Manuscript Collection, Library of Congress, Washington, D.C.

Account of Indian visit in Journal of Peter Boyd, Union Village, Ohio, March 1, 1805–December 15, 1850, Library of Congress, Washington, D.C.

Page 103. Photograph of apothecary chest by Martha H. Boice. Medicinal wine bottle, collection of Mary Ryan M. Allen.

Population of community listed in "A registry of Work performed by Second Family Sisters," recorded (1846–1849) by Sister Amy Slaters.

Wine industry described in *Shaker Community Wines. A treatise on Pure Wines,* Assistant Trustee William G. Ayer (Union Village, Ohio, n.d.), 11 pp., p. 4. Library of Congress, Washington, D.C.

Page 104. Photograph of Center Family dwelling, Hancock Shaker Village Collections.

Different drug plants and products listed in Botanical Catalogs (Union Village: Press of Richard McNemar, 1847, 1850), Library of Congress, Washington, D.C.

Page 105. Botanical Catalogs (Union Village: Press of Richard McNemar, 1847, 1850), Library of Congress, Washington, D.C.

Page 106. Photograph of Marble Hall by Martha H. Boice, Collection of Martha H. Boice.

Page 107. "Shaker Cough Syrup" broadside, Miller Collection.

Page 108. Boyd description of building cold frame in Manuscript journal, Peter Boyd, January 1833–September 1837, Library of Congress, Washington, D.C.

Boyd account of various activities in Manuscript journal, Peter Boyd, 1844, Library of Congress, Washington, D.C.

Page 109. Lupine drawn by Sister Cora Helena Sarle, Canterbury, photographed by Bill Finney; used by permission of Canterbury Shaker Village, Canterbury, New Hampshire.

Account book of Peter Boyd with copies of letters, 1851–1852. Library of Congress, Washington, D.C.

Page 110. Drawing of hardhack by Sister Cora Helena Sarle, Canterbury, used by permission of Canterbury Shaker Village, Canterbury, New Hampshire.

Page 111. The Influence of the Shaker Doctor, issued by Union Village Society, 1850, Cleveland, Western Reserve Historical Society.

Witch hazel drawn by Sister Cora Helena Sarle, Canterbury, photographed by Bill Finney; used by permission of Canterbury Shaker Village, Canterbury, New Hampshire.

Page 112. Mulberry drawn by Sister Cora Helena Sarle, Canterbury, photographed by Bill Finney; used by permission of Canterbury Shaker Village, Canterbury, New Hampshire.

Pages 113–114. Health of North Union Shakers described in James S. Prescott, *History of North Union,* 2nd ed. (Printed by North Union Society, 1880), Cleveland, Western Reserve Historical Society.

1856 description of Pleasant Hill in The Albany [N.Y.] *Cultivator,* September 1856, Library of Congress, Washington, D.C.

Page 115. Photograph of Pleasant Hill, Hancock Shaker Village Collections.

1843 garden activities in Diary of Dr. Benjamin Dunlavy, 1843–1868, Library at Shakertown, Pleasant Hill, Ky.

Daily activities 1843-1850 recorded in Family journal kept by Order of the Deaconesses of the East House, 1843–1871, Library of the Filson Club, Inc., Louisville, Ky.

Page 116. Photograph of Pleasant Hill herb garden, Collection of Shaker Museum at Pleasant Hill, Kentucky.

Page 117. Photograph of garden and gardener, Collection of Shaker Museum at Pleasant Hill, Kentucky.

Financial journal kept at Pleasant Hill, Library of the University of Southern Kentucky, Bowling Green, Kentucky.

Center Family herb industry described in Center family journal, Pleasant Hill, 1843–1869, Library at Shakertown, Pleasant Hill, Ky.

Page 118. Photograph of doors of East Family dwelling, Pleasant Hill: Robert F. W. Meader photo, Hancock Shaker Village Collections. "Pure and Reliable" advertisement, 1877, reprinted in 1972 calendar, Shaker Museum at Pleasant Hill, Kentucky.

Aromatic Elixir of Malt advertisement cited in Calendar, 1974, Library at Shakertown, Pleasant Hill, Kentucky.

Page 119. Photograph of Wash House, South Union: Robert F. W. Meader photo, Hancock Shaker Village Collections.

Journal of Thomas Jefferson Shannon, October 6, 1831–February 2, 1832, Library, University of Kentucky, Bowling Green, Ky.

Page 120. Photograph of herb garden and Centre House, Shaker Museum at South Union, Kentucky.

South Union history, *passim,* in *History of South Union Colony 1804–36,* vol. 1–A (1804–21), transcribed 1870 by Hervey L. Eades from original journals and diaries pertaining to South Union, Western Kentucky State College, Bowling Green, Ky.

Cholera remedy on herb label, Shaker Collection at Shaker Museum at South Union, Kentucky.

Page 121. Spider bite incident in *History of South Union Colony 1804–36,* vol. 1–A (1804–21), transcribed 1870 by Hervey L. Eades from original journals and diaries pertaining to South Union, Western Kentucky State College, Bowling Green, Ky.

Page 122. Account of Reconstruction period in Julia Neal, *By Their Fruits* (Chapel Hill, N.C.: University of North Carolina Press, 1947), p. 221.

Glossary

Abortive Capable of producing abortion.

Acrid Biting; caustic.

Adenagic Acting on the glandular system.

Affections Bodily conditions.

Ague A fever of malarial character marked by paroxysms of chills, fever, and sweating, which occur at regular intervals.

Ague cake The enlarged hard spleen of chronic malaria.

Alkaloid A nitrogenous organic base, usually of vegetable origin, toxic in effect.

Alterative Capable of producing a salutary change in disease through catalytic action when used with another substance; any drug used empirically to alter favorably the course of an ailment and to restore healthy body functions (now rarely used technically).

Alvine Cleansing the bowels.

Amenorrhea Absence or suppression of menstruation from any cause other than pregnancy or menopause.

Anaphrodisiac Capable of blunting the sexual appetite.

Anodyne Relieving pain or causing it to cease.

Anthelmintic Expelling or destroying parasitic worms, especially of the intestine.

Antibilious Correcting the bile and bilious secretions.

Antilithic Preventing the formation of calculous matter.

Antiperiodic Preventive of periodic returns of paroxysms or exacerbations of disease (as in intermittent fevers).

Antiphlogistic Counteracting inflammation.

Antiscorbutic Opposed to scurvy.

Antiseptic Opposed to putrefaction; checking the growth or action of microorganisms.

Antispasmodic Tending or having the power to prevent or relieve spasms or convulsions.

Antisyphilitic Acting against venereal disease.

Aperient A laxative agent.

Apothecary One who prepares and sells drugs or compounds for medicinal purposes.

Aromatic Fragrant, spicy.

Astringent Shrinking and driving the blood from the tissues.

Balsamic Mild, healing, and soothing.

Bright's disease Any of several forms of disease of the kidney.

Caked breast A localized hardening in one or more segments of a lactating breast caused by accumulation of fluid.

Calculus Any abnormal hard mass formed in the body.

Canker (obsolete) A spreading sore that corrupts and eats away body tissues.

Carminative An agent used to allay pain by expelling gas from the alimentary canal and relieve colic, griping, or flatulence.

Catarrh Inflammation of a mucus membrane characterized by congestion and secretion of mucus.

Cathartic A purgative, cleansing agent.

Cephalic Relating to the head.

Chlorosis An iron-deficiency anemia in young girls characterized by a greenish color of the skin, weakness, and menstrual disturbances.

Cholagogue Inducing a flow of bile.

Cholera infantum An acute, noncontagious intestinal disturbance of infants, formerly common in congested areas of high humidity and temperature but now rare.

Cholera morbus A gastrointestinal disturbance characterized by griping, diarrhea, and sometimes vomiting and usually resulting from overeating or from contaminated foods.

Chorea Any of various nervous disorders of organic or infectious origin.

Colic A paroxysm of acute abdominal pain localized in a hollow organ or tube and caused by spasm, obstruction, or twisting.

Cornine A bitter principle sometimes used as a mild astringent and stomachic.

Cornus The root.

Corrigent A substance added to a medicine to modify its action or counteract a disagreeable effect.

Corroborant Strengthening and giving tone.

Costiveness Constipation.

Croup A spasmodic laryngitis in infants and children.

Cutaneous Of or relating to the skin.

Decoction The act or process of boiling, usually in water, so as to extract the flavor or active principle; the extract thus obtained.

Demulcent A substance capable of soothing an inflamed or abraded mucus membrane or protecting it from irritation.

Deobstruent Removing obstructions.

Depurative Purifying or cleansing.

Detergent Cleansing parts of wounds.

Diaphoretic An agent inducing sweating.

Discutient Repelling or resolving tumors.

Diuretic Increasing the secretion of urine.

Drastic Operating powerfully on the bowels.

Dropsy An abnormal accumulation of watery fluid in body tissues or cavities.

Dysentery An often epidemic or endemic disease characterized by severe diarrhea, with passage of mucus and blood.

Dyspepsia A condition of disturbed digestion characterized by nausea, heartburn, pain, gas, and a sense of fullness due to local causes or to disease elsewhere in the body.

Emetic An agent that induces vomiting.

Emmenagogue An agent that promotes menstrual discharge.

Emollient Relaxing and softening inflamed parts.

Empiric A member of an ancient sect of physicians who based their practice on experience alone, disregarding all theoretical and philosophical considerations.

Erratic Having unpredictable results.

Erysipelas An acute febrile disease associated with intense local inflammation of the skin and subcutaneous tissues.

Excitant Stimulant.

Expectorant Facilitating or provoking discharge of mucus.

Febrifuge An agent that mitigates or removes fever.

Febrile Of or relating to fever.

Flux A flowing or discharge of fluid from the body; usually an excessive or abnormal discharge from the bowels.

Fomentation The application of hot moist substances (as wet cloths) to the body for the purpose of easing pain.

Gleet A chronic inflammation of a bodily orifice in man or animals, usually accompanied by an abnormal discharge from the orifice.

Gonorrhea Contagious inflammation of the genital mucus membrane.

Gout A metabolic disease occurring in paroxysms and marked by a painful inflammation of the fibers and ligamentous parts of the joints.

Gravel A deposit of small calculous concretions in the kidneys and urinary bladder.

Griping Causing a pinching spasmodic intestinal pain.

Herpatic Attacking cutaneous diseases.

Hydragogue Capable of expelling serum.

Hypnotic Promoting sleep, somniferous.

Indolent Causing little or no pain; growing or progressing slowly; slow to heal.

Infusion The introducing of a solution into a vein; the steeping or soaking, usually in water of a substance (as a plant drug) in order to extract its virtues; the liquid extract obtained by the latter process.

Inspissated Thickened by boiling.

Laxative Gently cathartic.

Lead colic Intestinal colic associated with obstinate constipation due to chronic lead poisoning, called also painter's colic.

Leukorrhea A white, yellowish, or greenish white viscid discharge from the vagina.

Lochia Discharge from the uterus and vagina following delivery.

Materia medica Material or substance used in the composition of medical remedies; a branch of medical science dealing with the sources, natures, properties, and preparation of the drugs used in medicine.

Menorrhagia Abnormally profuse menstrual flow.

Menstruum A substance that dissolves a solid or holds it in suspension.

Mordant A chemical that serves to fix a dye in or on a substance by combining with the dye to form an insoluble compound.

Mucilaginous Relating to the secretion of mucilage, a gelatinous substance that swells in water without dissolving, and forms a slimy mass.

Narcotic Having the property of stupefying.

Nauseant Exciting nausea.

Nephritic Relating to the kidney.

Nervine Acting in the nervous system.

Nutritive Relating to nutrition.

Nux vomica The poisonous seed of an Asiatic tree that contains several alkaloids but chiefly strychnine and brucine.

Ophthalmia An inflammation of the conjunctiva or of the eyeball.

Parturient Inducing or promoting labor.

Pectoral Relating to the breast.

Pharmacopoeia A book containing a selected list of drugs, chemicals, and medicinal preparations with descriptions of them, tests for their identity, purity, and strength, and formulas for making the preparations; especially one issued by official authority and recognized as a standard.

Phrenic Relating to the diaphragm.

Phthisis A wasting or consumption of the tissue.

Populin A sweet crystalline glucoside found in aspen bark and leaves and poplar buds.

Potherb An herb that is boiled for use as a vegetable.

Prolapsis ani Falling of the anus.

Prolapsis uteri Falling down of the uterus.

Purgative Operating on the bowels more powerfully than a laxative.

Quinsy An acute infection of the throat, especially when discharging pus or mucus.

Refrigerant Depressing the morbid temperature of the body.

Resinoid Plant material, soluble in organic solvents but not in water.

Rubefacient A substance for external application that produces redness of the skin.

Salicin A bitter, white crystalline beta-glucoside found in the bark and leaves of several willows and poplars; used as a tonic.

Salt rheum Eczema.

Scab head A Shaker term for a scalp affliction.

Scarlatina A term for scarlet fever.

Scorbutic Of or relating to scurvy.

Scrofula Swelling of the lymph glands of the neck.

Secernant Affecting the secretions.

Sedative Directly depressing the vital forces.

Senega The dried root of senega root containing an irritating saponin (a glycoside occurring in many plants, which foams when in a water solution).

Sialogogue Provoking the secretion of saliva.

Spermatorrhea Abnormally frequent or excessive involuntary emission of semen without orgasm.

Stimulant Causing a temporary increase in vital activity.

Stomachic Relating to stomach; exciting action of stomach.

Strangury Slow and painful discharge of urine drop by drop produced by spasmodic muscular contractions of the urethra and bladder.

Styptic Arresting hemorrhage; stopping bleeding.

Sudorific Provoking sweat.

Syphilis Chronic, contagious, usually venereal disease caused by a spirochete.

Tetter Any of various vesicular skin diseases (as ringworm eczema).

Tic douloureux Painful twitch; neuralgia.

Tonic Invigorating; bracing; refreshing.

Vermifuge Serving to destroy or expel parasitic worms, especially of the intestine.

Vesicant Inducing blistering.

Volatize To make volatile; to cause to exhale or evaporate.

Vulnerary Promoting healing of wounds.

Wen A cyst formed by obstruction of secreted material from a sebaceous gland.

Bibliography
for the History

Adrosko, Rita J. *Natural Dyes and Home Dyeing.* New York: Dover, 1971.

Andrews, Charles M. *The Colonial Period of American History.* New Haven: Yale University Press, 1934.

Andrews, Edward D. *The Community Industries of the Shakers.* New York State Museum Handbook, No. 15. Albany, N.Y.: University of the State of New York, 1933.

———. *The Hancock Shakers, 1780–1960.* New Haven: Carl Purington Rollins Press, Shaker Community, Inc., 1961.

———. *The People Called Shakers.* New York: Oxford University Press, 1953.

———, and Andrews, Faith. *Shaker Herbs and Herbalists.* New Haven: Carl Purington Rollins Press, Shaker Community, Inc.

Barker, R. Mildred. *Holy Land: A History of the Alfred Shakers.* Sabbathday Lake, Me.: The Shaker Press, 1986.

———. *The Sabbathday Lake Shakers: An Introduction to the Shaker Heritage.* Sabbathday Lake, Me.: The Shaker Press, 1985.

Beale, Galen, and Mary Rose Boswell. *The Earth Shall Blossom: Shaker Herbs and Gardening.* Woodstock, Vt.: Countryman Press, 1991.

Blinn, Henry Clay, ed. *The Life and Gospel Experience of Mother Ann Lee.* East Canterbury, N.H.: Shakers, 1901.

———. *The Manifesto, 1883–99.* Canterbury, N.H.

Boice, Martha, Dale Covington, and Richard Spence. *Maps of the Shaker West.* Dayton, Ohio: Knot Garden Press, 1977.

Bremer, Fredrika. *Homes of the New World,* vols. 1 and 2. Translated by Mary Howitt. New York: Harper & Brothers, 1853.

Brewer, Priscilla J. *Shaker Communities, Shaker Lives.* Hanover, N.H.: University Press of New England, 1986.

Briggs, Asa. *Victorian Cities.* New York: Harper & Row, 1963.

Brooklyn Botanical Garden. *Handbook on Herbs, Plants and Gardens,* vol. 14, no. 2, 1950.

Buchanan, Rita. *The Shaker Herb and Garden Book.* Boston: Houghton-Mifflin, 1996.

Burns, Deborah E. *Shaker Cities of Peace, Love, and Union: A History of the Hancock Bishopric.* Hanover, N.H.: University Press of New England, 1993.

Carter, Kate B. *Pioneer Medicines.* Salt Lake City: Daughters of Utah Pioneers, 1958.

Clark, Thomas D. *Pleasant Hill in Civil War.* Pleasant Hill, Ky: Pleasant Hill Press, 1972.

———, and Ham, F. Gerald. *Pleasant Hill and Its Shaker Community.* Pleasant Hill, Ky: Shakertown Press, 1968.

Clarkson, Rosetta E. *Herbs and Savory Seeds.* New York: Dover, 1972.

———. *Herbs, Their Culture and Uses.* New York: Macmillan, 1942.

———. *Magic Gardens.* New York: Macmillan, 1939.

Coleman, J. Winston, Jr., ed. *Kentucky, A Pictorial History.* Lexington, Ky.: University Press of Kentucky, 1971.

Coon, Nelson. *Using Plants for Healing.* Great Neck, N.Y.: Hearthside, 1963.

———. *Using Wayside Plants.* Great Neck, N.Y.: Hearthside, 1957.

Creevey, Caroline. *Flowers of Field, Hill and Swamp.* New York: Harper & Brothers, 1897.

Culpepper, Nicholas. *Culpepper's Complete Herbal.* London: W. Foulsham, n.d.

Desroche, Henri. *The American Shakers: From Neo-Christianity to Presocialism.* Translated by John K. Savacool. Amherst: University of Massachusetts Press, 1971.

Dioscorides. *The Greek Herbal.* Oxford: Oxford University Press, 1934.

Dixon, William Hepworth. *New America.* Philadelphia: Lippincott, 1867.

———. "Shakerism in the United States," *Westminster Review,* n.s. 3 (April 1861).

Doe, John E. *Beginning Again.* London: Hogarth Press, 1964.

Dwight, Timothy. *Travels in New England and New York.* New Haven: Timothy Dwight, 1822.

Earle, Alice Morse. *Old Time Gardens.* New York: Macmillan, 1901.

Elkins, Hervey. *Fifteen Years in the Senior Order of Shakers.* Hanover, N.H.: Dartmouth Press, 1853.

Evans, Elder Frederick W. *Autobiography of a Shaker.* New York: American News Co., 1888.

———. *Compendium of the Origin, History, Principles, Rules & Regulations, Government, and Doctrines of the United Society of Believers in Christ's Second Appearing.* New York: Appleton, 1859.

———, and Doolittle, Antoinette, eds. *Shaker and Shakeress, 1873–75.* Mt. Lebanon, N.Y.: n.d.

Felter, Harvey Wicker. *Genesis of American Materia Medica.* Cincinnati, 1927.

Fenton, William N. *Contacts Between Iroquois Herbalism and Colonial Medicine.* Washington, D.C.: Smithsonian Institution, 1941.

Freeman, Margaret B. *Herbs for the Medieval Household.* New York: Metropolitan Museum of Art, 1943.

Gibbons, Euell. *Stalking the Healthful Herbs.* New York: McKay, 1966.

Gray, Asa. *Manual of Botany.* 8th ed., rev. Merritt Lundon Fernald. New York: American Book Co., 1950.

Green, Calvin, and Wells, Seth Y. *A Summary View of the Millennial Church or United Society of Believers (Commonly Called Shakers).* Albany, N.Y.: 1823.

Grieve, Maude. *Modern Herbal: The Medicinal, Culinary, Cosmetic and Economic Properties, Cultivation and Folklore of Herbs, Grasses, Fungi, Shrubs and Trees.* New York: Harcourt, 1931.

Gunther, Robert T. *The Greek Herbal of Dioscorides.* New York: Hafner, 1959.

Hedrick, Ulysses Prentiss. *A History of Agriculture in the State of New York.* New York: Hill & Wang, 1966.

Henkel, Alice. *American Medicinal Leaves and Herbs.* U.S.D.A. Bulletin no. 219, Washington, D.C.: Government Printing Office, 1911.

Hobrook, Stewart H. *The Golden Age of Quackery.* New York: Macmillan, 1959.

Holloway, Mark. *Heavens on Earth.* New York: Dover, 1966.

Holmes, Oliver Wendell. *Medical Essays.* Boston: Houghton Mifflin, 1861.

In Memoriam. Henry Clay Blinn 1824–1905. Concord, N.H.: Rumford Printing Co., 1905.

Jarvis, D. C., M.D. *Folk Medicine.* New York: Henry Holt, 1958.

Johnson, Theodore E., ed. *The Shaker Quarterly 1961.* Sabbathday Lake, Maine.

Kadans, Joseph M. *Encyclopedia of Medicinal Herbs.* New York: Arco, 1972.

Kreig, Margaret B. *Green Medicine.* Chicago: Apollo, 1971.

Lamson, David R. *Two Years' Experience Among the Shakers.* West Boylston, Mass., 1848.

Lassiter, William Lawrence. *Shaker Recipes for Cooks and Homemakers.* New York: Greenwich, 1959.

Leighton, Ann. *Early American Gardens: For Meat or Medicine.* Boston: Houghton Mifflin, 1970.

Leyel, Mrs. C. F. *Culpepper's English and Complete Herbal.* London: Culpepper House, 1947.

———. *The Magic of Herbs.* London: Jonathan Cape, 1926.

———. *The Truth About Herbs.* London: Andrew Dakers Limited, 1943.

Lockwood, Alice G. B. *Gardens of Colony and State Before 1840.* New York: Charles Scribner's Sons, 1931.

Lomas, G. Albert, ed. *The Shaker, 1871–72.* Watervliet, N.Y.

———. *The Shaker, 1876–77.* Watervliet, N.Y.

———. *The Shaker Manifesto, 1878–1882.* Watervliet, N.Y.

Lossing, Benson John. "The Shakers of Lebanon, New York," *Harper's New Monthly Magazine,* vol. 15, no. 86 (July 1857).

MacLean, John P. *A Bibliography of Shaker Literature with an Introductory Study of the Writings and Publications Pertaining to Ohio Believers.* Columbus, Ohio: Fred J. Heer, 1905.

McNemar, Richard. *The Kentucky Revival.* Albany, N.Y.: E. and E. Hosford 1808.

Melcher, Marguerite F. *The Shaker Adventure.* Cleveland: The Press of Case Western Reserve University, 1960.

Meyer, Clarence. *American Folk Medicine.* New York: Crowell, 1918.

Meyer, Joseph E. *The Herbalist.* Hammond, Ind.: Indiana Botanic Gardens, 1934.

Millennial Laws, The. Orders and Rules of the Church at New Lebanon. Published by the Ministry and Elders, 1821.

Millennial Laws, The. Revised at New Lebanon, New York. Published by the Ministry and Elders, 1845.

Neal, Julia. *By Their Fruits, The Story of Shakerism in South Union, Kentucky.* Chapel Hill, N.C.: University of North Carolina Press, 1947.

———. *The Journal of Eldress Nancy.* Nashville: Parthenon Press, 1963.

Nordhoff, Charles. *The Communistic Societies of the United States.* New York: Harper & Brothers, 1875.

Noyes, John Humphrey. *History of American Socialisms.* New York: Dover, 1966.

Old Herb Doctor, The: His Secrets and Treatments: Over 1,000 Recipes. Hammond, Ind.: Hammond Book Co., 1941.

Pearson, Elmer R., and Julia Neal; Magda Gabor-Hotchkiss, ed., 2nd edition. *The Shaker Image.* Hancock, Mass.: Hancock Shaker Village, Inc., 1995.

Piercy, Carline B. *The Valley of God's Pleasure.* New York: Stratford House, 1951.

Redford, Arthur. *The History of Local Government in Manchester, England.* 2 vols. New York: Longmans, Green and Co., 1939.

Robinson, Charles Edson. *A Concise History of the United Society of Believers Called Shakers.* East Canterbury, N.H. Shaker Village, 1893.

Sarle, Cora Helena. *A Shaker Sister's Drawings.* New York: Monacelli Press, 1997.

Sears, Clara Endicott, ed. *Gleanings from Old Shaker Journals.* Cambridge, Mass.: Houghton Mifflin, 1916.

Shaker Heights Then and Now. Publication Committee, Shaker Heights Board of Education, Cleveland, 1938.

Shimko, Phyllis. *Sarsaparilla Encyclopedia.* Aurora, Ore.: privately printed, 1969.

Sigerist, Dr. Henry E. *The Great Doctors.* New York: Dover, 1971.

Silliman, Benjamin. *Peculiarities of the Shakers, Described in a Series of Letters from Lebanon Springs in the Year 1832.* New York: J. K. Porter, 1832.

———. *Remarks Made on a Short Tour between Hartford and Quebec.* New Haven: S. Converse, 1820.

———. "Shakers," *Christian Monthly Spectator* 6 (1824).

Smith, J. E. A. *The History of Pittsfield — 1880–1876.* Pittsfield, Mass.: Published by the author; n.d.

Stein, Stephen J. *The Shaker Experience in America.* New Haven: Yale University Press, 1992.

Taylor, Norman. *Plant Drugs That Changed the World.* New York: Dodd, Mead, 1965.

Testimonies of the Life, Character, Revelation and Doctrines of Mother Ann Lee. 2nd ed. Albany, N.Y.: Weed, Parsons and Co., 1888.

Webster, Helen Noyes. *Herbs. How to Grow Them and How to Use Them.* Newton: Charles T. Branford Co., 1939.

Wheelwright, Edith Grey. *The Physick Garden.* Boston: Houghton Mifflin, 1935.

Bibliography
for the Herbal Compendium

Bailey, Liberty Hyde, and Ethel Zoe, eds. *Hortus Second.* New York: Macmillan, 1940.

Barton, William C. P. *Vegetable Materia Medica of the United States.* Philadelphia: H. C. Carey and I. Lea, 1825.

Beale, Galen, and Mary Rose Boswell. *The Earth Shall Blossom: Shaker Herbs and Gardening.* Woodstock, Vt.: Countryman Press, 1991.

Bigelow, Jacob, M.D. *Florula Bostoniensis.* 2nd ed. Boston: Cummings, Hilliard and Co., 1824.

Buchanan, Rita. *The Shaker Herb and Garden Book.* Boston: Houghton-Mifflin, 1996.

Cobb, Boughton. *A Field Guide to the Ferns and their Related Families.* Boston: Houghton Mifflin, 1956.

Eaton, Amos C. *Manual of Botany for North America.* Albany, N.Y., 1829.

Gray, Asa. *Manual of Botany.* 8th ed. rev. Merritt Lundon Fernald, ed. New York: American Book Co., 1950.

Grieve, Maud. *A Modern Herbal.* Ed and introduction, Mrs. C. F. Leyel. London: Jonathan Cape, 1931.

House, Homer D. *Wild Flowers of New York.* Vols. 1, 2. Albany: New York State Museum, 1921.

Johnson, Laurence. *A Manual of the Medical Botany of North America.* New York: William Wood and Co., 1884.

Meyer, Joseph E. *The Herbalist.* Hammond, Ind.: Indiana Botanic Gardens, 1934.

Millspaugh, Charles F. *Medicinal Plants: An Illustrated and Descriptive Guide to Plants Indigenous to and Naturalizd in the United States in Medicine (One Thousand Medicinal Plants).* 2 vols. Philadelphia: John C. Yorston and Co., 1892.

Muhlenberg, Gothilf H. E. *General Catalog of the Plants of North America.* Lancaster, Pa., 1813.

Peterson, Roger Tory, and McKenny, Margaret. *Field Guide to Wildflowers.* Boston: Houghton Mifflin, 1994.

Petrides, George A. *A Field Guide to Trees and Shrubs.* Boston: Houghton Mifflin, 1996.

Rafinesque, C. S. *Atlantic Journal and Friend of Knowledge.* Philadelphia: printed for the author by H. Probasco, 1832–1833.

———. *A Life of Travels and Research in North America. 1785–1840.*

———. *Medical Flora and Manual of the Medical Botany of the United States.* Philadelphia: Atkinson & Alexandria. 1828.

———. *New Flora of North America.* Philadelphia, 1836.

Stearns, Samuel. *American Herbal or Materia Medica.* Walpole, N.H., 1801.

Torrey, John D. *Compendium of the Flora of the Northern and Middle United States.* New York, 1826.

Wherry, Edgar T. *Wild Flower Guide.* New York: Doubleday, 1948.

Botanical Index

A general index begins on page 212.

A

Abies balsamea, 153
Abscess, 126
Acer pensylvanicum, 161
Acer rubrum, 161
Achillea millefolium, 187
Aconite, 126
Aconitum napellus, 126
Acorus calamus, 180
Actaea pachypoda, 141
Actaea rubra, 141
Adder's violet, 168
Adiantum pedatum, 147
Agrimonia eupatoria, 126
Agrimony, 126
Agropyron repens, 145
Ague root, 132, 178
Ague weed, 133
Alcea rosea, 153
Alder, black, 126
Alder, red, 126
Alder, tag, 126
Alder dogwood, 134
Alder-leaved dogwood, 166
Alehof, 156
Aletris farinosa, 132, 178
All heal, 174
Allium sativa, 150
Alnus oregona, 126
Alnus rugosa, 126
Alpinia galangal, 150
Althaea officinalis, 160
Alum root, 126
Alumroot, 143
Amaranthus hybridus var.
   erythrostachys, 167
American colombo, 142

American dittany, 145, 163
American elder, 146
American hellebore, 153
American ipecac, 147
American larch, 180
American mezereon, 158, 162
American poplar, 169
American sanicle, 172
American thrift, 161
American tormentilla, 143
American valerium, 157
American wild, 181
Anaphalis margaritacea, 158
Anethum graveolens, 145
Angelica, 127
Angelica atropurpurea, 127
Anise root, 139
Anthemis arvensis, 138
Anthemis cotula, 162
Apocynum androsaemifolium, 13,
   131
Apocynum cannabinum, 155
Apple, 127, 181
Aralia hispida, 146
Aralia nudicaulis, 8, 84, 172
Aralia racemosa, 177
Arbutus uva ursi, 183
Archangel, 127
Arctium lappa, 134
Arctostaphylos uva-ursi, 183
Arisaema triphyllum, 146, 155
Aristolochia serpentaria, 176
Armoracia rusticana, 154
Arnica, 127
Arnica montana, 127
Arrow wood, 134
Arsmart, 185

Artemisia abrotanum, 177
Artemisia absinthium, 187
Artemisia vulgaris, 164
Arum triphyllum, 186
Asarum canadense, 151, 175
Asclepias incarnata, 155
Asclepias syriaca, 162
Asclepias tuberosa, 9, 13, 168
Ash, mountain, 127
Ash, prickly, 127
Ash, white, 127
Asparagus officinalis, 128
Asparagus root, 128
Aspen, 169
Aspen, quaking, 128
Aster novae-angliae, 178
Aster puniceus, 141
Asthma weed, 159
Athyrium filix-femina, 128
Atropa belladona, 130
Autumn-crocus, 142
Avens, water, 128

B

Backache brake, 128
Balm, lemon, 10, 128
Balm, Moldavian, 10, 128
Balm of gilead, 8, 129
Balmony, 129, 175
Balsam, 153
Balsam, sweet, 129
Balsamweed, 138
Banal, 133
Baneberry, 141
Bane berry, 141
Baptisia tinctoria, 155
Barberry, 129

Bardana, 134
Basil, 10, 129, 163
Basswood, 129
Bath flower, 182
Bayberry, 14, 130
Bean herb, 173
Bearberry, 183
Bear's bud, 163
Beaver poison, 139
Beaver root, 159
Beccabunga, 133
Bed straw, 140
Bee balm, 128, 166
Beech, American, 130
Beechdrops, 130
Beech drops, 135
Bee's nest seed, 137
Beggar lice, 144
Beggar's tick, 152
Belladona, 6, 130
Bellwort, 130
Benjamin bush, 148
Benne, 130
Berberis vulgaris, 129
Bergamot monarda, 166
Bethroot, 131, 182
Betony, wood, 131
Betula lenta, 131
Bidens connata, 152
Bidens frondosa, 144
Bilberry, 185
Bindweed, 156, 160
Birch, black, 131
Bird cherry, 134
Bird pepper, 131
Bird pepper chillies, 137
Bird's-foot violet, 183

Bird's nest, 148
Birth root, 131
Birthwort, 1
Bishops-cap, 142
Bitter bloom, 138
Bitter clover, 138
Bitter herb, 129, 131, 175
Bitteroot, 131
Bitter plantain, 168
Bitter root, 155
Bittersweet, 87, 132
Bittersweet, false, 132
Bitterworm, 134
Blackberry, 132
Black cherry, 138, 165
Black cohosh, 9, 27, 175
Black henbane, 6, 153
Blackroot, 144
Black snake root, 141
Blazing star, 132, 175
Blessed thistle, 136
Bloodroot, 44, 93, 132
Blooming spurge, 155
Blow ball, 144
Blue balm, 128
Bluebells, 126
Blueberry, 141, 185
Blueberry root, 166
Blue cardinal flower, 136
Blue cohosh, 166, 178
Blue curls, 174
Blue flag, 44, 132, 149
Blue lobelia, 136
Blue mountain tea, 151
Blue scullcap, 174
Blue vervain, 183
Bogbean, 134
Bog myrtle, 180
Bog onion, 155
Bohnenkraut, 173
Boneset, 10, 17, 133
Borage, 18, 133
Borago officinalis, 133
Botrychium lunaria, 142
Bouncing bet, 176
Bowman's root, 155
Boxberry, 133, 138
Boxwood, 10, 133, 146
Boy's love, 177
Brake root, 147
Bramble, 132
Brassica hirta, 164
Brassica nigra, 164
Bristlestem, 146

Bristly stem, 172
Broad-leaved dogwood, 166
Brook alder, 126
Brookline, 133
Broom, 133
Broom rape, 135
Brown wort, 174
Buckbean, 134
Buckhorn brake, 134
Buckthorn, 29, 71, 134
Budwood, 133
Bugbane, 141
Bugle, 12
Bugle, bitter, 29, 45, 134
Bugle, sweet, 134
Bugleweed, 12
Bugle weed, 134
Bugloss, 133
Bug myrtle, 134
Bullsfoot, 142
Burdock, 17, 134
Burdock root, 71
Burnet, great, 56, 133
Burning bush, 184
Burrage, 133
Burren myrtle, 185
Buttercup, 135
Butterfly weed, 52, 168
Butternut, 10, 17, 135
Butternut bark, 22, 44, 184
Butter weed, 149
Button snake-root, 12

C

Cabbage rose, 171
Calamus, 180
Calendula officinalis, 161
Canada maple, 161
Canada root, 181
Canada snakeroot, 151
Canada thistle, 181
Canadian hemp, 155
Canadian moonseed, 166
Cancer root, 135
Candle berry, 130
Canella, 135
Canella winterana, 135
Canker root, 135, 151
Canker weed, 135
Cankerwort, 144
Capsella bursa-pastoris, 174
Capsicum annuum, 137
Capsicum frutescens, 131
Caraway, 136

Cardamon, 136
Cardinal, blue, 136
Cardinal, red, 10, 136
Cardinal flower, 136
Cardus, spotted, 136
Carpenter's square, 136, 173
Carrot, wild, 137
Carthamus tinctorius, 172
Carum carvi, 136
Cassia marilandica, 174
Castanea dentata, 139
Castor bean, 137
Castor oil plant, 137
Catarrh root, 150
Catch weed, 140
Catmint, 137
Catnep, 137
Catnip, 70, 74, 137
Cat's-paw, 156
Caulophyllum thalictroides, 141, 166
Cayenne, 78, 137
Ceanothus americanus, 170
Cedar, red, 137
Celandine, garden, 137
Celandine, wild, 138
Celastrus scandens, 132
Centaurium erythraea, 131
Centaury, 1, 138, 139
Centaury, American, 138
Centaury, red, 138
Cetraria islandica, 154
Chamaelirium luteum, 182
Chamaemelum nobile, 138
Chamomile, 138
Chamomile, low, 138
Chamomile, Roman, 138
Checkerberry, 133, 138, 178, 186
Cheese plant, 160
Cheeses, 160
Chelidonium majus, 137
Chelone glabra, 129, 175
Chenopodium ambrosioides, 187
Chenopodium botrys, 165
Cherry, wild, 15, 138
Cherry birch, 131
Chestnut, 139
Chickentoe, 144
Chickweed, 139
Chicory, 139
Chillies, 131
Chimaphila umbellata, 168
Chinese seng, 151

Chocolate root, 128
Choke-cherry, 138
Cholic root, 9, 139
Christmas rose, 152
Chrysanthemum leucanthemum, 144, 185
Chrysanthemum parthenium, 148
Cicely, sweet, 139
Cichorium intybus, 139
Cicuta, 6, 10, 17, 139
Cimicifuga racemosa, 9, 141, 175
Cinchona, 140
Cinchona pubescens, 140
Cinnamomum zeylanicum, 140
Cinnamon, 140
Cinquefoil, 149
Cirsium arvense, 181
Citrullus lanatus, 185
Citrus sinensis, 165
Clammy sage, 140
Clarry, 140
Clary, 140
Cleavers, 22, 140
Clematis, 184
Clematis virginiana, 184
Cliff brake, 170
Climbing orange root, 132
Clivers, 140
Clorbur, 134
Cloud berry, 132
Clover, red, 6, 17, 140
Clover, white, 140
Clover, yellow, 140
Clover blows, 140
Cloves, 141
Cnicus benedictus, 136
Coakum, 150, 169
Cocash, 141
Cocash weed, 141, 159, 178
Cocculus carolinis, 142
Cockhold herb, 152
Cockleburr, 126
Cock-up-hat, 170
Cohosh, black, 9, 27, 44, 141
Cohosh, blue, 141
Cohosh, red, 141
Cohosh, white, 141
Coix lacryma-jobi, 156
Colchicum, 142, 162
Colchicum autumnale, 142, 162
Cold water root, 141
Colic root, 132, 139, 175, 178, 186

Collinsonia canadensis, 170, 179
Colombo, American, 142
Coltsfoot, 59, 142
Colt's tail, 149
Comfrey, 11, 142
Commiphora opobalsamum, 129
Common burnet, 135
Common plantain, 168
Common sorrel, 176
Common thyme, 181
Compass plant, 154, 171
Comptonia peregrina, 148
Cone-disk, 181
Cone-flower, 181
Conium maculatum, 11, 139
Consolida regalis, 158
Consumption brake, 142
Coolwort, 142
Coptis trifolia, 151
Corallorhiza odontorhiza, 144
Coral root, 144
Coriander, 143
Coriandrum sativum, 143
Corn chamomile, 138
Cornus alternifolia, 166
Cornus canadensis, 36
Cornus florida, *133*
Cornus rugosa, 166
Cornus sericea, 146, 186
Corydalis, 182
Corydalis sempervirens, 187
Cotton root, 143
Couch grass, 145, 157
Cough root, 131
Coughweed, 178
Coughwort, 142
Cow lice, 144
Cowparsnip, 10, 143, 161
Cowparsnip, royal, 143
Cramp bark, 143
Cramp weed, 174
Cranesbill, 126, 143
Crawley, 144
Creeping thyme, 181
Crosswort, 133
Crowfoot, 135, 143
Crown bark, 140
Cuckold, 144
Cucumber tree, 185
Cucurbita pepo, 170
Cud weed, 163
Culver's physic, 144
Culver's root, 144
Cunila origanoides, 145, 163

Curcuma domestica, 182
Cure-all, 128
Curled dock, 145
Cursed thistle, 181
Cypripedium acaule, 157
Cypripedium calceolus var. *pubes-
cens,* 157, 183
Cytisus scoparius, 133

D
Daffodil, 144
Daffy-downdillies, 144
Daisy, white, 144
Dandelion, 6, 10, 13, 17, 89,
144
Daphne mezereum, 162
Datura stramonium, 6, 181
Daucus carota, 137
Deadly nightshade, 10, 130
Deer berry, 138, 178
Devil's bit, 132, 173, 175
Dewberry, 132
Dicentra canadensis, 182
Digitalis purpurea, 149
Dill, 145
Dillseed, 145
Dilly, 145
Dioscorea villosa, 139, 186
Diplazium pycnocarpon, 177
Dirca palustris, 158
Dittany, 145
Dock, broadleaf, 145
Dock, water, 145
Dock root, yellow, 3, 17, 68, 69,
71, 145
Dogachamus, 166
Dogbane, 131
Dog fennel, 162
Dog grass, 145, 157
Dogsbone, 131
Dogwood, 133, 146
Double tansy, 180
Dovesfoot, 143
Dracocephalum moldavica, 128
Dragonhead, 128
Dragon root, 146, 155, 186
Dragon's claw, 144
Dragon turnip, 155
Drooping starwort, 182
Dropberry, 176
Dropsy plant, 128
Dropwort, 155
Dryopteris austriaca var.
spinulosa, 174

Dryopteris filix-mas, 147
Durfa grass, 145
Dutchman's pipe, 148
Dwale, 130
Dwarf elder, 172
Dysentery weed, 163
Dysentery-weed, 147

E
Earth smoke, 150
East India catarrh root, 150
Elder, 10, 11, 13, 146
Elder, dwarf, 146
Elecampane, 146
Elettaria cardamomum, 136
Elm, slippery, 9, 10, 83, 146
Emetic root, 155, 159
Endive, 139
Epifagus virginiana, 130
Epigaea repens, 12, 152
Epilobium angustifolium, 185
Erechtites hieracifolia, 148
Erect vervain, 183
Ergot, 147, 177
Erigeron canadensis, 149
Erigeron philadelphicus, 185
Eryngo-leaved liverwort, 154
Euonymous, 184
Euonymus atropurpurea, 184
Eupatorium, 133
Eupatorium perfoliatum, 69, 133
Eupatorium purpureum, 72, 170,
179
Euphorbia, 147
Euphorbia ipecacuanhae, 147, 155
European centaury, 131
European seneca, 162
Evans root, 128
Everlasting, 163
Eve's cup, 168
Eye balm, 151
Eyebright, 138
Eye-bright, 159

F
Fagus grandifolia, 130
Fake alder, 126
False gromwell, 156
False hellebore, 153
False jasmine, 150
False spikenard, 176
False valerian, 159
False wintergreen, 168
Featherfew, 148

Female fern, 128, 147
Female regulator, 159, 178
Fennel, 147
Fern, maidenhair, 147
Fern, male, 147
Fern, polypody, 147
Fern, sweet, 148
Fern gale, 148
Feverbush, 148
Fever bush, 177
Feverfew, 148
Fever root, 144, 155
Feverroot, 148
Fever twig, 132
Fever wood, 148
Feverwood, 177
Feverwort, 133
Field balm, 156
Field balsam, 158
Field sorrel, 176
Figwort, 136, 152, 173
Fireweed, 148
Fishmouth, 129
Fit plant, 148
Fitsroot, 148
Five-finger grass, 149
Five fingers, 151
Flag lily, 132
Flax, 149
Fleabane, 15, 17, 149
Fleur-de-lis, 132, 149
Flower de luce, 149
Flowering cornel, 133, 146
Flytrap, 131
Fly trap, 168
Fly-trap, 184
Foeniculum vulgare, 147
Foso bark, 140
Foxglove, 11, 17, 149
Fragaria virginiana, 179
Fraxinus americana, 127
Frog lily, 159
Frost plant, 149
Frostwort, 149
Fumaria officinalis, 150
Fumatory, 150
Fumitory, 150

G
Galangal, 150
Gale fern, 180
Galium aparine, 140
Garantogen, 151
Garden burnet, 135

Garden chamomile, 138
Garden nightshade, 6, 10, 132, 165
Garden thyme, 181
Garget, 150, 169
Garlic, 150
Gaultheria procumbens, 133, 138, 186
Gayfeather, 175
Gelsemium, 150
Gelsemium sempervirens, 150, 187
Genista, 133
Gentian, blue-fringed, 17, 150
Gentianopsis crinita, 150
Geranium maculatum, 143
Geum rivale, 128
Ghostflower, 148
Gillenia trifoliata, 155
Gill-go-over-the-ground, 156
Gill run, 156
Ginger, 151
Ginger, African, 151
Ginger root, 142
Ginseng, 151
Gipseywort, 134
Gipsy wort, 184
Glechoma hederacea, 156
Glycyrrhiza glabra, 159
Gnaphalium obtusifolium var. *polycephalum,* 129, 158
Gnaphalium uliginosum, 163
Golden alexanders, 143
Golden ragwort, 178
Goldenrod, 151
Goldenseal, 12, 44, 151
Golden senecio, 159
Goldthread, 151
Goodyera pubescens, 168
Goose-foot, 187
Goose grass, 140
Goose tansy, 174
Gossypium herbaceum, 143
Gout berry, 132
Gravel plant, 12, 152
Gravel root, 170, 179
Gravel weed, 152
Great celandine, 137
Greater plantain, 168
Great water dock, 145
Great wild valerian, 183
Greek valerian, 126
Green archangel, 134
Green ozier, 146

Gromwell, 156
Ground holly, 168
Ground joy, 156
Ground laurel, 152
Ground lily, 131
Ground moss, 163
Ground raspberry, 151
Ground squirrel pea, 182
Gum plant, 142

H
Hackmatack, 180
Hamamelis virginiana, 186
Hardhack, 110, 152, 178
Hardrock, 170
Harvest lice, 144, 152
Heal-all, 136, 152, 173, 174
Healing herb, 142
Heart's ease, 152
Heart snake root, 175
Heartweed, 185
Hedeoma pulegioides, 167
Hedge fumitory, 150
Helianthemum canadense, 149
Helianthus annuus, 179
Helianthus divaricatus, 179
Hellebore, black, 152
Hellebore, white, 48, 153
Helleborus niger, 152
Helmet pod, 182
Helonias, 182
Hemlock, 11, 153
Hemlock, poison, 6
Hemlock spruce, 11, 153
Hemp, Indian, 13
Henbane, black, 6, 10, 17, 153
Hepatica americana, 159
Heracleum sphondylium subsp. *montanum, 143*
Heuchera pubescens, 126
High angelica, 127
High balm, 166
High cranberry, 143
Hog physic, 136
Hogweed, 187
Hollyhock, 153, 170
Holy thistle, 136
Honey bloom, 131
Hoodwort, 174
Hop, 10, 17, 73, 153
Horehound, 17, 153
Horsefly weed, 155
Horse gentian, 148
Horsemint, 154, 163

Horseradish, 69, 154
Horse weed, 149
Horseweed, 170
Horse weed, 179
Humulus lupulus, 153
Hundred-leaved rose, 171
Huntsman's cup, 168, 184
Hydrangea, 154
Hydrangea arborescens, 154
Hydrastis canadensis, 12, 151
Hyoscyamus niger, 6, 153
Hypericum perforatum, 156
Hyssop, 11, 154
Hyssopus officinalis, 154

I
Iceland moss, 154
Ice plant, 148
Ilex verticillata, 126
Impatiens pallida, 138
Imperatoria ostruthium, 143, 161
Indian arrow-wood, 184
Indian balm, 131
Indian cup, 154
Indian cupweed, 154
Indian dream, 170
Indian elm, 146
Indian ginger, 175
Indian hemp, 13, 155
Indian lettuce, 142
Indian paint, 132
Indian physic, 155
Indian-physic, 155
Indian pink, 136
Indian pipe, 148
Indian poke, 153
Indian posey, 158
Indian posy, 129
Indian sage, 133
Indian tobacco, 159
Indian turnip, 146, 155
Indigo, wild, 155
Indigo broom, 155
Indigo weed, 155
Inkberry, 169
Ink root, 161
Inula helenium, 146
Ipecac, Carolina, 155
Ipecac milk, 155
Ipomoea jalapa, 156
Ipomoea pandurata, 160
Iris, 156
Iris sambucina, 149
Iris versicolor, 132

Iris x germanica var. *florentina,* 156
Ironweed, 156
Itch weed, 153
Ivy, ground, 156

J
Jack-in-the-pulpit, 146, 155, 186
Jacob's ladder, 126, 156
Jalap, 156
Jamaica ginger, 151
Jamestown weed, 181
Jeffersonia diphylla, 182
Jersey tea, 170
Jerusalem oak, 165
Jerusalem tea, 165
Jesuit tea, 165
Jewelweed, 138
Jimson weed, 6, 181
Job's tears, 156
Joepye, 170
Joe-pye, 179
Johnswort, 156
Juglans cinerea, 135, 184
Juglans nigra, 184
Juniper, 6, 157
Juniper bush, 157
Juniperus communis, 157
Juniperus sabina, 173
Juniperus virginiana, 137

K
Kalmia angustifolia, 158
Kassamak root, 150
Kidney liver leaf, 159
King's clover, 140, 157, 180
King's fern, 134
Knot grass, 157

L
Labrador tea, 157
Lactuca sativa, 158
Lactuca serriola, 158
Ladies' thump, 152
Lady fern, 128
Lady's mantle, 187
Lady's slipper, 15, 157
Lady's slipper, yellow, 157
Lambkill, 158
Larch, American, 180
Large fennel, 147
Larix laricina, 180
Larkspur, 158

Laurel, 158
Laurel, sheep, 158
Lavandula angustifolia, 158
Lavender, English, 10, 158
Lavose, 160
Leafy burr mangold, 144
Leatherwood, 158
Leather wood, 162
Ledum groenlandicum, 157
Lemon balm, 10, 93
Lemon walnut, 135
Leonurus cardiaca, 163
Leopardsbane, 127
Leptandra, 144
Lesser centaury, 131
Lettuce, garden, 10, 17, 158
Lettuce, wild, 10, 17, 158
Levisticum officinale, 160
Liatris spicata, 12, 175
Licorice, 159
Life everlasting, 129, 158
Life-of-man, 177
Life root, 141, 159, 178
Ligustrum vulgare, 169
Lily, white water, 159
Lily, yellow pond, 159
Lime tree, 129, 181
Limonium carolinianum, 161
Linden, 129, 181
Lindera benzoin, 148, *177*
Link, 133
Linseed, 149
Lint bells, 149
Linum usitatissimum, 149
Lion's tail, 163
Liquidambar styraciflua, 180
Liquorice, 159
Liriodendron tulipifera, 185
Liver leaf, 159
Liver lily, 132
Liverwort, 8, 159
Lobelia, 10, 11, 17, 24, 159
Lobelia cardinalis, 10, 42, 136
Lobelia inflata, 159
Lobelia siphilitica, 136
Locust plant, 174
London pride, 176
Loosestrife, 172
Lovage, 160
Lovely bleeding, 167
Lungwort, 160
Lupine, 109
Lycopersicon lycopersicum, 182
Lycopus americanus, 134

Lycopus europaeus, 134, 184
Lycopus virginicus, 12, 184
Lythrum salicaria, 172

M
Mad-dog, 174
Mahogany birch, 131
Male fern, 134
Male shield fern, 147
Maller, 160
Mallow, low, 160
Mallow, marsh, 160
Malus sylvestris, 127
Malva rotundifolia, 160
Mandrake, 10, 17, 160
Man-in-the-earth, 160
Man-in-the-ground, 160
Man root, 160
Maple, red, 161
Maple, striped, 161
Maple lungwort, 160
Mare's tail, 185
Marigold, 161
Marjoram, sweet, 161
Marrubium vulgare, 153
Marsh mallow, 10, 11, 13
Marsh rosemary, 161
Marsh trefoil, 134
Marsh turnip, 155
Marygold, 161
Masterwort, 127, 143, 161
Matico, 161
May apple, 160
Mayflower, 152
Mayweed, 138, 162
Meadow cabbage, 175
Meadow fern, 180
Meadow pride, 142
Meadow root, 161
Meadow saffron, 142, 162
Meadowsweet, 152, 178
Melilot, 157, 162, 180
Melilotus alba, 140
Melilotus officinalis, 157, 162, 180
Melissa officinalis, 128
Menispermum canadense, 166
Mentha spicata, 177
Mentha x piperita, 167
Menyanthes trifoliata, 134
Mezereum, 162
Milk ipecac, 131
Milk purslane, 147
Milk thistle, 136

Milk turnip, 155
Milkweed, 162
Milkwort, 162
Millefoil, 187
Mint, 10, 98
Mitchella repens, 178
Mitella diphylla, 142
Mitrewort, 142
Mohawkweed, 130
Monarda, 163
Monarda didyma, 166
Monarda punctata, 154, 163
Monkshood, 126
Monotropa uniflora, 148
Moonwort, 142
Moor grass, 174
Moose elm, 146
Moosewood, 158, 161
Morus rubra, 164
Moss, haircap, 163
Mother of thyme, 181
Motherwort, 163
Mountain balm, 166
Mountain box, 183
Mountain cranberry, 183
Mountain dittany, 145, 163
Mountain flax, 175
Mountain mint, 163
Mountain pink, 152
Mountain tea, 138
Mountain tobacco, 127
Mouse ear, 139, 163
Mouth root, 151
Mugwort, 164
Mulberry, 112, 164
Mullein, 164
Musquash root, 139
Mustard, black, 164
Mustard, white, 164
Myrica cerifera, 14
Myrica gale, 13, 180
Myrica pensylvanica, 130
Myrtle, 130

N
Nanny berry, 164
Nanny bush, 164
Narcissus pseudonarcissus, 144
Narrow dock, 145
Necklace weed, 141
Nepeta cataria, 137
Nerve root, 157, 183
Nettle, 165
New England aster, 178

New Jersey tea, 134, 170
Nightshade, 6, 10, 17, 132, 165
Ninsin, 151
Noah's ark, 141, 157
Noble liverwort, 159
Noble pine, 168
Noble yarrow, 187
Nuphar advena, 159
Nymphaea odorata, 159

O
Oak, black, 165
Oak, red, 165
Oak, white, 165
Oak Jerusalem seed, 187
Oak of Jerusalem, 165
Ocimum basilicum, 129
Oenothera biennis, 173
Ohio curcuma, 151
Oil nut, 135, 184
Old field balsam, 129
Old maid's pink, 176
Old man's tree, 177
One berry, 178
Opium poppy, 169
Orange, 165
Orange root, 151
Origanum majorana, 161
Orobanche uniflora, 135
Orris root, 156
Osier, green, 166
Osmorhiza longistylis, 139
Osmunda regalis, 134
Oswego tea, 166
Ova ova, 148
Oxalis acetosella, 176
Oxbalm, 170, 179
Ox eye daisy, 185
Ox-eye daisy, 144

P
Paeonia lactiflora, 167
Pale rose, 171
Panax quinquefolius, 151
Panicle elder sambucus, 146
Papaver somniferum, 169
Papoose root, 141
Papooseroot, 166
Parilla, yellow, 166
Pariswort, 131
Parsley, 166
Partridge berry, 178
Paul betony, 17, 134
Peach, 166

Pedicularis canadensis, 131
Pellaea atropurpurea, 170
Pennsylvania sumach, 179
Pennyroyal, 70, 167
Peony, 10, 167
Peppermint, 167
Pepper turnip, 155
Peru, 181
Peruvian bark, 140
Petroselinum crispum, 166
Petty morrel, 177
Phytolacca americana, 150, 169
Pigeon berry, 150, 169
Pilewort, 148, 167
Pine, white, 167
Pink lady's slipper, 157
Pink moccasin flower, 157
Pink root, 167
Pinus rigida, 153
Pinus strobus, 167
Pipe plant, 148
Piper angustifolium, 161
Pipsissewa, 98, 168, 186
Pitcher plant, 168, 184
Pitch pine, 153
Plantago major, 168
Plantain, 168
Plantain, downy rattlesnake, 168
Pleurisy root, 9, 13, 52, 168
Podophyllum peltatum, 160
Poison flag, 132
Poison hemlock, 6, 139
Poison ivy, 168
Poison parsley, 139
Poison root, 139
Poison vine, 168
Poke, 150, 169
Poke root, 150
Polar plant, 171
Polecat weed, 175
Polemonium caeruleum, 156
Polemonium reptans, 126, 183
Polygala lutea, 162
Polygala senega, 175
Polygonatum multiflorum, 176
Polygonum hydropiperoides, 185
Polygonum persicaria, 152
Polypodium vulgare, 147
Polytrichum juniperinum, 163
Pomegranate, 169
Pond lily, yellow, 159
Pool root, 172
Poplar, 169

Poppy, 10, 23, 169
Populus balsamifera, 8
Populus tremuloides, 128, 169
Potato, wild, 160
Potentilla anserina, 174
Potentilla canadensis, 149
Pot marigold, 161
Prairie dock, 154
Prenanthes alba, 135
Prenanthes serpentaria, 135
Pride weed, 149
Prim, 169
Primrose scabious, 173
Prince's feather, 167
Prince's pine, 168
Privet, 13, 169
Privy, 169
Prunella vulgaris, 152, 174
Prunus persica, 166
Prunus serotina, 138
Ptelea, 169
Ptelea trifoliata, 169
Pteris atropurpurea, 170
Pterospora, 8
Puke weed, 159
Pulmonaria officinalis, 160
Pumpkin, 6, 170
Punica granatum, 169
Purging berries, 134
Purple angelica, 127
Purple boneset, 170
Purple willow herb, 172
Pycnanthemum montanum, 163
Pyramid flower, 142
Pyrola, 168

Q
Queen Anne's lace, 137
Queen of the meadow, 72, 170, 179
Queen's delight, 170, 178
Queen's root, 170, 178
Quercus alba, 165
Quercus rubra, 165
Quercus velutina, 165
Quickens, 157
Quick grass, 145

R
Raccoon berry, 160
Ragged cup, 154
Ragweed, 187
Ragwort, 159
Rainbow weed, 172

Ranunculus acris, 135
Ranunculus ficaria, 135
Raspberry, 170
Rattle bush, 155
Rattle root, 141
Rattleroot, 175
Rattlesnake leaf, 168
Rattlesnake root, 135, 168
Rattle weed, 141
Red bark, 140
Red cardinal flower, 136
Red centaury, 138
Red clover, 6
Red cockscomb, 167
Red elm, 146
Red gum, 180
Red lobelia, 136
Red mulberry, 164
Red puccoon, 132
Red raspberry, 170
Red-rod, 186
Red root, 134, 170
Red stalked aster, 141
Red top sorrel, 176
Rhamnus cathartica, 134
Rheumatic weed, 168
Rheumatism root, 139, 182
Rheum rhabarbarum, 170
Rhubarb, 170
Rhus glabra, 179
Rhus toxicodendron, 168
Richweed, 170
Rich weed, 179
Ricinus communis, 137
Robin's eye, 163
Rock brake, 147
Rockbrake, 170
Rock parsley, 166
Rock polypod, 147
Rock rose, 149
Roman chamomile, 138
Roman motherwort, 163
Rosa centifolia, 171
Rosa damascena, 171
Rosaemifolium, 13
Rosa gallica, 171
Rosa x alba, 171
Rose, cabbage, 171
Rose, damask, 171
Rose, red, 24, 67, 171
Rose, white, 171
Rose bay, 185
Rose-colored silk weed, 155
Rosemary, 98, 171

Rose pink, 138
Rose willow, 146
Rosin weed, 154, 171
Rosmarinus officinalis, 171
Rough cleavers, 140
Round-leaved cornel, 166
Roundwood, 127
Royal cow parsnip, 161
Royal fern, 134
Rubus idaeus var. *strigosus,* 170
Rubus occidentalis, 132
Rubus spp., 132
Rudbeckia lacinata, 13
Rudbeckia laciniata, 181
Rue, 10, 11, 171
Rumex, 145
Rumex acetosella, 176
Rumex aquaticus, 145
Rumex crispus, 145
Rumex obtusifolius, 145
Ruta graveolens, 171

S
Sabatia angularis, 138
Saffron, 172
Sage, 10, 14, 68, 69, 72, 172
Sage willow, 172
Salix alba, 186
Salix discolor, 186
Salt rheum weed, 129
Salvia officinalis, 172
Salvia sclarea, 140
Sambucus canadensis, 146
Sanguinaria canadensis, 132
Sanguisorba officinalis, 135
Sanicle, black, 172
Sanicula marilandica, 172
Saponaria officinalis, 176
Sarracenia purpurea, 168, 184
Sarsaparilla, 6, 8, 13, 16, 84, 85, 87, 146
Sarsaparilla, American wild, 172
Sassafras, 172
Sassafras albidum, 172
Satureja hortensis, 173
Satureja montana, 173
Savin, 10, 13, 173
Savory, summer, 71, 173
Savory, winter, 173
Scabbish, 173
Scabious, 149, 173
Scabwort, 146
Scammony, wild, 160

Scarlet berry, 132
Scilla, 178
Scoke, 169
Scoke root, 150
Scokeroot, 169
Scratch grass, 145
Scrofula, 136, 173
Scrofula weed, 149
Scrophularia marilandica, 136, 173
Scullcap, 174
Scutellaria lateriflora, 174
Sea lavender, 161
Seal root, 176
Sea onion, 178
Sea thrift, 161
Secale cereale, 147, 177
Secale cornatum, 147
Self-heal, 152, 172, 174
Seneca root, 175
Senecio aureus, 159, 178
Senega root, 175
Senna, American, 174
September weed, 141
Sesamum indicum, 130
Seven barks, 154
Shagbarks, 184
Sheep berry, 164
Shell flower, 129, 175
Shepherd's heart, 174
Shepherd's purse, 174
Shield fern, 174
Shrubby trefoil, 169
Side-saddle flower, 184
Silk weed, 162
Silphium laciniatum, 171
Silphium perfoliatum, 154
Silver cinquefoil, 174
Silver leaf, 170, 178
Silver weed, 174
Simpler's joy, 183
Skole, 150
Skullcap, 174
Skunk cabbage, 15, 175
Skunk weed, 175
Slipperweed, 138
Slippery elm, 9, 10, 83, 146
Slippery root, 142
Small-pox plant, 184
Small spikenard, 172
Smart weed, 185
Smellage, 160
Smilacina racemosa, 176

Smooth alder, 126
Smooth sumach, 179
Smut rye, 147, 177
Snagrel, 176
Snakehead, 129, 175
Snake lily, 132
Snake root, 176
Snakeroot, black, 175
Snakeroot, button, 175
Snakeroot, Canada, 175
Snakeroot, seneca, 175
Snakeroot, Virginia, 176
Snake weed, 176
Snapping hazel, 186
Snapping hazel nut, 186
Snap wood, 148
Soapwort, 176
Soft maple, 161
Solanum dulcamara, 132
Solanum nigrum, 6, 165
Soldier's herb, 161
Solidago odora, 151
Solomon's seal, false, 176
Solomon's seal, giant, 176
Sorbus americana, 127
Sorrel, lady's, 176
Sorrel, sheep, 176
Sour dock, 145
Southernwood, 177
Sowberry, 129
Spanish needles, 144
Spanish pine, 167
Spatterdock, 159
Spearmint, 177
Speedwell, common, 177
Spice birch, 131
Spice bush, 148
Spicebush, 177
Spicey wintergreen, 186
Spigelia marilandica, 167
Spignet, 177
Spikenard, 177
Spindle tree, 184
Spiraea tomentosa, 152, 178
Spleenwort, silvery, 177
Spleenwort bush, 148
Splitrock, 126
Spoonwood, 129
Spotted alder, 186
Spotted cowbane, 139
Spotted geranium, 143
Spotted hemlock, 139
Spotted knot weed, 152

Spotted plantain, 168
Spreading spurge, 147
Spurge olive, 162
Spurred rye, 147, 177
Square stalk, 136, 173
Squawbush, 143
Squaw mint, 167
Squaw root, 141, 166
Squaw vine, 178
Squaw weed, 141, 159
Squaw-weed, 178
Squill, 178
Squirrel corn, 182
St. Johnswort, 83, 156
Staff tree, 132
Staffvine, 132
Stagger weed, 182
Starflower, 178
Stargrass, 132
Star grass, 178
Star-leaved gum, 180
Star root, 132, 178, 182
Starwort, 178, 182
Stave's acre, 158
Steeple bush, 152
Steeplebush, 178
Stellaria media, 139
Stickwort, 126
Stillingia, 170, 178
Stillingia sylvatica, 170, 178
Stinging nettle, 165
Stink weed, 181
Stone brake, 179
Stone mint, 145, 163
Stone root, 152, 170, 179
Storksbill, 143
Stramonium, 181
Strawberry, 179
Striped alder, 126
Succisa pratensis, 173
Succory, 139
Sumach, 179
Summer savory 14, 71
Sunflower, garden, 179
Sunflower, wild, 179
Suter berry, 127
Swamp beggar's tick, 144, 152
Swamp dogwood, 186
Swamp hellebore, 153
Swamp milk weed, 155
Sweating plant, 133
Sweet anise, 139
Sweet balm, 128

Sweet balsam, 158
Sweet birch, 131
Sweet bush, 148
Sweet clover, 140, 157, 162, 180
Sweet elder, 146
Sweet elm, 146
Sweet fennel, 147
Sweet fern, 148
Sweet flag, 180
Sweet gale, 13, 180
Sweet gum, 180
Sweet javril, 139
Sweet marjoram, 14
Sweet melilot, 140, 162
Sweet rush, 180
Sweet scabious, 173
Sweet scented goldenrod, 151
Sweet-scented water lily, 159
Sweet tansy, 180
Sweet viburnum, 164
Sweet white clover, 140
Sweet willow, 180
Symphytum officinale, 142
Symplocarpus foetidus, 175
Syzygium aromaticum, 141

T
Tabasco pepper, 131
Tag alder, 126
Tall speedwell, 144
Tall veronica, 144
Tamarack, 180
Tanacetum vulgare, 180
Tansy, 180
Taraxacum officinale, 144
Tarragon vinegar, 98
Tea balm, 128
Tea berry, 138
Tea berry plant, 186
Tetterwort, 132, 137
Thimble weed, 13, 181
Thistle root, 181
Thorn apple, 6, 10, 13, 181
Thoroughstem, 133
Thoroughwort, 69, 133
Throat root, 128
Throwwort, 163
Thyme, 14, 181
Thymus serpyllum, 181
Thymus vulgaris, 181
Tick weed, 167
Tilia americana, 129, 181
Tilia, 129, 181

Tinker's weed, 148
Toad flax, 149
Toad lily, 159
Tomato, 182
Toothache bush, 127
Touch-me-not, 138
Trailing arbutus, 152
Traveller's joy, 184
Tree primrose, 173
Trefoil, 134
Trembling aspen, 128, 169
Trembling poplar, 128, 169
Trifolium agrarium, 140
Trifolium pratense, 140
Trillium, purple, 182
Trillium erectum, 182
Trillium erectum var. *album,* 131
Triosteum perfoliatum, 148
Triticum, 145
Triticum repens, 157
Truelove, 131
Trumpet weed, 170
Tuber root, 168
Tulip poplar, 185
Tulip tree, 185
Turkey corn, 182
Turkey pea, 182
Turmeric, 137, 182
Turmeric root, 151
Turnhoof, 156
Turtlebloom, 129, 175
Tussilago farfara, 142
Twinleaf, 182

U

Ulmus fulva, 9, 10, 83
Ulmus rubra, *146*
Umbel, 157
Uncum, 159
Unicorn, 132
Unicorn root, false, 182
Upland cranberry, 183
Upland sumach, 179
Urginea maritima, 178
Urtica dioica, 165
Uva-ursi, 64, 183
Uvularia perfoliata, 130

V

Vaccinium myrtillus, 185
Valerian, American, 89, 183
Valerian, English, 89, 183
Valerian, Greek, 183

Valeriana officinalis, 183
Vandal root, 183
Vegetable antimony, 133
Veratrum viride, 95, 153
Verbascum thapsus, 164
Verbena hastata, 183
Vermont snake root, 175
Veronica beccabunga, 133
Veronica fasiculata, 156
Veronica officinalis, 177
Veronicastrum virginicum, 144
Vervain, 10, 11, 183
Viburnum lentago, 164
Viburnum trilobus, 143
Vine maple, 166
Viola pedata, 183
Viola rostrata, 184
Violet, 10, 183
Violet, canker, 184
Violet bloom, 132
Virginia cowslip, 160
Virginia prune, 138
Virginia scullcap, 174
Virgin's bower, 184

W

Wa-A-Hoo, 54, 184
Wafer ash, 169
Wake robin, 131, 146, 155, 186
Walnut, 184
Wandering milkweed, 131
Water bugle, 134, 184
Watercup, 184
Water flag, 132, 149
Water hemlock, 139
Water hoarhound, 134, 184
Water horehound, 134
Water lily, white, 159
Watermelon, 185
Water nerve root, 155
Water pepper, 185
Water pimpernel, 133
Water purslain, 133
Water shamrock, 134
Wax berry, 130
Wax myrtle, 130
Waxwork, 132
Whistle wood, 161
White balsam, 129, 158
White daisy, 185
White leaf, 152
White poplar, 169
White poppy, 169

White root, 9, 185
White turtlehead, 175
White walnut, 135, 184
White water lily, 159
White weed, 144, 185
White wood, 135
Whitewood, 185
Whortleberry, 185
Wickup, 185
Wild allspice, 148
Wild basil, 145, 163
Wild chamomile, 162
Wild cherry, 15
Wild citronella, 170
Wild coffee, 148
Wild elder, 146
Wild evening primrose, 173
Wild fennel, 147
Wild ginger, 151
Wild hydrangea, 154
Wild hyssop, 183
Wild ipecac, 148
Wild jalap, 160
Wild jessamine, 187
Wild lemon, 160
Wild licorice, 172
Wild mandrake, 160
Wild marjoram, 163
Wild potato, 160
Wild scammony, 160
Wild snowball, 170
Wild succory, 138, 139
Wild tobacco, 159
Wild turnip, 146, 155, 186
Wild woodbine, 150
Wild yam, 139, 186
Willow, pussy, 186
Willow, rose, 186
Willow, white, 186
Willow-herb, 185
Wind root, 168
Wind shamrock, 134
Wingseed, 169
Winterberry, 126
Winter bloom, 186
Winter clover, 178
Winter fern, 170
Wintergreen, 133, 138, 186
Winter pink, 152
Witch grass, 145, 157
Witch hazel, 90, 111, 186
Wolfsbane, 126
Woodbine, 187

Wood sorrel, 176
Woody nightshade, 132
Wormseed, 9, 165, 187
Wormwood, common, 69, 72, 187
Wormwood, Roman, 187
Wound wort, 174, 179

Y

Yarrow, 187
Yaw root, 170
Yellow broom, 155
Yellow clover, 162
Yellow dock root, 71
Yellow gentian, 142
Yellow jasmine, 150
Yellow Jessamine, 150, 187
Yellow lady's slipper, 183
Yellow moccasin flower, 157, 183
Yellow pond lily, 159
Yellow puccoon, 151
Yellow root, 151
Yellow sweet clover, 180
Yellow wood, 127

Z

Zanthoxylum americanum, 127
Zingiber officinalis, 151

General Index

Italicized numbers indicate that an illustration or photograph appears on that page. A botanical index begins on page 204.

A

Alfred, Me., Shaker community at
  descriptions of, 92–93
  establishment of, 91
  medicinal herb and seed business, 92–93
Architecture, Shaker
  barns, 6, *55*
  brick shops, *5*
  broomshops, *76*
  extract houses, *39*
  finishing rooms, *40*
  herb houses, *38, 67, 96*
  laboratories, *39*
  meetinghouses, 83, *94*
  trustees' offices, *78, 106*
Atherton, Simon T., 63, 65–66, 73
Ayer, William G., 103

B

Babbit, Tabitha, 64
Balm of 1000 Flowers, 17
Barker, Mildred, 92
Barns, Shaker, *6, 55*
Bates, Issachar, 101, 102
Bennett, D.M., 107
Bentley, Rev. William, 76
Bitters, 61
Blanchard, G.B., 78
Blinn, Elder Henry C., 74, 80, *81*, 81–82, 97
Boilers, 39
Borden's Milk Products Company, Inc., 39
Boyd, Peter, 102, 105, 108–11

Brackett, William C., 11
Brocklebank, Asa, 76–77
Brown, Samuel, 90
Brown's Extract of English Valerian, 89, 95
Buildings, Shaker. *See* Architecture, Shaker
Bullard, Marcia, 43
Bushnell, Elder, 37
Busro, Ind., Shaker community at, 101

C

Calver, Amelia J., 51
Canaan Society, 36
Canterbury, N.H., Shaker community at, 2, 3, 64
  Blinn, Elder Henry C., 80, *81*, 81–82
  buildings, *83*
  catalog pages, *86*
  catalogs, 84–87
  cookbooks, 87
  Corbett, Thomas, 81, 82–85
  Corbett's Compound Concentrated Syrup of Sarsaparilla, 84–87
  description of, 80
  gardens, *83*
  medicinal herb business, 82–83
  Parker, David, 81, 84–85, *86*
  Sarle, Cora Helena, 82, *82*
Carminative Salve, 15
Carr, Frances, 21, 90, 91, 96–100, 100, *100*
Cephalic pills, *8*

Cherry Water, 14
Circassian Balm, 15
Clough, Henry, 46–47, 51–52
Compound Concentrated Syrup of Sarsaparilla, 8, 84–87, 95
Compound Syrup of Black Cohosh, 9
Concentrated Syrup of Liverwort, 8
Cooking, Shaker, 87, 100
Copley, Harvey, 6
Corbett's Compound Concentrated Syrup of Sarsaparilla, 84–87
Corbett, Thomas, 73, 81, 82–85, 87
Cotton, John, 91

D

Dean, John, 37
Dickens, Charles, 20
Digestive pills, 8
Dioscorides, 1
Drawings
  plant, Cora Helena Sarle, *42, 48, 69, 82–84, 87, 109*
  spirit, 57, *57*
Duke of Portland's Powder, *1*
Dumont, Elder William, *95*
Duyckinck, Evert A., 25
Dyspepsia cure, 85

E

Eades, Hervey L., 120–22
Eastern Bishopric, 63
Eaton's Manual of Botany, 12

Enfield, Conn., Shaker community at, 3
  catalog pages, *61*
  catalogs, 61–62
  Church Family buildings, *60*
  description of, 55, 60
  dissolution of, 62
  seed business, 55, 60
Enfield, N.H., Shaker community at, 3
  Brown's Extract of English Valerian, 89
  catalogs, 90
  Church Family buildings, *88*
  description of, 88
  dissolution of, 90
  gardens, 88
  medicinal herb business, 89–90
Erickson, Larz, 101
Ervin, Anna, 62
Evans, Elder Frederick, 4, 19, 52
Evans, Ezekiel, 90
Extract house, 38, 39
Extracts, 6, 10, 13, 14, 17

F

Families, Shaker community, 4
"Floral Wreath," *57*
Fowler, Edward, 22, 25–26, 109

G

Gardens, *21*, 88
  family, 83
  flower, *93*
  herb, *98, 116, 120*
  kitchen, *19*

Gates, Benjamin, 31, 46–47, 96
Gathering plants
 depletion of wild botanicals, 21
 green *vs.* dried weight, 22
 plant beauty *vs.* function, 23–24
 rules, 6
Gift drawings, 57, *57*
Green, Elder Calvin, 30
Groveland, N.Y., Shaker community at
 buildings, *53*
 history of, 53
 medicinal preparations, 54

H

Hadd, Arnold, 95, 100, *100*
Hammond, Joseph, 65
Hampton, O.C., 102, 106
Hancock, Mass., Shaker community at
 buildings, *56*
 description of, 55
 dissolution of, 56
 seed business, 55, 56
Hancock Bishopric, 55
Hancock Shaker Village barns, *55*
Harlow, Eliab, 31–35
Harvard, Mass., Shaker community at, 2, 3, 64
 Atherton, Simon T., 65–66, 68, 73
 buildings, *63, 65*
 catalogs, 65–66
 Church Family buildings, *63*
 daybook accounts of life at, 68–72, 74
 description of, 64
 herb house, 67, *67*
 medicinal herb business, 64, 68–73, 75
Harvard Bishopric, 63
Healing Balm of 1000 Flowers, 17
Herbalism
 history of, 1–2, 5
 Native American, 47–48, 102
Herb houses, 38, *38, 96*
Herb industry, Shaker. *See* Medicinal herb industry, Shaker

Herbs
 gathering plants, 6, 21, 23–24
 names of, 28
 weight, green *vs.* dried, 22
Herrick, Darias, 58–59
Hibbard Co., 15
Hill, Isaac, 82–83, 88, 92–93
Hinckley, Barnabas, 34–35, *35,* 37, 41
Hippocrates, 1
Hocknell, John, 5
Hollister, Alonzo, 48
Holmes, James, 94–95
Holmes, J.P., 120
Hydraulic press, *38*

I

Indian spirit doctor, 78
Influence of the Shaker Doctor, The, 111
Inspissated juices, 13

J

Jewett, James, 88
Jewett, Sarah, 64
Johnson, Theodore, 97–100
Johnson, Willard, 59

K

Kaime, James S., 86

L

Lamson, David, 56
Laurus Eye Water, 9
Lawrence, Garrett Keatin, 31–35
Laxative Syrup, 88
Lee, Mother Ann
 arrival in America, 2
 founder of communities at Harvard and Shirley, Mass., 63–64
 and Maine Shakers, 91
 settlement of Watervliet, N.Y., 5
Lees, Ann. *See* Lee, Mother Ann
Liverpool, Eng., 2
Lossing, Benson J., 37–41

M

Manchester, England, 2
Manifesto, The, 3, 5, 75, 97

Mary Whitcher's Shaker House Keeper, 87
Mascoma Lake, N.H., 79
McNemar, Richard, 102
Meacham, John, 101
Medical care, Shaker
 advanced concepts, 114
 alliance with worldly doctors, 111–12
 Corbett, Thomas, 81, 82–85
 diary accounts of, 31–35
 first female physician, 64
 Harlow, Eliab, 31–35
 Influence of the Shaker Doctor, The, 111
 Lawrence, Garrett Keatin, 31–35
 medical procedures, 64, 121
 use of medical professionals, 4
Medicinal herb industry, Shaker
 extract houses, 38–39, *39*
 finishing rooms, 40, *40*
 herb houses, 38, *38*
 laboratories, 38–39, *39*
 production process, 37–41
 productivity of, 41–42
 profitability, 3
Medicinal preparations, Shaker, 8–9, 43–47, 54
Medicine shop, 37
Medicines, patent, 12, 15
Meeting Houses, Shaker, *94*
Millennial Laws, 3–4
Miller, Chauncey, 17–18, 69, 110
Mother Ann's Work, 57, 61
Mother Seigel's Syrup, 47, 88
Mount Lebanon, N.Y., Shaker community at. *See* New Lebanon, N.Y., Shaker community at
Munson, Abigail, 4
Myrick, Elijah, 64, 68, 73
Myrick, Elisha, 67–72
Myrick, Isaac, 68

N

Native Americans, 2, 5
Neal, Emma J., 38
New Gloucester, Me., Shaker community at, 93. *See also* Sabbathday Lake, Me., Shaker community at

New Lebanon, N.Y., Shaker community at, 64
 almanacs, 49–50
 book of extracts, 30
 Canaan Society, 36
 catalog excerpts, 30
 catalog pages, *29, 30*
 catalogs, 27–30, 50
 descriptions of, by visitors, 20, 25, 37
 diary accounts of life at, 23, 25, 31, 32–33, 34–35, 36, 37
 dissolution of, 52
 fires, 48–49
 Fowler, Edward, 22, 25–26
 gardens, *19, 21*
 Harlow, Eliab, 31–35
 Hinckley, Barnabas, 34–35, *35,* 41
 Lawrence, Garrett Keatin, 31–35
 medical care, 31–35
 medicinal herb business, 25–26, 34–35, 37–42, 45–47, 51–52
 medicinal preparations, 43–47
 and Native Americans, 47–48
 North Family buildings, *21*
 Norwood's Veratrum Viride, 43, *43*
 plant gathering activities, 21–24
 plant production, 25–26
 settlement of, 19
 Seven Barks, 44, *44*
Newton, Agnes, 79
Niskeyuna, 2
Nordhoff, Charles, 4
North Union, Ohio, Shaker community at, 113–14
Norwood, W.C., 43
Norwood's Veratrum Viride, *20,* 43, *43*

O

Oils, 6, 9
Ointments, 59
Onion juice, 78
Orcutt, Daniel, 60

P

Pain King, 44–45
Parker, David, 81, 84–85, 86, 110

Parker, James, 78
Patent medicines, 12, 15
Peach Water, 6, 10, 14
Pelham, Richard W., 108
Plant gathering, 6
  depletion of wild botanicals, 21
  green *vs.* dried weight, 22
  plant beauty *vs.* function, 23–24
  rules, 6
Pleasant Hill, Ky., Shaker community at
  buildings, *115*
  Centre House buildings, *101*
  description of, 114–15
  East Family buildings, *118*
  gardens, *116*
  herb drying room, *102*
  impact of Civil War on, 119
  journal accounts of life at, 115–17
  medicinal herb business, 118
Pohatton, Indian spirit doctor, 78
Poisonous plants, 5
Powder of Whiteroot, 9
Prescott, Elder James, 113
Pumpkin seed, oil of, 6

Q
Quincy House, Boston, 73

R
Rafinesque's Medical Flora, 11, 15
Randall, Joanna, 76
Rankin, Elder John, 108
Reed, Allen, 37
Robinson, Homer, 32–33
Roots, 6
Rose Water, 6, 9, 14, 67, 73
Ryan, Kitty Jane, 117

S
Sabbathday Lake, Me., Shaker community at
  catalogs, 94–95
  Church Family buildings, *91*
  descriptions of, 93
  establishment of, 91, 93
  gardens, *93, 98*
  Herb House, *96*
  medicinal herb business, 94–95

medicinal herb business revival, 97–100
  Meeting House, *94*
  Shaker Tamar Laxative, 95–97, *97*
Sabbathday Pond, Me. *See* Sabbathday Lake, Me., Shaker community at
Sarle, Cora Helena
  biography of, 82, *82*
  plant drawings, *42, 48,* 69, *82–84, 87, 109*
Sarsaparilla syrup, 6, 8, 16, 27, 84–87, 95
Sawyer, Elder Otis, 95
Sears, Clara Endicott, 77
Sears, Endicott, 75
Second Bishopric, 55
Serrette, David, 99
Seven Barks, 44, *44,* 95
Shain, John, 115
Shaker Asthma Cure, 44
Shaker communities, establishment of, 101–2
Shaker Hair Restorer, 45
Shaker Quarterly, The, 97
Shakers
  dependence on herbal remedies, 2
  as historians, 3–4
  importance of good health, 4
  origin and growth of, 2
Shaker Tamar Laxative, 95–97, *97*
Shaker Your Plate: Of Shaker Cooks and Cooking, 100
Shannon, Thomas Jefferson, 119–20
Shaw, Levi, 36
Shirley, Mass., Shaker community at
  broom shop, *76*
  catalogs, 77
  description of, 76
  medicinal herb business, 77
  seed business, 76–77
  trustees' office, *78*
Silliman, Benjamin, 20
Singerland, J.R., 111–12
Smith, Eldress Betsy, 37, 93
South Union, Ky., Shaker community at
  business ventures, 119–20
  Centre House buildings, *120*

dissolution of, 122
  gardens, *120*
  impact of Civil War on, 119, 121–22
  journal account of life at, 120–22
  Wash House, *119*
Spirit drawings, 57, *57*
Stewart, Philemon, 25, 30
Syrup of Black Cohosh, 84
Syrup of Liverwort, 8, 84
Syrup of Sarsaparilla, 6, 8, 16, 84–87, 95

T
Taylor, Leila, 60
Tamar Laxative, 95, *97*
Taraxacum Blue Pills, 13
Thomas, Elisha, 114
Thomson, Samuel, 114
Thomsonianism, 114
Tilden, Elam, 26
Tripure, William, 80
Turner, Louis, 111–12
Tyringham, Mass., Shaker community at
  Church Family buildings, *58*
  description of, 55
  seed business, 55, 59

U
Union Village, Ohio, Shaker community at, 2, 3, 64
  Boyd, Peter, 102, 105, 108–11
  broadsides, 107
  catalogs, 103–7
  Center Family buildings, *104*
  description of, 102
  dissolution of, 102, 112
  fire, 106
  journal account of life at, 102, 103
  medicinal herb business, 109–12
  North Family buildings, *102*
  trustees' offices, *106*

V
Vail, James, 48
Vegetable Balsam, 8
Vegetable Bilious Pills, 8, 84
Vegetable Family Pills, 15
Vegetable Rheumatic Pills, 84

W
Watermelon, medicinal, 105
Watervliet, N.Y., Shaker community at, 2, 3, 64
  barns, *6*
  brick shop, *5*
  catalog excerpts, 8–9, 12–13, 15, 16, 17–18
  catalog pages, *7, 14*
  catalogs, 7, 10, 13–18
  dissolution of, 18
  diversity of products, 7
  early marketing efforts, 6
  flyers and broadsides, 16
  Hocknell, John, 5
  Lee, Mother Ann, 5
  marketing to physicians, 12–13
  medicinal herb business, 10–12
  medicinal preparations offered, 8–9
  sarsaparilla syrup, 16
  settlement of, 5
Watervliet (Dayton), Ohio, Shaker community at, 101
Wells, Seth, 30
West, Arthur T., 67
West Gloucester, Me., Shaker community at. *See* Sabbathday Lake, Me., Shaker community at
Whitcher, Benjamin, 79
Whitcher, Mary, 87
White, A.J., 45, 49–50, 96
White, Eldress Anna, 21, 60
White, Jefferson, 3, 61–62
Whiteley, John, 65, 73
White Water, Ohio, Shaker community at, 101
Whitney, George B., 68
Whittaker, Father James, 53, 91
Wild Cherry Bitters, 15
Williams, John S., 97
Wood, Jonathan, 37
Wright, Elder Grove, 55
Wright, John, 56
Wright, Mother Lucy, 77

Y
Youngs, Benjamin S., 101

ILLUSTRATORS

Numerous artists have contributed illustrations to this book. In the Herbal Compendium they are identified by their initials, and their full names are listed below, followed by the additional page numbers where their illustrations appear in the History.

Sister Cora Helena Sarle's artwork is owned by Canterbury Shaker Village and may be found in *A Shaker Sister's Drawings: Wild Plants Illustrated by Cora Helena Sarle* (New York: The Monacelli Press, Inc., 1997).

Abbreviation	Illustrator
BA	Bobbi Angell
PD	Pat Dailey
BD	Beverly Duncan — 9, 12, 22, 27, 31, 47, 49, 71 (top), 99, 113, 117
RH	Regina Hughes — 13 (top)
AK	Alison Kolesar
CJ	Charles Joslin — 50, 51, 70 (bottom), 71 (bottom), 74, 77, 108
ML	Mallory Lake — 8, 13 (bottom), 41, 64, 70 (top)
LR	Louise Riotte
HS	Hyla Scudder
ES	Elayne Sears

Other Storey Titles You Will Enjoy

At Home with Herbs, by Jane Newdick. Provides more than 100 herbal craft projects for all types of enthusiasts. 224 pages. Hardcover. ISBN 0-88266-886-2.

From Seed to Bloom, by Eileen Powell. Easy-to-understand plant-by-plant format that includes information on hardiness zones, sowing seeds indoors and out, germinating times, spacing, light and soil needs, care, and propagation techniques. 320 pages. Paperback. ISBN 0-88266-259-7.

A Garden of Wildflowers, by Henry W. Art. Provides botanical drawings of more than 100 native species and includes growing information for each. 304 pages. Paperback. ISBN 0-88266-405-0.

Growing and Using Herbs Successfully, by Betty E. M. Jacobs. Teaches readers how to plant, propagate, harvest, dry, freeze, and store 64 of the most popular herbs. 240 pages. Paperback. ISBN 0-88266-249-X.

Growing Your Herb Business, by Bertha Reppert. Offers practical advice on establishing budgets, choosing locations, writing business plans, developing products, packaging, maintaining inventory, hiring staff, and setting prices. 192 pages. Paperback. ISBN 0-88266-612-6.

The Herbal Home Remedy Book, by Joyce A. Wardwell. Discover how to use 25 common herbs to make simple herbal remedies. 176 pages. Paperback. ISBN 1-58017-016-1.

The Herbal Palate Cookbook, by Maggie Oster and Sal Gilbertie. Offers 150 simple yet elegant recipes featuring fresh herbs as their central ingredient. An herb identification section contains color photographs and instructions for growing herbs in containers. 176 pages. Paperback. ISBN 1-58017-025-0. Hardcover. ISBN 0-88266-915-X.

The Herbal Tea Garden, by Marietta Marshall Marcin. Describes how to select, grow, and create special tea blends from 70 specific herbal tea plants. 224 pages. Paperback. ISBN 0-88266-827-7.

The Herb Gardener, by Susan McClure. Provides complete instructions on every conceivable aspect of herbs in the home and garden. 240 pages. Paperback. ISBN 0-88266-873-0. Hardcover. ISBN 0-88266-910-9.

The Gardener's Weed Book, by Barbara Pleasant. Explains how to understand, identify, and control weeds using earth-safe methods. Includes an encyclopedic section of common weeds and their characteristics as seedlings and as mature plants. 144 pages. Paperback. ISBN 0-88266-921-4. Hardcover. ISBN 0-88266-942-7.

Keeping Life Simple, by Karen Levine. Provides seven guiding principles to assess what is really satisfying and then offers hundreds of ideas about how to create a lifestyle that is more rewarding and less complicated. 160 pages. Paperback. ISBN 0-88266-943-5.

These and other Storey books are available at your bookstore, farm store, garden center, or directly from Storey Books, Schoolhouse Road, Pownal, Vermont 05261, or by calling 800-441-5700. Visit our website at www.storey.com.

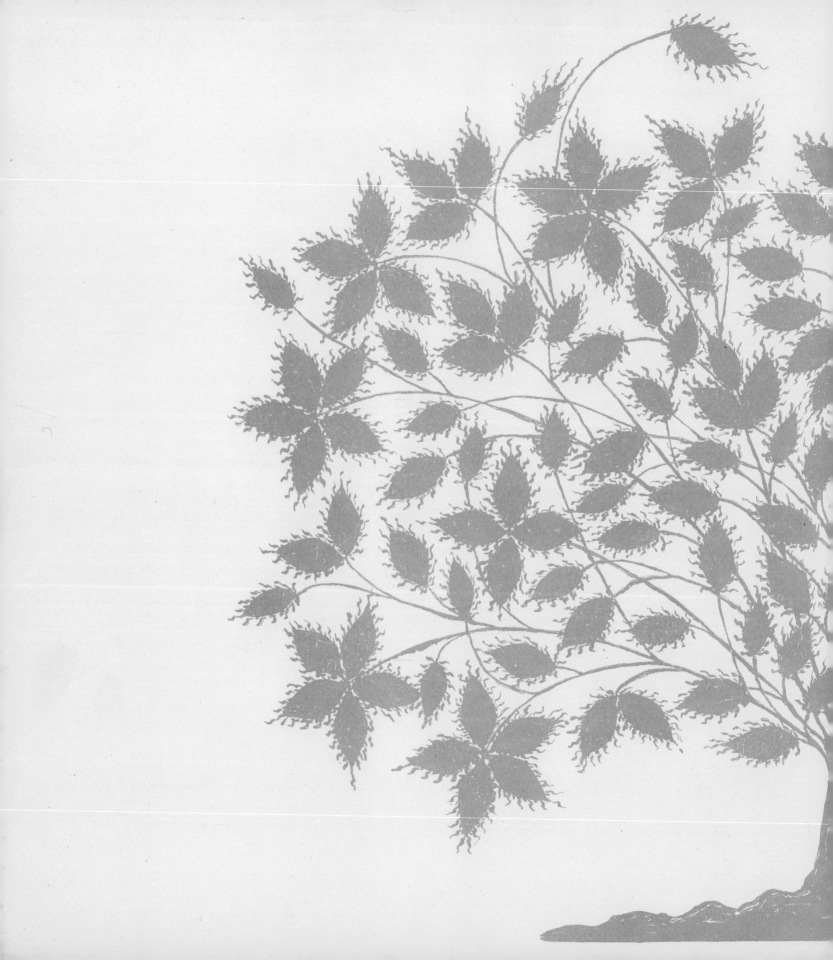